# Essentials of Toxicology for Health Protection

a handbook for field professionals

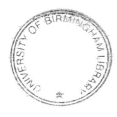

**Front cover images from top:**

Landfill, England. Courtesy of Chemical Hazards and Poisons Division, Health Protection Agency.

Cigarette smoke. Courtesy of Health Protection Agency.

Decontamination equipment, England. Courtesy of Chemical Hazards and Poisons Division, Health Protection Agency.

Fire and chemical spill at factory, England, 2006. Courtesy of Chemical Hazards and Poisons Division, Health Protection Agency.

Burn due to tetrachloroethylene. Courtesy of Chemical Hazards and Poisons Division, Health Protection Agency.

Smoke from the Buncefield fire, England, 2005. Courtesy of Hertfordshire Constabulary and Chiltern Air Support Unit.

Designed and printed by Cambridge University Press.
www.cambridge.org/printing

# Editors

## Professor David Baker

Consultant Medical Toxicologist, Chemical Hazards and Poisons Division, London, Health Protection Agency, UK
Consultant Anaesthesiologist, SAMU de Paris, Hôpital Necker – Enfants Malades, Paris, France

## Dr Robin Fielder

Head of General Toxicology Unit, Chemical Hazards and Poisons Division, Chilton, Health Protection Agency, UK

## Dr Lakshman Karalliedde

Consultant Medical Toxicologist, Chemical Hazards and Poisons Division, London, Health Protection Agency, UK
Visiting Senior Lecturer, Department of Public Health Sciences, School of Medicine, King's College London, UK
Post-graduate Supervisor, South Asian Clinical Toxicology Research Collaboration, Faculty of Medicine, Peradeniya, Sri Lanka

## Professor Virginia Murray

Consultant Medical Toxicologist, Head of London Unit of Chemical Hazards and Poisons Division, Health Protection Agency, UK
Visiting Professor in Health Protection, Department of Public Health Sciences, School of Medicine, King's College London, UK

## Norman Parkinson

Senior Lecturer, Department of Public Health Sciences, School of Medicine, King's College London, UK

# Assistant Editors

## Karen Hogan

Training Administrator, Chemical Hazards and Poisons Division, London, Health Protection Agency, UK

## Catherine Keshishian

Researcher, Institute of Psychiatry, King's College London, UK
Chemical Hazards and Poisons Division, London, Health Protection Agency, UK

# Acknowledgements

The editors wish to acknowledge the comments and input from all the participants of the courses held in the past two years which have guided us in presenting this book in a form which would be considered most appropriate, relevant and useful for future participants and other health professionals from different educational backgrounds.

The editors thank Penelope Dixey for her excellent secretarial help and assistance in formatting chapters which was rendered in a pleasing manner with great commitment.

Much of the information for the appendix was adapted and modified from *An Introduction to Human Physiology* by JH Green*. The editors thank Professor Robert Maynard for his input to the appendix.

We thank Dr Anne Jones for the support provided at the start of this activity.

Invaluable graphical help was provided by Jon White, with Henry Landon and Jamie Griffin contributing diagrams for the appendix, for which the editors are truly grateful.

The editors thank Ivan House for assisting with the chapter on toxicity and heavy metals.

Without exception, all the staff at CHaPD (London) helped in innumerable ways to ensure that the deadlines for publication were met.

Finally thanks go to the administration of the HPA and the staff of the Publication Department of the HPA for guidance, assistance and encouragement.

* Green, JH. (1976) *An Introduction to Human Physiology.* 4th edition. Oxford University Press, London.

# Contributors

**Dr Charlotte NB Aus**

Senior Environmental Epidemiologist, Chemical Hazards and Poisons Division, London, Health Protection Agency, UK

**Dr Diane Benford**

Senior Consultant Toxicologist, Food Standards Agency, UK

**Dr Simon FJ Clarke**

Consultant Emergency Physician, Frimley Park NHS Foundation Trust, UK Honorary Consultant in Emergency Response and Medical Toxicology, Chemical Hazards and Poisons Division, London, Health Protection Agency, UK

**Dr John Gray**

Consultant: Water Safety and Security Formerly Deputy Chief Inspector (Operations) with the Drinking Water Inspectorate, UK

**Robie Kamanyire**

Toxicology Scientist, Chemical Hazards and Poisons Division, London, Health Protection Agency, UK

**Dr Giovanni Leonardi**

Consultant Environmental Epidemiologist, Chemical Hazards and Poisons Division, Chilton, Health Protection Agency, UK

**Dr Timothy C Marrs OBE**

Edentox Associates, University of Central Lancashire, National Poisons Information Service, Birmingham Centre, UK

**Professor Robert L Maynard CBE**

Senior Medical Officer, Chemical Hazards and Poisons Division, Chilton, Health Protection Agency, UK

**Sarah McCrea**

Toxicology Scientist, Chemical Hazards and Poisons Division, London, Health Protection Agency, UK

**Dr Richard Mohan**

Environmental Scientist, Chemical Hazards and Poisons Division, London, Health Protection Agency, UK

**Dr Ovnair Sepai**

Senior Scientist, Chemical Hazards and Poisons Division, Chilton, Health Protection Agency, UK

**Dr James Wilson**

Senior Environmental Scientist, Chemical Hazards and Poisons Division, London, Health Protection Agency, UK

# Foreword

The Health Protection Agency (HPA) plays a critical role in protecting people from hazards involving **chemicals, poisons** and **radiation**. Every day in the UK, serious chemical incidents occur which threaten people's health. These might arise from accidents at home, in the workplace, or on the road or rail networks. They might involve industrial explosions, chemical fires, chemical contamination of the environment, or the deliberate release of chemicals and poisons.

The HPA Chemical Hazards and Poisons Division, part of our Centre for Radiation, Chemical and Environmental Hazards, provides guidance to government departments and round the clock advice to the NHS, local authorities, the emergency services, and other agencies, on the human health effects of chemicals in water, air, soil and waste. We also provide expert scientific support to the government's independent expert health advisory committees, advise on the potential health effects of proposed developments, and provide, through the National Poisons Information Service, guidance to doctors and nurses on the best way to manage patients who may have been poisoned.

The Division's Strategic Goal is *to anticipate and prevent the adverse effects of acute and chronic exposure to hazardous chemicals and other poisons.* To do this, we need a highly trained, multi-disciplinary staff that constantly strives to keep up to date with scientific and engineering advances. That is why I so strongly welcome the training courses and events offered by the Division in partnership with universities, and now, the publication of this new book *Essentials of Toxicology for Health Protection*.

But, this book is not just a manual for HPA staff. It is designed for all the various field professionals, from many different professional backgrounds, that are involved in health protection. The various agencies need to work together to provide reliable, effective and timely response to incidents and possible threats. The book draws heavily on the Division's experience and expertise in dealing with real incidents and problems. It will act both as a course reader and a reference manual. In appendices it provides some underpinning science and a glossary that will be particularly useful to those without a medical background. I feel sure that it will be of great value to all who read it.

**Justin McCracken,**
Chief Executive of the Health Protection Agency

# Introduction

## Norman Parkinson

### Background

The establishment of the *Health Protection Agency* (HPA) in 2003 has undoubtedly created a new focus for skills development and training in environmental public health. This book is a product of this emphasis on education and training.

In a review of existing training provision, the HPA has found that most existing masters courses in public health are generic in nature, and may not provide the depth of specialist health protection knowledge, skills and competencies needed to enable HPA staff to immediately fulfil their roles in advising and supporting local authorities, the NHS, the emergency services and other agencies, staff, whether in reacting to incidents and local concerns, or as consultees, for example, in relation to Integrated Pollution Prevention and Control. There is also a continuing need for specialist training of environmental public health personnel in other agencies, such as local authority environmental health practitioners and emergency planning officers.

The HPA sees a need for a comprehensive and structured national approach to the provision of such education and training, within the framework of continuing professional development and a national scheme of accredited masters level modules and programmes in health protection. The HPA also recognises the need to support trainers with suitable materials – including texts and case studies (Hawker, 2005).

Spiby (2006) developed a model of core competencies required of those working in environmental public health that reflects the need for a 'coming together of the knowledge and skills base of environmental science, public health, clinical toxicology and environmental epidemiology'. This model was broadly similar to that of Hawker (2005).

Spiby saw two main competency domains:
1. specialist environmental public health knowledge and skills, and
2. generic organisational skills.

**Domain 1.** Specialist environmental public health knowledge and skills contains five competency areas:

    A. Toxicology
    B. Environmental Science
    C. Environmental Epidemiology
    D. Risk Assessment and Risk Management
    E. Environmental Public Health – through organised efforts of society.

**Domain 2**. Generic organisational skills:

A. Teaching
B. Research
C. Management and Leadership.

The HPA Chemical Hazards and Poisons Division (CHaPD) responded by running courses, in partnership with universities, that map with these competency domains: an *Introduction to Environmental Epidemiology* module at the London School of Hygiene and Tropical Medicine, and two modules at King's College London: *Essentials of Environmental Science for Health Protection*, and *Essentials of Toxicology for Health Protection*.

These modules were available both to public health postgraduates at the university as part of their degree programmes, and to HPA staff and staff of other environmental public health agencies as part of their training portfolio or Continuing Professional Development programmes.

## The need for this book

In developing the *Essentials of Toxicology for Health Protection* module it became clear that there was no suitable reader. The Chemical Hazards and Poisons Division has published many advisory leaflets and case studies, and there are many good academic toxicology texts, and also texts that deal with environmental technologies and environmental management and administration, but nothing was available which brought together the various disciplines and focussed and applied them to UK situations.

In addition, in a study of London health protection professionals by Paddock (2006), it was found that 89% (33/37) of respondents did not feel confident about their knowledge of toxicology, and most had had limited experience of chemical incidents.

It was therefore decided to produce this book to meet the need for a single text that not only covers the basics of toxicology, but also its application to issues of topical concern such as contaminated land, food additives, water and air pollution, and emerging issues such as 'traditional' medicines.

The book is intended as both a course reader and a handbook for all health protection field professionals.

## Readership

The book is aimed at a wide range of professionals in environmental public health, including: health protection consultants; specialists and trainees; public health practitioners; environmental health practitioners; environmental scientists; and staff of the emergency services, the water and waste industries, and other industrial and regulatory bodies.

Most readers will be graduates with a good knowledge of public health sciences. We have tried to make the book accessible and readily understood by all field practitioners.

Also, we found, when running the *Essentials of Toxicology for Health Protection* course, that some students from non-medical backgrounds lacked sufficient understanding of basic human sciences, and so in an appendix we have included some underpinning physiology, pathology and general medicine, and there is a useful glossary.

## The scope of the book

Each chapter of the book has been written by an invited expert in that topic.

**Section 1.** *Fundamentals of Toxicology* provides a general introduction to the subject and explains how toxicological information is derived.

**Section 2.** *Applications of Toxicology* addresses exposure assessment, susceptible populations, and the medical management of chemical incidents. It also provides valuable pointers to sources of toxicological data.

**Section 3.** *Environmental Toxicology* considers pollutants in air, water, and land, and food contaminants and additives. In Occupational Toxicology, it considers exposures to toxic agents in the workplace.

**Section 4.** *A Review of Some Toxic Agents* addresses in detail a selection of important toxic agents: carbon monoxide; pesticides; heavy metals and trace elements as well as the emerging issues of traditional medicines and the deliberate release of toxic agents in warfare and terrorism.

A chapter on basic concepts of human science, and a glossary are included as appendices for those readers, for example environmental engineers, who don't have a background in medicine, biology or the health sciences.

## 'Environmental public health'

In the book we use the new term 'environmental public health'. In fact, this is synonymous with 'environmental health', but we use the new term to recognise and reflect the re-convergence of environmental health and public health, and the emerging partnerships between the HPA, local authorities, primary care trusts, and other agencies in the protection of public health from environmental hazards, and in achieving sustainable development.

## References

Hawker J. (2005) Postgraduate Academic Qualifications in Health Protection. Health Protection Agency (unpublished).

Paddock R. (2006) Chemical Incident Training Assessment Via a Health Professional Questionnaire. Chemical Hazards and Poisons Report (6):56–57. Health Protection Agency, Didcot.

Spiby J. (2006) Developing Competencies in Environmental Public Health. Chemical Hazards and Poisons Report (6) 57–59. Health Protection Agency, Didcot.

# Contents

*Editors*                                           *iii*
*Assistant Editors*                                 *iii*
*Acknowledgements*                                   *iv*
*Contributors*                                        *v*
*Foreword – Justin McCracken*                        *vi*

**Introduction** *Norman Parkinson*                 *vii*

**Section 1    Fundamentals of Toxicology**          **1**

1.1    Introduction to toxicology                      2
       *Lakshman Karalliedde, Sarah McCrea, Virginia Murray, Norman Parkinson*

1.2    Target organs                                  19
       *David Baker*

1.3    Experimental methods for investigating the toxicity of chemicals    35
       *Robin Fielder*

1.4    Introduction to human biomonitoring in public health    50
       *Ovnair Sepai*

**Section 2    Applications of Toxicology**          **61**

2.1    Sources of toxicological information           62
       *Robie Kamanyire*

2.2    Medical management of chemical incidents       71
       *Simon FJ Clarke*

2.3    Concept of susceptibility to environmental hazards    87
       *Charlotte NB Aus*

2.4    Exposure assessment using environmental monitoring and modelling    97
       *Richard Mohan, Giovanni Leonardi*

**Section 3    Environmental Toxicology**           **107**

3.1    Occupational toxicology                       108
       *Sarah McCrea, Virginia Murray, Norman Parkinson*

3.2    Air pollution and health in the UK            122
       *Robert L Maynard*

3.3    Contaminated land assessment                  130
       *James Wilson*

3.4    Management of incidents affecting drinking water quality    144
       *John Gray*

3.5    Food additives and contaminants               157
       *Diane Benford*

**Section 4     A Review of Some Toxic Agents**                                             **163**

  4.1   Carbon monoxide poisoning                                                            164
        *Lakshman Karalliedde, Catherine Keshishian*

  4.2   Toxicity of some heavy metals and trace elements                                     174
        *Robin Fielder, Lakshman Karalliedde*

  4.3   The toxicology of pesticides                                                         193
        *Lakshman Karalliedde, Timothy C Marrs*

  4.4   Toxicology associated with traditional medicines                                     201
        *Lakshman Karalliedde*

  4.5   Chemical weapons: deliberate release of chemical agents                              217
        *David Baker*

**Appendix**                                                                                 **235**

        Basic medical concepts                                                               236
        *David Baker, Lakshman Karalliedde, Virginia Murray, Norman Parkinson*

        Glossary and Abbreviations                                                           285

        Index                                                                                307

# Section 1

Fundamentals of Toxicology

# Section 1.1

# Introduction to toxicology

Lakshman Karalliedde, Sarah McCrea, Virginia Murray and
Norman Parkinson

## Learning outcomes

At the end of this chapter and any recommended reading the student should
be able to:

1. explain the commonly used terms and definitions in toxicology;
2. explain the role of toxicology in health protection;
3. classify toxicological agents and toxins,
    a) based on physico-chemical properties, and
    b) based on mode of toxic effects;
4. discuss and describe the routes of exposure;
5. describe the fate of toxins in the body;
6. describe the principles of risk assessment; and
7. apply their knowledge in the analysis and management of hazardous
   situations.

## 1 Introducing toxicology as a speciality

Simply and concisely, toxicology is the study of the nature and mechanism(s) of
toxic effects of substances on living organisms and other biological systems. Toxins,
commonly known as poisons, have the ability to cause harm or damage (toxicity) to
living organisms. Toxins or toxic substances vary in their origin, chemical structure, and
physical properties and most importantly in the manner in which they cause toxicity.

Toxicology is thus essentially the science of toxins or poisons. It is a speciality in
medicine which studies the manner in which toxins cause harmful effects to living
organisms, the amounts (doses) that cause such harm, the consequences of harm (e.g.
disordered function, disease, death), the manner in which such harm can be prevented
and the methods by which the harmful effects can be treated.

It is necessary to be aware that harmful effects may not be immediately visible or
detectable as effects such as the ability to cause cancers or abnormalities in the
development or function of organs may only occur months or years after the toxin had
entered the living organism. This is known as the lead time.

The discipline of toxicology has several essential components:

- Scientific and experimental toxicology: the study of basic toxic effects using animal and other models.
- Medical toxicology: the application of medical knowledge (diagnosis, treatment and prevention) to patients who have had toxic exposures and to chemical population exposure assessments.
- Clinical toxicology: direct provision of clinical toxicological care.
- Occupational toxicology: the study of toxic effects as a direct consequence of occupation.
- Environmental toxicology: the study of toxic effects on man as a result of release of toxic substances into his habitat.

All of these approaches to toxicology are linked by the common pathway of the effects of chemical substances on the systems/organs within the human body which enables an individual to maintain good health.

When a reference to toxicity of a substance is made, it is fundamental to consider the concept introduced by the father of toxicology, Paracelsus, in the 16th century –"No substance is a poison by itself. It is the dose that makes a substance a poison". Thus the dose differentiates a poison and a remedy.

The dose is the critical factor in the consideration of the potential toxicity of a substance. This means the amount (e.g. weights or volumes  – milligrams, micrograms, litres or millilitres or the concentrations in air in units such as milligrams per cubic metre (mg/m³) taken at a particular time (with a single exposure) or the amounts in total taken over a specified period of time. Thus the quantity of the substance and the duration during which the toxic exposure has taken place (orally, skin contact (dermally) or by inhalation) is critical in the assessment of the harmful effects a substance would produce in the human body.

**Box 1** Toxicity is the association between dose and exposure

> Dose (single or repeated) × exposure (single or repeated) = toxic effect

## 1.1    History

The development of toxicology has a colourful history. Early cave dwellers through personal experience knew of the dangers that some plants could cause to man. It is stated that as early as 1500 BC there were written recordings of the effects of hemlock, opium and animal poisons used to smear arrows to kill or immobilise animals for food and clothing. Also the harmful effects of some heavy metals have been recorded in ancient crypts associated with Traditional Medicines.

Poisons were used from the times of the origin of man to kill fellow human beings – be they enemies or relatives – and of course as punishment for crimes by the state or governing authorities. Amongst the historical persons fatally poisoned were Socrates, Cleopatra and Claudius. However, during the Renaissance, the study of poisons began to emerge as a science. Paracelsus (c.1500 AD) is considered by many to be the father of toxicology. He is reported to have said '*Sola dosis facit venenum*' (only the dose makes the poison), and thus developed the concept of dose-response.

Considering a universally used substance – alcohol or ethanol – the fundamental concept of Paracelsus can now be illustrated scientifically. The non-toxic or the beneficial dose of ethanol would produce a blood level of 0.05%, a toxic dose would produce a blood level of 0.1% and a lethal dose would produce a blood level of 0.5%.

A Spanish physician Matteo Orfila is considered by many to be the founder of toxicology as he developed a description of the relationship between chemicals and the effects each of these chemicals produced in the human body. He studied the harmful changes of a toxin on an organ/s in the human body and demonstrated the nature of damage caused by that particular poison.

## 2    Role of toxicology in health protection

Ill health due to chemicals present in the environment has become a worrying feature in medical practice, particularly in industrialised countries but also in developing countries that may be using cheaper substances that are potentially more toxic.

Industrialisation has resulted in the production of chemicals beneficial to man in diverse ways and in diverse situations. However, they all have the potential to cause harm to human health. There are over 34 million chemicals which have been allocated Chemical Abstract Service (CAS) numbers; these are chemicals which are in existence, in stable form (not intermediates). It has to be noted that there is scant information on the potential toxicity or toxicology for the majority of these (see Table 1).

Chemicals have specific uses and are intended to be used in a specific manner but it is to be expected that there are many instances where there have been misuse, overuse, or inappropriate use. As most of these chemicals have the ability to cause toxicity or harm to human health, it is necessary to ensure that the chemicals are properly manufactured, stored and used, with appropriate safeguards at each stage. Even some of those chemicals that have been introduced to destroy lower organisms (e.g. pesticides) are not selective in their toxicity, and can adversely affect humans. As a result of this, there is a need to ensure that production is to agreed specifications of purity, concentration and devoid of toxic contaminants. It is necessary to ensure that workers, those involved in production or manufacture and those using the chemicals (e.g. those that spray insecticides or use them in sheep dipping), are supplied with guidance in the safe handling of the particular chemical or chemical mixtures. These include the use of Personal Protective Equipment (PPE), health and safety actions to take in the event of an accident, and occupational health and hygiene guidance for periods where exposure to the industrial agent should be limited.

**Table 1** Numbers of chemicals and amount known to have reliable medical toxicology knowledge

| Numbers of chemicals and amount known to have reliable medical toxicology knowledge | Information source |
| --- | --- |
| Over 34,000,000 chemicals assigned CAS numbers | Chemical Abstract Service (March 2008) |
| 640,018 commercially available chemicals | Chemfinder (Cambridge Soft Corporation) |
| About 70,000 chemicals routinely transported in UK | National Chemical Emergency Centre (UK) |
| About 500 new chemicals introduced to UK market each year | Health and Safety Executive (UK) |
| About 5,000 chemicals have registered toxicology information for acute and chronic exposure | European Commission, 2001 |

In health protection activities, there are many scenarios where the potential of chemical substances to cause ill health to exposed populations are a concern. These include:

1. The entry of chemicals to the water supplies.
2. The effects of toxic vapours contaminating the environment of public places and housing complexes.
3. The presence of chemicals in land where buildings or recreational activities are planned – the problem of land contamination.
4. Instances where there would be deliberate release of toxic chemicals – either during warfare or as acts of terrorism.

Toxicology essentially involves the study of the potential of these chemicals to cause harm to the various systems/organs of the human body, in relation to concentration, duration and route of exposure. Thus the role of toxicology, essentially, is to reduce or prevent the incidence of ill health due to exposure to chemicals. Another related role is in the investigation and treatment of exposures, and to document these aspects for other medical disciplines, public health and government. Yet another aspect is to advise or provide governments or regulatory bodies with the appropriate information to facilitate policy and regulation in relation to import, export, manufacture and use of potentially harmful chemicals.

## 3   Types of toxic agents

Toxic agents can be classified according to their properties (Box 2) and their effects on human health (Box 3).

**Box 2**  Chemical classification based on physico-chemical properties
Adapted from Illing, 2001

| Physical | Chemical | Biological Agents |
|---|---|---|
| Ionising radiation | Human medicines | Vaccines |
| Non-ionising radiation | Veterinary medicines | Allergens |
| Noise | Consumer products | Endotoxins |
| Vibration | Industrial chemicals | |
| Synthetic pesticides | | |
| Food additives | | |
| Chemicals of natural origin | | |
| Warfare agents | | |

**Box 3**  Chemical classification of toxic agents based on toxic effects

| Class of substance | Toxic Effects |
|---|---|
| Irritant | Causes inflammation of the skin and mucous membranes (skin, eyes, nose, or respiratory system). Skin (dermal) irritants cause irritant contact dermatitis (acute inflammation of the skin), symptoms of which include itching and skin changes ranging from reddening to blistering or ulceration. Examples: dilute solutions of acids, alkalis and some organic solvents. Respiratory irritants cause injury to the nose, mouth, throat and lungs. Materials that are very water soluble affect mainly the nose and throat. Less water soluble materials act deeper in the lungs. |
| Corrosive | A material that can destroy human tissue. Includes both acids and alkalis and may be a solid, liquid or gas. |
| Asphyxiant | A material that deprives tissues of oxygen and causes suffocation by displacing oxygen or interfering chemically with oxygen absorption, transport or utilisation. |
| Asphyxiant *simple* | A simple asphyxiant displaces oxygen from the atmosphere, which prevents its absorption. Examples: carbon dioxide, methane, and nitrogen. |
| Asphyxiant *chemical* | A chemical asphyxiant prevents the uptake of oxygen by the cells. Examples: carbon monoxide combines with haemoglobin and prevents it transporting oxygen to the cells; hydrogen sulphide prevents uptake of oxygen by the cells by inhibiting the action of enzymes – cytochromes – which are necessary for this process. |

**Box 3** continued

| | |
|---|---|
| Sensitisers | A chemical that causes an allergic reaction, such as urticaria or breathing problems. Examples: nickel, colophony. |
| Systemic effects | A response to chemical exposure that affects the whole body. Systemic illnesses may cause symptoms in one or two areas, but the whole body is affected. |
| Anaesthetic | Depresses the central nervous system. Examples: alcohols, halogenated hydrocarbons. |
| Pulmonary toxin | Irritates or damages the lungs. Examples: asbestos, silica ozone, chromium. |
| Neurotoxin | Affects the nervous system. Examples: mercury, lead, carbon disulphide. |
| Cardiotoxin | Affects the heart. Example: carbon disulphide. |
| Hepatotoxin | Causes liver damage. Example: carbon tetrachloride, dimethyl sulphate, chloroform. |
| Haematopoietic toxin | Affects the function of the cellular components of blood. Examples: benzene, ethanol, 2,4,6-Trinitrotoluene . |
| Nephrotoxin | Causes kidney damage. Examples: chloroform, mercury, lead. |
| Carcinogen | A material which can cause cancer. Examples: asbestos, benzene, acrylonitrile, 1-2 naphthylamine, vinyl chloride monomer. |
| Mutagen | Anything which causes a change in the genetic material of a living cell. Many mutagens are also carcinogens. |
| Reproductive toxins | Causes impotence or sterility in men and women. Examples: lead, dibromodichloropropane. |
| Teratogen | A material which interferes with the developing embryo when a pregnant female is exposed to that substance. Examples: lead, thalidomide. |

## 4    Routes of exposure to toxic substances

A potentially harmful substance may enter a living organism by:

A. **Ingestion (Orally):** by mouth, when absorption of the administered dose usually occurs in the gastro-intestinal tract (i.e. stomach, intestines). On occasions, absorption may occur in the mouth through the mucous membrane of the mouth (particularly

**Figure 1** Summary of routes of exposure, absorption, distribution and excretion of toxins in the body.

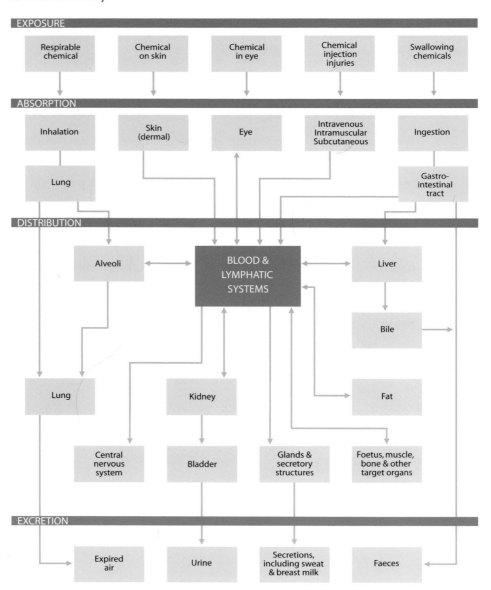

under the tongue when absorption is said to take place sublingually). Some drugs are prescribed for use sublingually (e.g. tablet placed under the tongue).

B. **Injection**: A potentially harmful substance can be administered directly into the blood stream, usually into a vein (intravenous injection), sometimes (rarely) into an artery. Injections are also given into a muscle (intramuscular), when absorption into the blood stream would depend on the blood flow to the muscle and therefore the time taken for entry into the blood stream would be slower than when the route of administration is intravenous. Substances are also injected into the superficial layers of the skin (intradermally or subcutaneously), into joints (intra-articular) or into fluids and spaces surrounding certain structures or organs within the body (e.g. intrathecally, when a substance is injected in the space between the layers covering the spinal cord which contains cerebrospinal fluid).

C. **Dermal:** One of the most common routes of exposure is when the potentially harmful substance is absorbed through the layers of the skin. In such instances, the vehicle or substances in which the toxin may be dissolved would influence the rate of absorption as such agents could either facilitate or decrease penetration of the skin layers.

D. **Inhalational**: This is also a common route of exposure, particularly in occupational settings. The harmful substances are inhaled via the nose and breathing tubes (bronchi and bronchioles) into the lung and finally into the thinly lined air cells (alveoli), which are surrounded by blood vessels. The harmful substances easily, albeit to varying degrees, diffuse across the thin lining of the alveoli into the blood stream. Figure 1 summarises routes of exposure and pathways of absorption, distribution and excretion of toxic chemicals in humans.

E. **Through mucous membrane:** Substances may also enter the body following absorption through the mucous membrane of the rectum or vagina (as with suppositories).

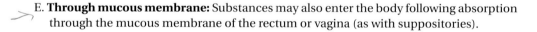

| 5 | Fate of a toxic substance that enters the body |
|---|---|

When a toxic substance enters the human body, it is subjected simultaneously to a number of processes, which results either in the total elimination of the toxic substance with no ill health, or ill-effects or altered function (of biological systems) or death of cells or enzyme systems. The fate of a toxic substance in a human body, i.e. the processes to which a toxin is subjected, e.g. metabolism, excretion or binding to tissues or cells or blood components such as proteins, is referred to as **toxicokinetics.** Similarly, when drugs used in the treatment of disease are considered, the term used is pharmacokinetics. What the toxin does to the structures in the human body e.g. cells or organs such as heart or brain, is referred to as **toxicodynamics.** The parallel term in drug therapy is pharmacodynamics.

Some factors influencing toxicokinetics are discussed below.

Most toxic substances have chemical and physical properties which determine the manner in which they are handled by the human body, and the nature of the harmful effects they produce. For example, if a substance is volatile (i.e. has a strong tendency to evaporate), it will usually be preferentially absorbed by inhalation. Substances which are lipophilic (dissolve easily in fat) will enter cells more easily than those which are essentially water soluble, because cell membranes have high lipid (fat) contents. The size of a molecule (usually described in terms of molecular weight) influences both its absorption and excretion (e.g. large molecules are absorbed less readily than small molecules; large molecules are poorly excreted by the kidneys).

When a toxic substance enters the body by mouth (orally), it is usually absorbed from the gut (gastro-intestinal system) and this may occur in the stomach or in the small or large intestines. Once absorbed, the toxic substance is taken by the blood vessels draining the intestine to the liver where the enzymes present in the cells of the liver either make them non-toxic (inactivated) or more toxic. The former, fortunately, is the more common occurrence. Amongst the enzymes present in the liver, the most important group is referred to as the cytochrome enzymes – notably the cytochrome P 450 enzymes. There are many components to this enzyme complex and each of the components has a specific affinity or ability to change the toxicity of the absorbed toxic agent. Amongst the constituents are CYP2C8 and CYP2C9, and these enzymes are best known as metabolisers or inactivators of drugs used in treatment of disease. What is important is that these enzymes can either increase in activity or decrease in activity, independently of the toxic substance. These changes to enzyme activity are predominantly brought about by other agents, usually drugs, but also by alcohol and cigarette smoking; those agents that increase the activity of the metabolising enzymes are called inducers and those that decrease the activity of the enzymes are called inhibitors. Thus it is necessary to know whether the metabolising enzymes of the liver (such enzymes are also present in the intestine and kidney and at some other sites) are induced or inhibited, for this information will influence the adverse effects that could be caused by the toxic substance.

It is now established that there are agents that facilitate the entry of substances from the gut (intestine) and also the loss of substances in the gut, kidney and bile. These are P-glycoproteins (P-gp) and organic anion transporting polypeptides (OATPs). These active transport systems play an important role in the elimination of drugs and also of toxins. These systems are affected by genetic factors and also by foods and drugs. The importance of these transport systems is that they influence the amount or concentration absorbed – be it a drug or toxin in the blood – by altering absorption or loss (excretion) from the intestine (gut), loss through the kidney (proximal renal tubular excretion) and loss through bile. A net result is that the amount of a substance that would be available to produce effects in the human body by acting at various sites or target organs will be affected by the relative contributions of the transport agents that promote removal or exit /efflux (i.e. the P-gp) and influx or entry (i.e. OATP mechanisms). What makes toxicity a complex process is that most agents that influence efflux and influx also affect the metabolising enzymes in the liver and intestine and kidney.

How chemicals may enter, be absorbed, become metabolised and are excreted from the body is illustrated in Figure 2; this illustrates toxicodynamics and toxicokinetics diagrammatically.

**Figure 2** Possible fates of a toxin in the body.

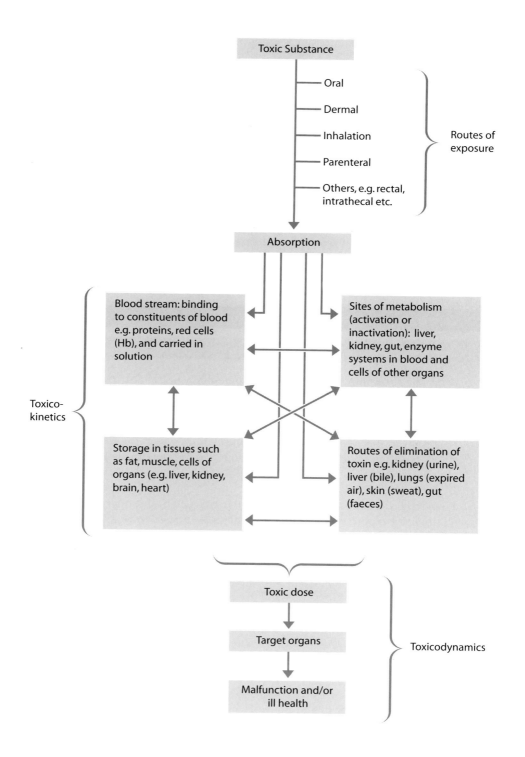

As stated earlier, the toxic effect or the harmful effect of a potentially toxic substance on an organ is determined primarily by the dose of the toxic substance that reaches the organ. Thus, if we consider an organ as being particularly susceptible to the effects of a toxic substance we would refer to that organ as a target organ. The dose of the potentially toxic substance that reaches the target organ is known as the target dose.

The target dose depends not only on the dose which reaches the body by inhalation, following ingestion, through the skin or by any other exposure route, but also by the processes that take place within the body once the potentially toxic substance gains entry into the body. These processes include:

- the rate of absorption – e.g. rate of absorption from the gut if intake is oral, rate of breathing if intake is inhalational, blood flow if intake is by intramuscular injection or intravenous injection.
- binding to proteins (especially in the blood), to fat and other tissues.
- metabolism (whereby a substance is usually made less harmful or toxic but the opposite may occur) by processes usually in the liver, kidney or intestine.
- excretion, that is removal of the potentially toxic substance from the body which is usually in the urine or in the faeces or in the bile or breath or through the skin.

## 6     Commonly used terminology in toxicology

### 6.1     Doses

*Dose:* The concentration of mass of the potentially harmful substance that is administered at one time – or the amount that enters the living organism at a given time.

*Exposure Dose:* The concentration of mass of the potentially harmful substance that is present in the environment or the source from which the harmful substance can enter the living organism – i.e. the amount of the potentially harmful substance in contaminated air, water, food and liquids.

*Absorbed Dose:* The exact amount of the potentially harmful substance, which is usually a proportion of the exposure dose that enters the living organism.

*Administered Dose:* The amount of the potentially harmful substance that is given (administered) to a living organism. A harmful substance may be administered by mouth or injected or applied to the skin or given by inhalation as an aerosol or spray.

*Total Dose:* The sum of all individual doses, from all routes.

*Toxic Dose (TD):* The dose that causes adverse or harmful effects:
- $TD_0$ is the dose that would cause harmful effects to 0% of the population.
- $TD_{10}$ is the dose that would cause harmful effects to 10% of the population.
- $TD_{50}$ is the dose that would cause harmful effects to 50% of the population.
- $TD_{90}$ is the dose that would cause harmful effects to 90% of the population.

*LOAEL*

*Threshold Dose:* The dose at which a toxic effect is first observed or detected.

*$LD_{50}$ (Lethal Dose 50%):* The statistically derived dose at which 50% of the individuals exposed will be expected to die (based on experimental observations, mostly in animals). This is the most frequently used estimate of toxicity of substances.

*$LC_{50}$ (Lethal Concentration 50%):* The calculated concentration of a gas lethal to 50% of a group when considering inhalational exposure. Occasionally $LC_0$ and $LC_{10}$ are also used.

*Effective Dose (ED):* This term indicates the effectiveness of a substance. In most instances, the effective dose refers to a beneficial effect, for example relief of pain. For certain drugs, e.g. muscle relaxing drugs which are used in anaesthesia to facilitate surgery, the effective dose of the substance would cause an effect which would be harmful in an uncontrolled setting (i.e. cause muscle paralysis). Thus depending on the nature of use of a substance, the effective dose could either indicate a beneficial effect or a harmful effect. A dose effective for 0% of the population would be indicated as $ED_0$, a dose effective for 10% of the population would be $ED_{10}$ and so forth.

The importance of knowing the toxic doses and the effective doses is that an indication of the safety of an agent could be understood. If the effective dose and the toxic dose for 50% of the population are similar the margin of safety with which the agent can be used is very small. In contrast, if there is a relatively large difference between the effective dose and the toxic dose for 50% of the population, the margin of safety would be greater.

## 6.2   Dose-response curve

This is a fundamental concept in the discipline of toxicology and has evolved from the speciality of pharmacology (the study of effects, actions and adverse effects of therapeutic agents or drugs used in treatment or prevention of disease).

The dose–response curve is an illustration indicating the effect or response to a particular dose of a drug used in treatment of disease or a chemical which has the potential to cause beneficial as well as harmful effects. It is an illustration which provides an indication of the doses at which a particular harmful effect is likely to occur, as well as information on when a maximal beneficial effect would occur.

A dose-response curve is calculated by using the lowest possible dose and noting the response, then increasing the dose at consistent increments and determining the response. These are then plotted on a graph, as in Figure 3.

The curve is a very valuable tool as it provides a visual guide as to the nature of responses for different doses of a particular substance. From such a curve one could obtain a basic concept of toxicity or harmful effect – e.g. death – and calculate the LD50, the dose at which 50 % of the subjects exposed are likely to die. The graph also provides information on what an effective dose or $ED_{50}$ of a substance would be – i.e.

**Figure 3** Dose-response curve.

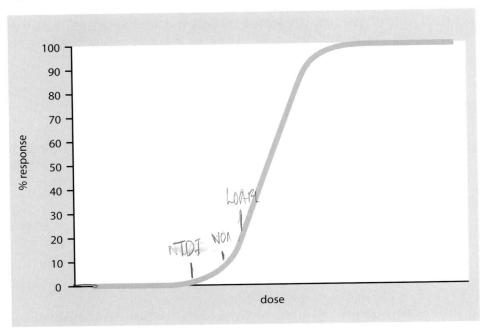

the dose at which an effective, usually beneficial, response would be obtained in 50% of the subjects exposed. The graph therefore gives an indication of the safety profile of a substance.

## 6.3   Other toxicology terms

*NOAEL/LOAEL:*
Following human and animal studies with substances that have the potential to cause harm, it is possible to obtain values or doses at which no harm would be expected. The highest level or dose at which there was no observed harmful or adverse effect is referred to as **No Observed Adverse Effect Level** (NOAEL). The lowest dose at which a harmful or adverse effect was observed is referred to as LOAEL – **Lowest Observed Adverse Effect Level**. As with effective doses, the terms NOAEL and LOAEL would be applicable for harmful or adverse effects as well as for desired therapeutic or clinical effects. In order to be more conservative, the **No Observed Effect Level** (NOEL) or **Lowest Observed Effect Level** (LOEL) are sometimes used to reassure the public of perceived toxicity with regards to substances that are frequently encountered in food or for domestic use (e.g. pesticides).

*Therapeutic Index:*
This term is used to compare the dose which produces a beneficial or therapeutic effect and the dose which causes harmful or toxic effects – the toxic dose.

*Half-Life:*

The elimination half-life of any xenobiotic agent (foreign substance) refers to the time course necessary for the quantity of the xenobiotic in the body (or plasma concentration) to be reduced to half its original level through various elimination processes.

Half-life is influenced by individual variations in genetic make up, state of health, age and several other factors.

This concept is important as it provides a timescale during which toxic effects may decrease due to the fall in concentration in the body, and also indicates how long a xenobiotic is likely to remain within the body. The half-life is also dependent on the medium in which the xenobiotic is found. For example with cadmium, the half-life in the blood is measured in days (approximately 5–7 days), whilst in the liver it is measured in months (7 months or so) and in the kidney it is measured in years (15 years or so).

The half-life is also important for biomonitoring for it indicates the peak time to take samples and carry out analyses.

## 7     Toxicity and target organs

The process(es) by which harm is done to a living organism by a xenobiotic is a complex phenomenon which is affected or influenced by several factors. Of these, as Paracelsus stated, dose is the most important.

Xenobiotics cause many types of toxicity by different mechanisms. Some chemicals are themselves toxic. Others may have to be metabolised (changed usually chemically in the body, usually by organs such as the liver) to become toxic.

Xenobiotics may affect only specific structures – i.e. organs or parts of cells. These sites which are affected by the xenobiotic to produce adverse effects are referred to as target organs. In contrast, some chemicals or xenobiotics can damage any cell or tissue they reach and come into contact with. The target organs affected may vary depending on the route of exposure and, of course, also the dose. It could be that a dose is sufficient to reach only certain tissues or cells rather than all tissues or cells.

Another important consideration is the duration of exposure. Here too, if the duration is short, possibly only the most vulnerable organs or tissues would be affected. If the duration is sufficiently long, all vulnerable tissues would be reached to cause adverse effects.

These aspects are dealt with in detail in Chapter 1.2 on target organs.

## 8     An introduction to risk assessment

A **hazard** is something (in the context of this book, a chemical) with the potential to cause an adverse, or 'harmful', effect. **Harm** may be physiological or psychological.

While psychological harm is a controversial issue, it shouldn't be underestimated when risks are communicated to the public.

**Risk** is usually defined as a measure of the likelihood of the occurrence of a particular adverse effect. It is therefore a probability, a number between zero and one, such as $10^{-6}$. This might sometimes be expressed as a ratio, e.g. one in a million.

The public usually seeks an assurance of zero risk, but this is rarely, if ever, possible. A lifetime risk of $10^{-6}$ (about the same as the risk of being struck by lightning) is often considered to be 'acceptable', but public acceptability often depends on whether the risk arises from a hazard that is perceived as pleasurable (such as alcohol consumption) or beneficial (such as a pharmaceutical). The public also more readily accepts risk when it is a matter of personal choice (such as smoking) rather than an imposition (food additives, water treatment chemicals). There are also emotional factors such as when children are exposed to risks.

'Safe' and 'dangerous' are imprecise and subjective terms, that are best avoided. They could be defined as 'risk which is acceptable/unacceptable to a particular individual or population'.

*Relative risk* is the ratio of the risk of the particular adverse effect in the population exposed to the hazard, to the risk to the population not exposed to the hazard.

*Risk* may also be defined as the product of the probability of the adverse effect and the magnitude of the effect.

In managing risk, setting standards, and in communicating with the public about hazards, public health agencies and regulatory bodies must balance the risks with the benefits to society of the chemical. To do this effectively, they need sound **Risk Assessment** procedures, and this in turn must be based upon good toxicological data. Unfortunately, there are many uncertainties and gaps in scientific knowledge and these have to be taken into account. Some of the methods and models used involve multiple assumptions, approximations and scientific judgements. Somewhat arbitrary 'safety factors', and 'uncertainty factors' may have been used in the extrapolation from animal studies to humans, in allowing for variations in animal and in human populations, and in reliance on small samples. These are all open to challenge. Risk assessment is certainly *not* an exact science!

Most models for risk assessment are based on the 4 steps listed below, whose origins are believed to be the National Research Council (1983).

> Hazard Identification;
> Dose-Response Assessment;
> Exposure Assessment, and
> Risk Characterisation.

*Hazard Identification*, in the context of chemicals, would involve the extensive search of published scientific evidence of adverse effects associated with exposure to the particular chemical, and similar substances. More than one hazard may result from exposure to a single substance.

The *Dose-Response Assessment* involves detailed study of available toxicological data; an understanding of the dose-response curve, threshold effects, elimination half-lives, $LD_{50}$s, NOAELs and LOELS etc. There may be other relevant data, such as epidemiological studies and incident reports.

*Exposure Assessment* includes a study of the frequency, duration, magnitude, concentrations and doses of chemicals to which humans will be exposed. The possible pathways and routes of entry will be analysed, and it will be remembered that the individual may be exposed to more than one source of the chemical. Both acute and chronic exposures will be considered.

*Risk Characterisation* brings together the other three steps to estimate risk and make recommendations for ***risk management***, including the setting of exposure standards and industrial codes of practice. It will include a detailed consideration and analysis of the robustness of the toxicological data, the appropriateness of analytical procedures and modelling techniques, the reasonableness of assumptions, including the magnitude of uncertainty and safety factors. With so many assumptions, uncertainties and subjectivity, outcomes are generally very conservative, usually using upper confidence limits. Risk assessors are mindful that their decisions are open to scrutiny and criticism and need to be constantly reviewed in the light of new or better information.

## 9     Further reading

Ballantyne B, Marrs T, Syversen T. (Eds.) (1999) *General and Applied Toxicology.* 2nd edition. MacMillan, London.

European Commission. (2001) White Paper on the Strategy for a Future Chemicals Policy. COM(2001) 88 final, Brussels.

Gilbert SG. (2004) *A Small Dose of Toxicology: The Health Effects of Common Chemicals.* CRC Press, New York.

Illing P. (2001) *Toxicity and Risk; Context, Principles & Practice.* Taylor & Francis, London & New York.

Klaassen C. (Ed.) (1996) *Casarett & Doull's Toxicology: The Basic Science of Poisons.* 5th edition. McGraw Hill, New York.

National Research Council. (1983) *Risk Assessment in the Federal Government: Managing the Process.* National Academy Press, Washington DC, USA.

Rodricks JV. (2007) *Calculated Risks.* Cambridge University Press, Cambridge.

Timbrell JA. (2002) *Introduction to Toxicology.* 3rd edition. Taylor and Francis, London.

*Useful internet links:*
Chemical Abstract Service: www.cas.org
Chemfinder: http://chemfinder.cambridgesoft.com/
Health and Safety Executive: www.hse.gov.uk
National Chemical Emergency Centre: www.the-ncec.com

# Section 1.2

## Target organs

David Baker

### Learning outcomes

At the end of this chapter and any recommended reading the student should be able to:

1. explain the normal structure and function of the human body systems, and the concept of target organs and systems;
2. explain, with the use of examples, how dysfunction in each of the important body systems may occur following exposure to toxic agents;
3. describe and discuss the manifestations of dysfunction in each of the important systems of the human body;
4. demonstrate awareness of the common chemicals causing ill health and the associated symptoms and signs, and
5. apply their knowledge in the analysis and management of hazardous situations.

## 1   Body systems and target organs

The human body can be regarded as a number of systems operating in parallel with each other to maintain normal life. The nervous, cardiovascular (heart and circulation), digestive and urinary systems are examples. Each system contains a number of key structures which are essential for its function. These are vulnerable to injury by foreign substances and in this context are termed target organs, since they are the clinical target of the toxic assault.

Target organs and systems will be discussed in this chapter using a standardised approach. This is:
1. the definition of the system in terms of its anatomy and physiology;
2. a brief description of normal function;
3. the medical expressions of abnormal function.

Note that medical expressions in terms of overall signs and symptoms (Box 1) are the final pathway of many biochemical processes that are covered by the science of biochemical toxicology. Such examples are provided in Table 1.

**Box 1**  Definition of signs and symptoms

A symptom is an indication of disease, illness, injury, or that something is not right in the body. Symptoms are felt or noticed by a person, but may not easily be noticed by anyone else. For example, chills, weakness, aching, shortness of breath, and a cough may be symptoms of pneumonia.

A sign is also an indication that something is not right in the body. But signs are defined as things that can be seen by a doctor, nurse, or other health care professional. Fever, rapid breathing rate, and abnormal breathing sounds heard through a stethoscope may be signs of pneumonia.

Our analysis will include key chemical changes (for example in disturbance of chemical transmitters in the body) but will emphasise the overall somatic disturbances produced by the toxic exposure. This is the role of medical toxicology.

The normal function of each target organ and system will only be presented in outline. The non-medical reader is advised to read this chapter in conjunction with the basic medical concepts appendix where the normal function of the body is described in more detail.

## 2    The nervous system

The nervous system controls all aspects of body function. It consists of the central nervous system, which includes the brain and spinal cord, and the peripheral nervous system, which transmits messages from the brain to all the organs of the body and also receives messages about the body and about the environment from the sensory system. The nervous system is made up of nerve cells and fibres which carry electrical impulses from the brain, and also chemical transmitters which amplify these electrical impulses at relay stations called synapses. The peripheral nervous system is subdivided into the voluntary system, which controls all muscular movements, and the autonomic system, which is not under voluntary control and ensures the function of all organs except the muscular system. There are many chemical transmitters involved in both the central and peripheral nervous system. One of the most important is acetylcholine, which is the chemical transmitter between the end of the motor nerves and muscle fibres, and also in the end synapses of the parasympathetic nervous system.

### 2.1    The central nervous system

*Key targets:  brain (including cerebrum, cerebellum hindbrain)*

**Table 1** A few symptoms and some possible chemical causes

| Symptoms | Substance |
| --- | --- |
| Alopecia (loss of hair on the head) | Arsenic, barium, bismuth, borates, carbon monoxide, gold compounds, lead, thallium |
| Amnesia (forgetfulness) | Bromides, ethanol, hydrogen sulphide, methyl bromide |
| Aplastic anaemia (lack of blood cells due to failure of production by the bone marrow) | Arsine, benzene, carbon tetrachloride, lindane, nitrous oxide |
| Chest pain (heart-attack like) | Cocaine, carbon disulphide |
| Convulsions (fits) | Carbon monoxide, cyanide, lindane, opiates, arsenic, lead |
| Diplopia (double vision) | Bromide, carbamates, carbon dioxide, carbon disulphide, carbon monoxide, ethanol, ethylene glycol, lead, mercury, methanol, methyl bromide, methyl chloride, organophosphate, trichloroethylene, triethyl tin |
| Eye irritation or redness | Chlorine (and similar e.g. hydrogen chloride), crowd control agents (e.g. CS gas) |
| Fasciculations (visible involuntary twitching of muscles) | Organophosphates, carbamates |
| Hallucinations | Methyl chloride, some solvents, thiocyanates |
| Hearing loss | Bromates, carbon monoxide aminoglycosides such as kanyamycin, toluene |
| Haematemesis (vomiting of blood) | Acetone, acids, alkalis, fluoride, formaldehyde, hypochlorites, phosphorus |
| Miosis (small or pinpoint pupils) | Acetone, carbamates, organophosphates, opiates |
| Mydriasis (large or dilated pupils) | Benzene, carbon dioxide, chloroform, cyanide, ethyl bromide, ethylene glycol, fluoride, methyl bromide, thallium, toluene |
| Nystagmus (jerky movements of the eyeball) | Arsenic, carbon disulphide, carbon monoxide, ethanol, ethyl bromide, ethylene glycol, gold compounds, manganese, methyl bromide, methyl chloride, organophosphates, toluene, xylene |
| Photophobia (intolerance of or hypersensitivity to light by the eyes) | Bromide, carbon dioxide, methanol, mercury |

**Table 1** continued

| Skin irritation with defatting of skin and/or rashes | Acids, alkalis, alcohols, chlorinated compounds, ketones, nickel, phenol, trichloroethylene |
|---|---|
| Tinnitus (ringing in the ears) | Arsenic, ethanol, trimethyl tin, toluene |
| Upper respiratory tract irritation | Oxides of nitrogen, oxides of sulphur, crowd control agents (e.g. CS gas) |
| Wheezing | Chlorine, phosgene, oxides of nitrogen or sulphur (asthmatics), organophosphates (inhalation), acrolein, asbestos, chromium, hydrogen sulphide, nickel, nitrogen dioxide, ozone, silica |

### 2.1.1  Normal function

The brain is a complex array of neurons grouped to control motor, sensory, posture and higher cognitive function. The brainstem controls much of the essential physiological activity such as breathing. See section 3.1 of the Appendix for more information on the normal functioning of the central nervous system.

### 2.1.2  Abnormal function

Toxic effects on the central nervous system have profound effects both on higher cerebral functions including consciousness and also on the movements of the body and their control. Examples of manifestations of toxic damage or injury to the brain are coma, convulsions, impairment of memory and disturbances in gait.

## 2.2  The peripheral nervous system

*Key targets: Sensory, autonomic and motor nerves*

### 2.2.1  Normal function

*Sensory nerves.* These are of varying sizes and transmit information about the body such as pain and temperature from special receptors.

*Acetylcholine.* Acetylcholine (ACh) is a major chemical neurotransmitter. It is released in small packets or vesicles from the nerve terminal and creates an amplified electrical response on the other side of the synapse. When this has happened the transmitter is very rapidly broken down by an enzyme called acetyl cholinesterase which is present throughout the cholinergic nervous system.

*The cholinergic nervous system.* The control of the concentrations of ACh is essential to the functioning of the cholinergic nervous system. This includes:

- Voluntary motor nerves: Acetylcholine transmission at the neuromuscular junction.
- The autonomic nervous system: This comprises the parasympathetic and sympathetic systems. The parasympathetic system uses ACh as a transmitter whereas the sympathetic system uses noradrenaline. In general, the sympathetic system causes stimulation of body systems whereas the parasympathetic has the reverse effect. A good example is found in the nervous control of the heart.

Cholinergic effects are divided into muscarinic and nicotinic effects. These terms were derived from the actions of the compounds muscarine and nicotine during the early research into the cholinergic system. Muscarinic ACh receptors are found in the gut, heart (vagus) and the pupil and accommodation muscles of the eye. The actions are blocked by atropine. Nicotinic ACh receptors control the voluntary nerve endings to muscle.

See section 3.2 of the Appendix for more information on the normal functioning of the peripheral nervous system.

## 2.2.2   Abnormal function

Failure of the peripheral nervous system affects both the sensory and motor systems. The autonomic nervous system can also be affected. A direct toxic effect on nerves is called toxic neuropathy. This causes failure of nerve transmission due to the dysfunction of motor and large sensory fibres.

1. *Failure of nerve conduction*
   Toxic neuropathy affects nerve conduction by toxic effects on the myelin sheath of the nerve which is essential for normal function. Many chemical substances cause damage to nerve conduction, a condition called toxic peripheral neuropathy. Examples include some organophosphate pesticides (no longer used in the UK) and industrial substances such as lead, thallium, triorthocresyl phosphate, carbon disulphide, n-hexane and acrylamide. Nerve conduction can also be affected by toxins. These are naturally occurring compounds which are produced by plant, animal and aquatic organisms and bacteria. Examples are tetrodotoxin and saxitoxin, which interrupt nerve conduction by blocking essential sodium ion channels in the nerve.

   Finally, nerve conduction can also be interrupted by an inappropriate immune reaction from the body. An example is the Guillain Barré syndrome (acute idiopathic inflammatory polyneuropathy), which may be caused by a cell-mediated hypersensitivity (see section 8.2).

2. *Failure of chemical transmission*
   If the acetyl cholinesterase at the cholinergic synapses fails, this causes an **increase** in ACh at cholinergic synapses, causing poisoning by over-stimulation of the voluntary and autonomic cholinergic nervous systems. This is the case in organophosphate (OP)

and carbamate pesticide poisoning. Increases in the ACh concentrations cause effects at all cholinergic synapses, both peripheral and in the central nervous system (Box 2). Further information on OP poisoning is found in Chapter 4.3 on pesticides.

**Box 2** Classic signs and symptoms of organophosphate anticholinesterase poisoning

- Pin point pupils
- Excess salivation
- Lachrymation
- Urination
- Involuntary defaecation
- Muscle fasciculation and paralysis
- Central nervous stimulation and fitting
- Failure of respiratory control in the brain stem

Cholinergic synaptic transmission can also be affected by a **reduction** in the release of ACh. This is the case following intoxication by botulinum toxin as a result of food poisoning. In botulism, there is muscle weakness, but the clinical picture is one of failure of cholinergic transmission rather than overstimulation, as in the case of pesticide poisoning. The muscles of the shoulder girdle, respiration and of swallowing are particularly affected, creating the classic syndrome of botulism. The onset of paralysis is much slower than with anticholinesterase poisoning and the weakness can be overcome to an extent in the early stages by extra voluntary effort.

Alterations in transmission of impulses at cholinergic synapses have far reaching effects on other body systems and target organs which are considered below.

## 3    The cardiovascular system (the heart and circulatory system)

Blood is transported through the body via a continuous system of blood vessels. This comprises arteries, capillaries and veins. Arteries carry oxygenated blood away from the heart into capillaries supplying tissue cells. Veins collect the blood from the capillary bed and carry it back to the heart. The main purpose of blood flow through body tissues is to deliver oxygen and nutrients to the cells and to remove waste products. Circulation besides the heart and pulmonary circulation is known as the systemic circulation.

The cardiovascular system forms the transport system of the body. As such it carries:
1. oxygen from the lungs to the tissues;
2. carbon dioxide from the tissues to the lungs so that it may be eliminated during the expiration phase of breathing;
3. food components from the digestive tract to the cells to provide nutrition for growth and energy;
4. waste products from cells in the body to the kidneys to be removed in the urine;

5. hormones from the glands that produce them (endocrine glands) to other organs of the body;
6. heat produced in other parts of the body to the skin so that the surplus heat can be given off.

## 3.1    The heart

*Key targets: Heart (including nerve control, conducting system, heart muscle)*

### 3.1.1   Normal function

See section 4.1 of the Appendix for information on the normal functioning of the heart.

### 3.1.2   Abnormal function

#### Direct toxic effects
The heart beats by contraction of its individual muscle fibres or myocytes. The heart muscle itself can be a target for toxic attack. Toxic effects may occur on:

- **the conducting system.** The conducting system carries impulses from the sino atrial node in the atria through to the ventricles and controls the timing and synchronisation of the heart. Interference with this system may be either direct or indirect and lead to irregular heart beats or dysrhythmias.
- **myocytes** (the heart muscle fibres). Many toxic substances such as inhaled hydrocarbons, including volatile anaesthetics, produce atrial and ventricular ectopic beats. These compounds can also affect conduction at the junction between the atria and the ventricles.

#### Indirect toxic effects
These are mediated via the autonomic nervous system. The heart is controlled by the vagus nerve which is cholinergic and also by sympathetic nerves. Stimulation of these nerves causes:

- slowing of the heart via stimulation of the vagus nerve muscarinic receptors. This is most commonly seen in pesticide poisoning. The effect can be blocked by atropine which causes block of the vagal impulses. In poisoning by *Atropa belladonna* (Deadly Nightshade), tachycardia is a key sign.
- acceleration of the heart via stimulation of the sympathetic nervous system and noradrenaline receptors. This is seen in cases of adrenaline overdose.

## 3.2    The arterial system

*Key targets: veins, arteries*

### 3.2.1  Normal function

See section 4.2 of the Appendix for information on the normal functioning of the arterial system.

### 3.2.2  Abnormal function

In addition to the heart, the arterial system can be a target organ. Both constriction and dilation of vessels can occur, as with ergotamine poisoning (from the fungus *Claviceps purpurea*) and vasodilators such as nitrites and alcohol. Vasodilation is also a beneficial effect on the coronary arteries when drugs such as glyceryl trinitrate are used. Overdose with vasodilators can lead to a major fall in blood pressure.

## 4     The gastro-intestinal system

*Key targets: small intestine, large intestine, stomach, mouth, oesophagus*

**Figure 1** Blood supply to the liver comes from both the arterial supply and from the portal system from the gut. Courtesy of Timbrell J

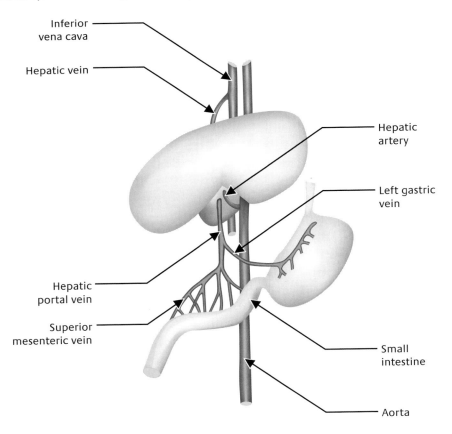

## 4.1    Normal function

See section 6 of the Appendix for information on the normal functioning of the gastro-intestinal system.

## 4.2    Abnormal function

### *Toxic actions on the gut mediated by nervous control*
The gut is controlled by the parasympathetic autonomic nervous system. Toxic effects begin at the mouth where there may be hyper- and hypo-salivation caused by OP and atropine respectively. Intestinal motility may be increased by OP or carbamate pesticides leading to colic and diarrhoea, or decreased by morphine and related compounds.

### *Direct effects*
Direct effects on the gut may occur through:
- corrosive effects on the stomach (e.g. by acids);
- acute toxic effects on gut absorption (e.g. by enterotoxins); and
- chronic effects such as neoplasia, carcinoma of the mouth, tongue and oesophagus (e.g. by chillies, betel nuts, tobacco).

# 5    The liver

*Key target: Liver*

## 5.1    Normal function

The liver is a major target organ which is associated with the alimentary system. It has an essential role in the body in nutrition and in the removal of a number of toxic substances. Normal biochemical detoxification functions are part of balanced excretion and detoxification. The liver is a key target organ for a large number of toxic substances such as alcohol and carbon tetrachloride and a number of general anaesthetic agents. Although liver cells are capable of regeneration, toxic actions cause a breakdown in the cellular structure of the organ and a failure of its biochemical functions, as occurs in cirrhosis.

The liver is a key target organ for many toxic substances because:

- it receives a rich blood supply from the gut where toxic substances may be absorbed (Figure 1);
- it has a unique structure based upon hepatocytes which are metabolically very active, and
- it has a major metabolic and excretory role.

The liver receives 25% of the blood supply from the heart. Toxic substances absorbed from the gut are transported directly to the liver which is therefore the first target organ exposed after the gut itself. Hepatocytes are cells that make up most of the structure of the liver and are very metabolically active. Normally they are involved in many essential biochemical processes such as removal of nitrogen as urea, synthesis of glycogen as a glucose store and lipid metabolism. Many toxic substances inhibit protein synthesis because of their action in the liver. Apart from metabolising the body's own waste products, the liver also has a key role in removing external poisons (xenobiotics) such as carbon tetrachloride and alcohol. Carbon tetrachloride blocks protein synthesis through a free radical mechanism.

See section 7 of the Appendix for more information on the normal functioning of the liver, including the excretion of bilirubin.

## 5.2   Abnormal function

Failure to excrete bilirubin gives rise to a yellowish discolouration of the whites of the eyes, the skin and nails and mucosal membranes, known as jaundice. Several toxic compounds such as some pesticides, solvents such as carbon tetrachloride and dry cleaning fluids damage the liver cells and prevent them from functioning normally. There are many drugs used in the treatment of medical conditions which also damage the liver cells and are termed hepatotoxic. For example, very high doses of the common drug paracetamol can cause liver damage, liver failure and jaundice.

Therefore in **liver failure**, jaundice occurs, the blood urea falls (as urea is no longer formed from ammonia), there is insufficient production of proteins, of which albumin is the most important, which may lead to swelling of ankles or oedema (as proteins are essential to maintain plasma osmotic pressure which keeps fluid within capillaries) and blood clotting will be impaired. The most important effect is that the blood will not have sufficient glucose for the cells to function normally. In addition, when the liver cells fail to function properly, their ability to make foreign substances less toxic by metabolic enzymes fails and the toxicity of some drugs used in medicine such as morphine is increased.

## 6     The respiratory system

Respiration involves transport of oxygen from the atmosphere to the cells of the body and carbon dioxide in the opposite direction. It is divided into external respiration, which describes the passage of oxygen to the red blood cells in the lung sacs (alveoli), and internal respiration, which describes the carriage of oxygen from the lungs to the cells and carbon dioxide back to the lungs.

## 6.1 External respiration

*Key targets: Brainstem (respiratory control), lungs (airways and alveoli)*

## 6.1.1   Normal function

The respiratory centres in the mid brain and brain stem control cyclical active inflation and passive deflation of the lungs, commonly called breathing. Breathing ensures passage of oxygen to alveoli and removal of carbon dioxide to the atmosphere via upper and lower airways. The exchange of gases to and from the blood in the alveoli takes place at the alveolar membrane (where internal respiration starts). Normal external respiration is designed to maintain the oxygen and carbon dioxide levels in the blood at levels that allow the body cells to operate normally. The thin membrane between the alveolar sac and the pulmonary capillary is highly vulnerable to direct attack by inhaled toxic compounds.

In addition to its role in exchanging gases, the pulmonary capillary bed acts as an active filtration and detoxification system. This makes it very vulnerable to a number of toxic substances.

See section 5 of the Appendix for more information on the normal functioning of the external respiratory system.

## 6.1.2   Abnormal function

*Depression of central control of respiration*
Many toxic substances act on the brain and depress breathing, for example opioids and organophosphates. This leads to a build up of carbon dioxide in the lung sacs and in the blood causing hypoxia and respiratory acidosis. If breathing depression is not reversed or artificial ventilation started, the hypoxia will worsen followed by cardiac arrest (stoppage of the heart beat due to lack of oxygen to the heart muscle).

*Effects on lung parenchymal tissue*
The air sacs of the lung (the alveoli) have many functions apart from exchange of gases. They are very fragile and susceptible to toxic attack either directly by inhaled toxic substances, for example phosgene, causing toxic pulmonary oedema, or indirectly as a result of filtering out toxic substances such as paraquat (a weedicide), which attacks the pulmonary capillaries.

The outcome of toxic effects on the lung and airways may be divided into:
- acute respiratory failure. Failure of breathing and ventilation of the lungs leads to increasing carbon dioxide levels and hypoxia in the alveoli. Hypoxic myocardium leads to secondary cardiac arrest.
- chronic respiratory failure where there is fibrosis and adult respiratory distress syndrome.
- neoplastic effects including carcinoma of the bronchus from tobacco smoke and mesothelioma from the inhalation of asbestos particles.

## 6.2   Blood and internal respiration

*Key targets: red blood cells, mitochondria*

### 6.2.1   Normal function

The red cells of the blood contain haemoglobin which carries oxygen from the lungs to the cells of the body. In the cells, oxygen is delivered to the mitochondria – intra-cellular structures which are the 'powerhouses' of the cells. Mitochondria have cytochromes which generate energy in the form of adenosine triphosphate (ATP) which ensures normal life function.

### 6.2.2   Abnormal function

#### *Red cells*

Haemoglobin can be a target if the oxygen carrying capacity is blocked by toxic gases. This is the case in carbon monoxide (CO) poisoning, where CO combines with haemoglobin more easily than oxygen (see Chapter 4.1 on carbon monoxide for more information).

#### *Mitochondria*

The other key targets in the internal respiratory system are the mitochondria in the cells. The interaction of oxygen with the cytochrome system in the mitochondria can be blocked leading to a failure of internal respiration. This is the case in cyanide poisoning and is also considered to follow exposure to carbon monoxide.

## 7    The haematopoietic system

*Key target: Bone marrow, white blood cells*

### 7.1   Normal function

The bone marrow is the source of both white and red blood cells. White cells have an essential role in inflammatory, coagulation and immune function. Red cells, as noted above, have an essential role in the carriage of oxygen. See section 4.3 of the Appendix for more information on the normal functioning of the haematopoietic system.

### 7.2   Abnormal function

The bone marrow is a major target for many toxic substances. As a result of failure of generation of new cells, there may be failure of the red cell system (aplastic anaemia), failure of the white cell system causing both overwhelming infection due to absence of granulocytes (agranulocytosis), and failure of the immune system from a total reduction of the white cell count, including lymphocytes (pancytopaenia).

Failure of cellular development can be caused by a number of toxic agents including drugs, mustard gas and heavy metals. Toxic effects on the bone marrow may cause generation of a type of cancer called leukaemia.

## 8    The immune system

*Key targets: Immune reactions are mediated by a number of cell types in the body, each of which may be regarded as a system in its own right*

### 8.1    Normal function

See section 10 of the Appendix for information on the normal functioning of the immune system.

### 8.2    Abnormal function

Toxic reactions involving the immune systems may involve direct or indirect immunotoxicity.

#### Direct immunotoxicity

Direct effects are caused by immunosuppression or immunostimulation. In immunosuppression, the toxic agent reduces the activity of the immune system causing malfunction. This may be due to an effect on a target organ of the system such as the thymus, which produces B lymphocytes, or the bone marrow which produces blood cells. Examples of substances causing immunosuppression include dioxin and polonium 210.

In immunostimulation, the immune system is stimulated by a challenge from an administered protein which is similar to that found in humans but is treated by the body as an antigen. Examples include drugs derived from recombinant DNA.

#### Indirect immunotoxicity

Indirect effects include hypersensitivity, allergic reactions or autoimmunity. These are caused by a toxic substance presenting a challenge to the immune system as an antigen. Most toxic chemicals are too small to do this and have to combine with a larger molecule such as a protein (called a hapten) to be able to create an effective foreign antigen.

Immune reactions which result from indirect immunotoxicity are classified as type 1 – type 4.

##### Type 1 reactions

In this reaction, free antigen fixes to IgE antibody which then attacks mast cells releasing vasodilator mediators (e.g. 5 HT). This type of reaction causes acute collapse following a prior sensitisation (anaphylaxis) or pulmonary sensitisation/ asthma-like effects. Examples include drugs such as penicillins, or industrial compounds such as toluene di-isocyanate.

### Type 2 reactions

In this reaction there is a break-up of the cell (cytolysis). Antigen bound to cell membranes associates with free antibodies (IgG, IgM, IgA) to produce agglutination with complement fixation and cell lysis. Examples include drugs such as aminopyrine.

### Type 3 reactions

In this reaction there is free soluble antigen in excess of antibody, which combines with free antibody. This then causes a complex known as precipitin to be deposited in the inner lining of blood vessels (the vascular endothelium). An example is the drug hydralazine, sometimes used for the emergency reduction of high blood pressure.

### Type 4 reactions

These are cell-mediated hypersensitivity reactions. In this reaction, part of the cell membrane becomes an antigen. This then combines with killer T lymphocytes causing death of cells. An example is the familiar nickel contact dermatitis.

## 9   The urinary system

*Key targets:  Kidney, bladder*

### 9.1   Normal function

See section 8 of the Appendix for information on the normal functioning of the kidney.

### 9.2   Abnormal function

The kidney, like the liver, has a high blood supply and metabolic activity, but its major role is in excretion of urea and maintenance of the somatic acid-base balance, rather than metabolic activity. Substances that cause kidney damage are those which are concentrated in the organ. This accumulation may produce acute and chronic toxic effects on the tubule system which can lead to acute and chronic renal failure. Examples include heavy metals such as ionised mercury, lead and the antibiotic gentamycin.

In addition to the kidney, other parts of the urinary tract may be the target of toxic attack, such as the neoplastic effects on the bladder of aniline dyes.

## 10   The reproductive system

*Key targets: Ovaries, testes, oocytes, spermatozonia*

## 10.1 Normal function

The reproductive system comprises the ovaries in the female which release oocytes and spermatozonia in the male which are involved in fertilisation of the oocyte.

## 10.2 Abnormal function

Toxic effects on the reproductive system may be manifest as effects on fertility or on development of offspring. Impaired fertility has been noted with chemicals but only following prolonged exposure, whereas developmental toxicity may occur following a single exposure. Teratogenicity, the production of congenital malformations following exposure during pregnancy, is a particular concern. The actions of certain drugs as teratogens are well-known since the problem was first highlighted by thalidomide in the 1960s. The foetus is very vulnerable to teratogenic effects during the first trimester of pregnancy, and during the second and third trimesters drugs may affect growth and functional development. Since the 1960s, detailed rules for prescribing have been published (see British National Formulary), which underline the fact that drugs should only be prescribed in pregnancy if the expected benefit to the mother is thought to be greater than the risk to the foetus. All drugs should be avoided if possible during the first trimester except for life-threatening conditions.

## 11    The epithelial system

*Key targets: eyes, skin and mucous membranes*

## 11.1 Normal function

The epithelial system includes the skin, the mucous membranes which line the mouth and the eyes. The system has an important role in the body's defences. The skin is not usually regarded as an organ (some consider the skin to be the largest organ in the body) but it should nevertheless be included as a toxic target organ. The skin, like the liver and the alimentary tract, is constantly under renewal with new cells being created in the dermis and migrating outwards to the epidermis. This process of cellular renewal is a target for a number of toxic pathways.

## 11.2 Abnormal function

### The eye
The pupil is a good indicator of toxic effects. The constrictor muscle is cholinergic (muscarinic) and is affected by toxic agents with an action on this system. Pupils may be small (pin point pupils) as a result of OP pesticide poisoning. Morphine also causes the same result but by a different central mechanism.

The pupil may also be dilated following a blocking of the constrictor muscle as in the case following atropine (deadly nightshade) poisoning. The cornea of the eye is very vulnerable to attack by corrosive and vesicant agents such as mustard gas (see Chapter 4.5 on chemical warfare agents).

### The skin

A number of toxins have a direct effect on the skin. Ricin acts due to a generalised inhibition of protein synthesis and leads to a multiple breakdown of body organ systems prior to death (multiple organ dysfunction syndrome). *Clostridium welchii*, the organism causing gas gangrene, produces dramatic clinical effects on the skin with widespread necrosis due to the action on phospholipase C. There are possibilities that this toxin may have been considered for development as an agent of chemical warfare.

There may be direct toxic effects on the DNA structure of the dermis leading to DNA cross-linking that is thought to be behind the vesicant effects of mustard gas. Mustard gas causes damage presenting as severe blistering and ulceration. Equally, corrosive substances such as strong acids cause chemical burning by direct chemical disruption of the cells.

The skin may also be affected by allergic reactions leading to eczema – dermatitis (as in the case of nickel contact  – see type 4 immune reactions above) and also through urticaria produced as a result of a generalised allergic reaction.

## 12    Conclusions

A wide variety of toxic substances produce a medical expression through target organs and systems in the body. Effects may be considered in terms of normal and abnormal function of organs and systems. Expression of toxicity may be acute and chronic through pharmacological, physiological, immune, teratogenic and carcinogenic mechanisms. Target organ toxicology provides the link between biochemical toxicology and overall signs and symptoms which are the end stage of toxic exposure.

## 13    Further reading

British National Formulary (BMF) www.bnf.org

Lu FC, Kacew S. (2002) *Lu's Basic Toxicology*. 4th edition. Taylor and Francis, London.

Timbrell J. (2002) *Introduction to Toxicology*. 3rd edition. CRC Press, London.

# Section 1.3

# Experimental methods for investigating the toxicity of chemicals

Robin Fielder

## Learning outcomes

At the end of this chapter and any recommended reading the student should be able to:

1. explain how toxicological data is produced and be able to describe some of the methods used;
2. understand the limitations of the data and its use in the setting of standards;
3. take a critical and analytical approach to the application of standards set by advisory and regulatory bodies, and
4. apply their knowledge in the analysis and management of hazardous situations.

## 1 Introduction

For most chemicals there are little if any sound human data from experience in use on which to base an assessment of their health effects. Thus such assessments must largely be based on results of toxicological studies in animals. Despite considerable research into alternatives to animals, there are only a few specific areas of toxicology where reliable data may be obtained from *in vitro* methods. These relate to assessing mutagenic potential (basically the ability to damage DNA or genetic material), or local effects (severe skin and eye irritants and sensitivity to light-photoirritancy).

For assessing general toxicological effects of single and repeated exposure to chemicals, mainly rodents have to be used in laboratory studies. Every effort is made to ensure that tests are carried out using the minimum number of animals with minimal distress to the test animals. EU member states have a legal requirement to observe what is often referred to in the animal welfare context as the 3 Rs (Reduction, Refinement and Replacement when practical and validated alternatives are available) (Council Directive, 1986).

The key guidelines for methods for investigating the toxic effects of chemicals are those produced under the auspices of the Chemicals Programme of the Organisation of Economic Cooperation and Development (OECD Guidelines). These are internationally recognised and have done much to reduce the needless duplication of studies to satisfy specific requirements of different countries/regulatory agencies. They are updated both with regard to advances in science and animal welfare considerations.

It is recognised that there are uncertainties in extrapolating from animal data to humans. This is taken into account by dividing the critical no observed adverse effect level (NOAEL) in animal studies by Uncertainty Factors (or Assessment Factors). A value of 100 is commonly used comprising 10 to account for inter-species differences and 10 for intra-individual variability (IPCS, 1999). This value may be modified to account for incomplete data sets or severity of effects. Recent reviews give more details of the use of Uncertainty Factors and their possible replacement by chemical specific factors if sufficient data are available, but this is rarely the case (IGHRC, 2003; IPCS, 2005).

The approach described above of estimating a safe exposure level is appropriate for toxicological effects that have a threshold. This is true for most toxic effects but there is one important exception. Compounds that are mutagenic, namely those that damage DNA which may be expressed as carcinogenicity or induction of heritable mutations, may not have a threshold. Any exposure to a mutagenic compound may be associated with an adverse effect, although this may be very small. This is because one 'hit' on DNA may result in a mutation that can, after clonal expansion, lead to tumour formation. Although in practice there may be a threshold, due for example to rapid detoxification of the chemical, this is difficult to convincingly demonstrate, and the prudent assumption to make is that such compounds do not have a threshold. For these compounds a risk management approach of reducing exposure to as low as reasonably practicable or 'ALARP' is generally adopted.

Guidance on general principles for assessing chemical carcinogens is provided in an IGHRC document (IGHRC, 2002).

In order to draw up a reasonably complete toxicological profile of a chemical, information from the following studies would be expected:

- acute toxicity;
- skin and eye irritancy and skin sensitisation;
- repeated dose toxicity (28 or 90 days);
- mutagenicity (and hence potential carcinogenicity);
- toxicity to the reproductive system.

In addition, information from chronic toxicity/carcinogenicity bioassays may be available for a more complete dataset.

Toxicity test methods for each area are considered in the following sections.

## 2    Acute toxicity

The aim of an acute toxicity study is to investigate effects following a single exposure for a period of up to 24 hours using the oral, dermal or inhalation route as appropriate. Normally three dose levels are used except for relatively non-toxic compounds when a single limit dose is acceptable (2000 mg/kg bodyweight/day by the oral route). In the past, emphasis was on calculation of an $LD_{50}$ value with confidence limits. The $LD_{50}$ approach has been heavily criticised however, because of animal welfare considerations and also as being scientifically unnecessary. The methods now recommended place emphasis on noting signs of toxicity (onset and duration) rather than calculating an $LD_{50}$ value. One approach, first proposed by a working group of the British Toxicology Society and now recognised as an OECD guideline, does not use death as an endpoint, the maximum dose level used being designed to produce 'evident toxicity' i.e. clear signs of toxicity such that the next higher dose level would be expected to produce mortality or severe pain and distress (van den Heuval *et al.,* 1990).

In all acute toxicity studies animals are observed carefully during the first four hours post dosing, and then on a daily basis for at least 14 days. Animals are then subject to autopsy at termination, when all gross pathological changes are recorded together with microscopic examination of organs showing gross pathology.

Results from these studies are used for hazard assessment and for classification of chemicals on the basis of acute toxicity.

## 3     Skin and eye irritancy and skin sensitisation

Knowledge of the direct irritant properties of a chemical on skin and eyes, and also the potential to produce an allergic reaction in the skin, is important in hazard assessment particularly with regard to occupational exposure and also exposure of the general public to consumer products. There are well established animal models to investigate such effects, the results of which are used to classify chemicals on the basis of their irritant or sensitisation properties.

Methods for investigating irritancy are based on the rabbit model. There have been major changes in how such studies are conducted over recent years and these are reflected in the updated OECD guidelines in these areas, which were adopted in 2002. It is now possible by consideration of various factors (physico-chemical properties/pH, results from validated *in vitro* tests for skin corrosivity/severe irritation of eyes) to predict severe effects without using live animals. The animal tests are used to confirm lack of irritancy or to grade mild to moderate irritation. If there is any doubt, tests are carried out on a single animal in the first instance.

Investigating skin sensitisation is another area where there have been significant changes over the past few years. For many years, the guinea pig was the animal of choice and the preferred method was referred to as the Guinea Pig Maximisation Test. The initial dose to induce sensitisation was given intradermally (into the skin), together with Freunds Complete Adjuvant (water-in-oil emulsion of inactivated and dried mycobacteria) to enhance the response. This was followed by a rest period of about two weeks to allow the immune response to develop. A non-irritant challenge dose was then applied topically to the skin and any skin response observed over the next few days was compared to that seen in the control animals.

However, more recently a mouse model has been developed which offers the advantage of a more objective endpoint than visual examination of the skin reaction. It also has distinct animal welfare advantages (use of fewer animals and not involving induction of a dermal (skin) hypersensitivity response).The new test is referred to as the Local Lymph Node Assay (LLNA). The underlying principle that forms the basis for this test is that sensitisers induce primary proliferation of lymph nodes, draining the site where the chemical was applied, in this case the ear. This proliferation is proportional to dose and potency of the allergen and this provides an objective, quantitative measure of sensitisation. Cell proliferation is measured in the lymph nodes draining the ear by preparing a suspension of lymph node cells from animals that have been pre-treated with tritiated methylated thymidine. The incorporation of the radioactive tritium is measured by scintillation counting. Results are compared to a control group and expressed as the stimulation index (Kimber *et al.,* 1994). The OECD adopted a test guideline for the LLNA as a method for investigating skin sensitisation in 2002.

Chronic Toxicity

## 4    Repeated dose toxicity study (28 or 90 day)

Assessment of the possible health hazards arising from repeated exposure is usually determined by either a 28 day or a 90 day study in rodents. There are OECD guidelines for such studies by the oral, dermal and inhalation routes. The 28 day study is designed for use with chemicals for which a 90 day study would not be warranted, for example because of low production volume and limited potential for human exposure.

Many aspects of the 28 day and 90 day studies are common. At least three dose levels are used, together with a control group, using five males and five females per group in the 28 day study, and double these numbers in the 90 day study. The highest dose is chosen with the aim of inducing toxic effects but not death or severe suffering. Lower doses are selected with a view to demonstrating any dosage related response and a NOAEL. Dose levels are usually selected from a small range-finding study. For essentially non-toxic compounds, a single limit-dose of 1000 mg/kg/day may be used.

Both the 28 day and the 90 day study have been revised in recent years to provide more information on neurotoxicity (toxicity to the nervous tissue-nerves, neurones) and also effects on immunological systems and reproductive organs.

The need for careful clinical observations throughout the exposure period is important so as to obtain as much information as possible. In addition to the general clinical observations daily (with observations for morbidity/mortality twice daily), detailed clinical observations are made outside the home cage in a standard arena before exposure, and then weekly thereafter. In the last week of exposure, what is referred to as a functional observation battery is carried out. This involves testing sensory reactivity to stimuli (auditory-hearing, visual, proprioceptive-touch), grip strength and motor activity. Haematology and clinical chemistry studies are carried out at the end of the test period, with interim samples being taken in the 90 day study during the course of the experiment.

Full gross autopsies are carried out on all animals at the end of the exposure period with a wide range of organs/tissues being observed (slightly more in the 90 day study than the 28 day). Full histopathology is carried out on all the preserved organs/tissues from animals in the high dose group, together with tissue/organs from any group showing gross lesions.

A well designed repeated dose toxicity study should provide valuable information on the cumulative toxicity of a substance and the NOAEL, a critical factor in risk assessment. Such studies provide an efficient way of detecting a wide range of adverse effects potentially affecting any one of numerous potential target organs, often resulting from complex interactions (e.g. metabolism) in the animal. This is one reason why it is so difficult to replace animal studies for investigating the general toxicity of a chemical. The repeated dose study is an efficient way of obtaining general information on the toxicity of a chemical, target organs etc. *In vitro* studies may however have a role in investigating the mode of action of the chemical whose target organ(s) are known.

For most chemicals information will not be available from studies of longer than 90 days, and for risk assessment purposes there will be a need to extrapolate the findings to more prolonged exposure. It is recognised that the NOAEL in a 90 day study in the rat will be higher than the NOAEL for the same end-point in a chronic or essentially lifetime study (two years in the rat), although this is not always the case and the variability is often in the range 2–4 fold but may be higher (Doe *et al.*, 2006). Account for this may be made in extrapolation to essentially lifetime exposure by dividing the NOAEL by an additional Uncertainty Factor.

## 5    Mutagenicity

Mutagenicity is the ability to induce a permanent change in the amount or structure of the genetic material (DNA) in an organism or cell.

Data on the mutagenicity of a chemical is important both because of concerns about heritable effects due to mutations in germ cells and also as a screen for carcinogenicity because of mutations in somatic cells.

There is no convincing evidence that any chemical has produced heritable mutations in humans. However this would be very difficult to demonstrate due to few suitable genetic endpoints, the rarity of individual mutations which may also not be manifest at birth, inadequate base line data and the need for a large group size. It is known that mutations contribute significantly to human health detriment, especially reproductive problems, being a major cause of foetal death and spontaneous abortion. Also, chemical mutagens can produce heritable effects in insects and mice. It is thus prudent to assume that mutagenicity itself is a cause for concern.

The crucial role of mutagenesis in carcinogenicity is also well established. It is known that certain dominant inherited conditions predispose to cancer, for example retino-blastoma (a malignant tumour within the eye), and familial adenomatous polyposis coli (finger like outgrowths or polyps with a stalk within the lumen of the intestine).

Furthermore there is a good correlation between chemicals shown to be *in vivo* mutagens and those that are carcinogenic in animal bioassays. This evidence was sufficient for the Committee on Mutagenicity of Chemicals in Food, Consumer Products and the Environment (COM) and its sister committee on carcinogenicity (COC) to conclude that it is prudent to assume that a chemical capable of producing *in vivo* somatic mutations in mammals has carcinogenic potential (Department of Health, 1989; Department of Health, 1991). But it was noted that mutagenicity studies provide no information on potency or tissue specificity of carcinogens nor would such data provide information on chemical carcinogens whose mechanism of action did not relate to mutagenicity. An example of the latter would be a chemical that induced cancer by sustained cell proliferation in a particular tissue due to hormonal effects. It is thus important to recognise that not all chemical carcinogens induce cancer specifically by a mutagenic effect; such compounds are generally referred to as non–genotoxic carcinogens.

## 5.1   Strategy for investigating mutagenicity of chemicals

There are well established strategies for the investigation of the mutagenicity of chemicals. The COM produced guidance in 1989 which was updated in 2000 by their publication Guidance on a Strategy for Testing Chemicals for Mutagenicity (Department of Health, 2000). The overall strategy was very similar in both cases with initial testing *in vitro* to assess the mutagenic potential of a chemical, followed by *in vivo* testing of positive compounds in somatic cells *in vivo* to assess whether the activity can be expressed in the whole animal, and finally, and if appropriate, testing in germ cells *in vivo* for potential inheritable effects. The 2000 guidance did put more emphasis on the need to detect aneugens in the initial screening, and also more guidance on possible *in vivo* assays in somatic cells was provided with the need for a flexible approach being emphasised. The overall strategy being recommended is considered in the following sections.

Before any testing is carried out some idea as to whether a chemical would be expected to have any mutagenic potential can be provided by considering whether it has any structural alerts for DNA reactivity (Ashby and Paton, 1993).

### 5.1.1   Stage 1. *In vitro* testing

The initial testing *in vitro* needs to cover all the three types of mutation, namely gene mutation (alterations in DNA involving a single gene), clastogenicity (structural chromosome aberrations) or aneuploidy (numerical chromosome aberrations). There is no single validated test that can provide information on all three end-points. The initial testing *in vitro* is based on use of a limited number of well validated and informative tests. Three tests are recommended and for each there are OECD test guidelines which were updated in 1997. They are considered below.

#### Bacterial Reverse Mutation Test

The bacterial assay for gene mutation uses *Salmonella typhimurium* (this test was developed by Professor Bruce Ames and is often referred to as the Ames test). This has the most extensive database of any of the *in vitro* tests. These special strains of salmonella require an essential amino acid, histidine, for growth. A reverse mutation to the wild type caused by the chemical being tested removes this dependency and the revertant bacteria may be detected by growth on medium deficient in histidine.  A range of bacterial strains are available that measure different types of point mutation (base-pair or frame-shift, both of which result in addition or deletion of one or a few DNA base pairs).The following five strains of *Salmonella typhimurium* are routinely used: TA 1535, TA 1537 (or TA 97 or TA 97a), TA 98, TA 100, and TA 102. Testing is carried out in the presence and absence of an appropriate exogenous metabolic activation system since it is known that many chemical mutagens are only able to react with DNA following metabolic activation by enzymes present in the liver and other tissues of mammals. At least five concentrations are tested up to a level producing toxicity (or a maximum concentration of 5 mg/plate). Negative and appropriate positive controls are used and all results confirmed in an independent experiment.

### Test for clastogenicity and indications of aneuploidy in mammalian cells

The second *in vitro* test is for clastogenicity and indications of aneugenicity. One of two options is possible. The most widely used approach is metaphase analysis for chromosome damage. Either cell lines e.g. Chinese hamster ovary (CHO) or alternatively primary cultures of human lymphocytes (stimulated by addition of mitogen) are used. At least three concentrations of test compound are investigated at levels up to those causing marked cytotoxicity (effects on mitotic index). Cells are harvested for metaphase analysis at a time equivalent to about 1.5 normal cell cycle lengths after the beginning of treatment. Testing is carried out both in the presence and absence of an exogenous metabolic activation system. Negative and appropriate positive controls are employed. This may involve sampling cells at a time interval of longer than 1.5 cell cycle lengths. Results are confirmed in an independent experiment.  Chromosome damage is recorded using standard methods. Some information on aneugenicity is obtained from the incidence of hyperdiploidy, polyploidy or modification of the mitotic index.

An alternative approach recommended by the COM was the recently developed *in vitro* micronucleus test. It was recognised that there was no internationally agreed method at the time but it was felt that work on the validation of this approach should be encouraged. This assay measures micronuclei in interphase cells rather than chromosome aberrations in metaphase cells. These micronuclei may arise either from acentric fragments (chromosome fragments lacking a centromere) or whole chromosomes that are unable to migrate with the rest of the chromosomes during the anaphase of cell division. The assay thus detects both clastogenic and aneugenic chemicals. The endpoint (i.e. whether or not a cell contains micronuclei) is more easily measured than examining chromosomes and recording subtle damage as in metaphase analysis. Also since micronuclei may contain whole (lagging) chromosomes there is the potential to detect aneuploidy inducing agents that are more difficult to study in the conventional chromosome aberration test using metaphase analysis. Either primary human peripheral lymphocytes or cell lines such as CHO may be used. Testing is carried out in the presence or absence of an exogenous source of metabolic activation. At least three concentrations are used, the highest producing around 50% cytotoxicity. After addition of the test chemical, cell cultures are grown for a period sufficient to allow chromosome or spindle damage to lead to the formation of micronuclei in interphase cells and to trigger the aneuploidy sensitive stage (G2/M). The interphase cells are then harvested and stained for the presence of micronuclei. Ideally micronuclei should only be scored in cells that have completed nuclear division following exposure to the test chemical. This is most readily achieved by use of a cytokinesis blocking agent (e.g. cytochalasin B) and scoring only binucleate cells. As noted above this is a relatively new assay and only recently have sufficient validation data become available to consider the development of an OECD test guideline; a draft guideline is now available. This is now being progressed and it is anticipated that this approach will become more widely used once there is an internationally agreed test method.

### Mammalian Cell Gene Mutation Test

The third *in vitro* test is another assay in mammalian cells, the mouse lymphoma assay. This has the advantage of detecting both gene mutations and various sizes of chromosome aberrations. The assay uses L5178Y mouse lymphoma cells and measures mutations at the thymidine kinase (TK) locus. Cells deficient in TK due to the mutation are resistant to the cytotoxic effects of the pyrimidine analogue trifluorothymidine (TFT). TK proficient cells are sensitive to TFT. Thus mutant cells are able to proliferate in the presence of TFT whereas normal cells are not. As in the other mammalian cell assays, studies are carried out in the presence and absence of an appropriate exogenous metabolic activation system and a range of concentrations are investigated up to appreciable cytotoxicity. Negative and appropriate positive controls are employed. Results are confirmed in an independent experiment.

### Implication of results from the three in vitro tests

A clear positive result in any one of the three *in vitro* tests described above is sufficient to define the chemical as an *in vitro* mutagen. There is then the need to proceed to Stage 2, i.e. *in vivo* testing.

The three tests should detect almost all compounds with mutagenic potential, and indeed most will be detected by the first two tests. Chemical mutagens that have shown activity only *in vivo* are very rare and it is thus possible to test for mutagenic potential using *in vitro* studies (Tweats and Gatehouse, 1988).

In order for a compound to be considered to have no significant mutagenic potential, negative results are normally required from all three tests. However for added reassurance for compounds where there is likely to be high, or moderate and prolonged levels of direct exposure to humans (e.g. most medicines), then an *in vivo* assay is also recommended. At the other extreme of exposure, for compounds where little or no human exposure is expected, results from the third test may not be required.

### 5.1.2    Stage 2. *In vivo* studies in somatic cells

*In vivo* studies in animals are not justified for routine screening of chemicals for mutagenicity. Their main purpose is to ascertain whether mutagenic potential seen *in vitro* can be expressed *in vivo*. There are numerous reasons why activity seen *in vitro* may not be observed *in vivo*, for example lack of absorption, inability of the active metabolite to react with DNA, rapid detoxification and elimination. Data from *in vivo* studies are thus essential before any definite conclusions can be drawn regarding the potential mutagenic hazard to humans from chemicals which have given positive results in one or more *in vitro* tests.

When undertaking *in vivo* testing, it is important that a flexible approach is adopted with consideration of the nature of the chemical, the results from the initial mutagenicity tests and its toxicokinetic profile. For compounds that have shown mutagenic potential *in vitro*, negative results from *in vivo* studies from at least two different tissues will be needed before adequate reassurance is provided that activity cannot be expressed *in vivo*. In most cases the first test will involve the bone marrow as this tissue is readily assessable to chemicals present in the blood.

Most data are available from the bone marrow micronucleus test and there is an OECD guideline outlining the methodology. The micronucleus test indirectly detects clastogens by measuring micronuclei in newly formed cells in the bone marrow. It can identify the induction of both structural and numerical aberrations by appropriate staining techniques. Micronuclei containing whole chromosomes (as opposed to fragments) can be identified by use of kinetochore or centromeric staining techniques. The mouse is usually used for this assay since in this species (and unlike the rat) the spleen does not remove micronucleated erythrocytes. Three dose levels are used up to the maximum tolerated dose (i.e. one that produces signs of toxicity such that higher dose levels would be expected to produce lethality) together with a negative and positive control group. Either multiple dosing is used with a single harvest time, or a single dose with multiple harvest times is used.

Alternatively chromosome damage in bone marrow may be measured by metaphase analysis. The rat is usually used for these studies. A single dose is administered at three dose levels up to the maximum tolerated dose defined as above for the bone marrow micronucleus test. Bone marrow is harvested at two different time intervals. Both negative and positive control groups are used.

A positive result in the bone marrow assay will indicate that the compound should be regarded as an *in vivo* mutagen. A negative result however will not be sufficient to conclude that the compound is not an *in vivo* mutagen and further testing in at least one additional tissue *in vivo* will be required. The appropriate additional test needs to be considered on a case-by-case basis taking into account the structure of the compound, its toxicokinetic properties, the results from earlier studies and also the available expertise. There are a number of possible approaches that the COM document recommends be considered. This is a difficult area as in most cases the methods have not been developed to a level where there is international agreement on methodology. There is one important exception to this, namely the assay to detect unscheduled DNA synthesis (UDS) in liver cells obtained from treated animals. This is important as the liver is often the most appropriate second tissue in which to investigate *in vivo* activity. The endpoint UDS is indicative of DNA damage and subsequent repair in liver cells. Studies are usually in the rat. UDS is measured by determining the uptake of labelled nucleocides, usually tritiated thymidine by autoradiography, in liver cells that are not undergoing scheduled (S phase) DNA synthesis.

Although the liver is often an appropriate second tissue this will not be the case for short lived reactive mutagens where assays using site-of-contact tissue(s) should be considered. The following types of study are possible:

- measurement of induction of DNA lesions or adducts potentially in any tissue using one of the following approaches:
  - the Comet assay (single cell gel electrophoresis), which measures DNA strand breaks.
  - the $^{32}$P post-labelling assay for DNA adducts.
  - detection of DNA adducts by measurement of covalent binding to DNA using radio-labelled material or Accelerator Mass Spectrometry.

There are commercially available transgenic animal models that have the potential for measuring gene mutations in any tissue provided that sufficient DNA can be isolated (e.g. Muta ™ Mouse and Big Blue™). In general these are less sensitive than methods measuring DNA adducts. There has been relatively little published work to date on the validation of these assays and further work is needed on optimising methodology for particular tissues.

Consideration of the results from testing *in vivo* in somatic cells may lead to the conclusion that the compound is an *in vivo* somatic cell mutagen and hence a potential carcinogen and possible germ cell mutagen, or alternatively that it is not an *in vivo* mutagen.

### 5.1.3    Stage 3. *In vivo* germ cell assays

There is no need to screen for germ cell mutagens in the initial stages of investigating mutagenic hazard as all established germ cell mutagens have also been shown to produce positive results in bone marrow assays and there is currently no evidence for germ cell specific mutagens (Shelby, 1996). The reverse is not true and not all somatic cell mutagens can be demonstrated to be germ cell mutagens.

*In vivo* data on mutagenic effects in germ cell DNA are needed before drawing definite conclusions regarding heritable effects. However in most cases such testing will not be justified since once established as an *in vivo* somatic cell mutagen, the compound will be assumed to be a potential genotoxic carcinogen and appropriate risk management procedures adopted. In some cases germ cell studies may be undertaken for the specific purpose of demonstrating whether an *in vivo* somatic cell mutagen is, or is not, a germ cell mutagen. There are two possible approaches for which there are methods in the OECD guidelines. These are listed below.

#### *The Dominant Lethal Assay in rodents.*
A dominant lethal mutation is one occurring in a germ cell which does not cause dysfunction of the gamete but which is lethal to the fertilised egg or developing embryo. The assay measures embryo-lethal genetic changes (mainly chromosomal) expressed as death of the conceptus as a blastoma or soon afterwards.

*A*

*n assay for structural chromosome aberrations in rodent spermatogonia.*
This is an *in vivo* cytogenetic assay that detects chromosome aberrations in spermatogonial cells of rodents.

## 6    Carcinogenicity

As noted above, almost all *in vivo* somatic cell mutagens are also animal carcinogens when adequately tested and it is thus prudent to assume that they are also potential human carcinogens. However mutagenicity tests do not detect non-carcinogens whose mechanism is not primarily related to mutagenicity, for example carcinogens that act by sustained cell proliferation, e.g. due to hormonal effects on certain tissues or to sustained cytotoxicity. When knowledge of carcinogenicity is essential, animal carcinogenicity bioassays are needed.

In the introduction to this chapter it was noted that in most cases there will be few sound toxicology data directly from use in humans. It is pertinent to note here a particular problem in this regard with respect to chemical carcinogens. This relates to the long latent period from first exposure to the development of tumours. This may well be 20 years or more (in the case of asbestos it is know to be 20–40 years or more). Thus it is essential that we have experimental methods for the detection of chemicals with carcinogenic potential. It is possible to screen for genotoxic carcinogens using mutagenicity studies. This is a particularly important category of carcinogen as it is for these compounds that we make the prudent assumption that there is no threshold to their effects and that any exposure is associated with some increase in risk, although this may be very small. Nearly all the chemical carcinogens that are recognised as human carcinogens are in fact genotoxic carcinogens, the exceptions being those that act by hormonal mechanisms e.g. post-menopausal oestrogen therapy or tetrachlorodibenzodioxin ('dioxin').

There are well established methods for investigating the carcinogenicity of chemicals. Because of the long latent period it is essential to expose the animals to the chemical for a high proportion of their life span, namely two years in the rat or 18 months for mice. Also because of the need, as far as practical, to detect low incidence effects, large numbers of animals have to be used. Hence the carcinogenicity bioassay requires a major commitment in animal resources, time and expense, and should only be carried out when justified by the very real need to ascertain whether a chemical is a carcinogen. There are short term tests (based on mutagenicity assays) that can be used to screen for genotoxic carcinogens but not for carcinogens that may act by other mechanisms.

The general principles governing these assays have not changed over the past two decades or so. In addition to carcinogenicity, information may also be obtained on chronic (essentially lifetime) toxicity. There are OECD guidelines for both the carcinogenicity bioassay and a combined chronic toxicity/carcinogenicity bioassay. In the latter case satellite groups are used for investigating clinical chemistry and haematology.

The objective of the carcinogenicity bioassay is to dose and observe animals for a major proportion of their lifespan for the development of tumours. Full autopsies are carried out on all animals that die or are killed during the test or at termination, with detailed histopathology. For pragmatic reasons testing is limited to rats, mice or hamsters (the latter are rarely used). Three dose levels are used, the highest being the Maximum Tolerated Dose. This is described as being sufficient to elicit signs of minimal toxicity (e.g. slight depression of body weight gain, less than 10%), without substantially altering lifespan. For pragmatic reasons, group size is usually 50 males and 50 females, with higher numbers in the control groups. Exposure is from shortly after weaning for at least two years in the rat and 18 months in the mouse. It is important to have good knowledge of the spontaneous incidence of tumours at specific sites in test animals (i.e. good historic control data).

## 7    Toxicity to the reproductive system

There are two different endpoints on which reproductive toxicity data are necessary: (i) developmental toxicity, namely the effects on developing offspring following in-utero (inside the uterus) or neonatal exposure; and (ii) effects on reproduction over one or more generations including effects on male and female fertility. There are established animal studies to provide information on these endpoints which are described below.

### 7.1    Developmental toxicity

The OECD guideline in this area, entitled Prenatal Developmental Toxicity Study, has recently been updated (it used to be called the Teratogenicity Study). Pregnant animals (rodents or rabbits) are exposed from implantation to one day prior to the day of scheduled sacrifice which is as close as possible to the normal day of delivery. In the past, exposure was only for the period of organogenesis (i.e. day 5–15 in rodents) but the need to cover a wider range is now recognised. Shortly before caesarean section, the animals are killed and uteri and contents are evaluated for soft tissue and skeletal effects. Key endpoints noted are death of offspring, resorptions, embryonic development, foetal growth, morphological variations and malformations. This study does not detect functional deficiencies in the offspring, but these are covered in the studies considered later. Guidance on group size is that each test and control group should contain a sufficient number of females to result in approximately 20 animals with implantation sites at necropsy. At least three dose levels and a concurrent control group are used. The top dose is chosen so as to produce some evidence of toxicity in the maternal animal, but not death or marked suffering, the intermediate dose to have minimal observable toxic effects, and the lowest dose no maternal or developmental toxicity.

### 7.2    One and two generation reproductive toxicity study

These studies are designed to provide general information on the effect of the test substance on integrity and performance of the male and female reproductive system, including gonadal function, the oestrous cycle, mating behaviour, conception, gestation, parturition, lactation and weaning, and growth and development of offspring. The test substance is given in graduated doses (at least three plus controls) to several groups of male and female animals. Group size is such as to give not less than 20 pregnant females. Males of the parent generation are dosed for at least one complete spermatogenic cycle (circa 70 days in rats, the preferred species) prior to mating. Females are dosed for several oestrogenic cycles before mating. The test substance is then administered to the parental animals throughout the mating period and the resultant pregnancies, and through weaning of first generation (F1) offspring. In the second generation study the administration of substance is continued during their growth into adulthood, mating and production of the F2 generation, until the F2 is weaned. Clinical observations and pathology/histopathology examinations at autopsy are carried out with emphasis on the integrity and performance of reproduction and growth and development of offspring.

## 7.3   Reproductive/developmental toxicity screening test in the rat

Both the developmental toxicity study and the one or two generation reproductive toxicity study are relatively expensive with regard to number of animals used, time and costs involved.  Reproductive toxicity data is also the most common gap in a chemical's toxicological profile. This has been clearly shown in the OECD High Production Volume (HPV) chemicals programme. In this voluntary programme manufacturers agree to provide the minimum information for any meaningful hazard assessment (referred to as screening information data sets or SIDS). In this context, the OECD have agreed on a Reproductive/Developmental Screening test in the rat that can be used to provide initial information on possible effects on reproduction and developmental toxicity.

In this test, the chemical is given in graduated doses to groups of male and female animals (at least ten with the aim of at least eight pregnancies), with three dose levels being used. The males are dosed for two weeks prior to mating, during mating and approximately two weeks post-mating, followed by sacrifice and detailed histopathology of the testes. Females are dosed for same period as the males and for at least four days after delivery, and are killed and necropsied one day later.  Observations are made in particular on the effects on fertility, pregnancy outcome, maternal and suckling behaviour and the development of the offspring to day four post-partum. It is recognised that the study only provides limited data particularly on post-natal effects, and it is not used where there is a regulatory requirement for testing for toxicity to the reproductive system. However in the absence of any other data, the study has been shown to provide useful preliminary information on reproductive toxicity and may contribute to decisions with respect to the need for further testing.

## 7.4   *In vitro* approaches to investigating reproductive toxicology

Considerable research is ongoing into the development of *in vitro* methods to investigate aspects of reproductive toxicology (Bremer *et al.*, 2005).  Clearly in view of the complexities of mammalian reproduction it is most unlikely that complete replacement of animal tests will be possible. *In vitro* tests are however likely to play an important role in identifying priority compounds for investigating reproductive toxicology in animal studies and also for mechanism of action studies. One particularly promising area is in the development of *in vitro* assays for embryotoxicity (Scholz *et al.*, 1999). The embryonic stem cell test (EST) can measure differentiation of stem cells into cardiac myocytes (heart muscle cells), neuronal cells (nerve cells or neurones) and chondrocytes (bone-forming cells). Effort is currently concentrating on developing a metabolic activation system that can be used with this assay as the standard systems that have been developed for use in mutagenicity assays cannot be used because of their high toxicity to stem cells.

## 8    References

Ashby J, Paton D. (1993) The influence of chemical structure on the extent and sites of carcinogenesis for 522 rodent carcinogens and 55 different human carcinogen exposures. *Mutat Res* 286(1):3–74.

Bremer S, Cortvrindt R, Daston G, Eletti B, Mantovani A, Maranghi F, Pelkonen O, Ruhdel I, Spielmann H. (2005) Reproductive and development toxicity. *Altern Lab Anim* 33 Suppl 1:183–209.

Council Directive of 24 November 1986 on the approximation of laws, regulations and administrative provisions of the Member States regarding the protection of animals used for experimental and other scientific purposes (86/609/EEC). *Official Journal of the European Communities* L358:1–29.

Department of Health. (1989) Guidelines for the testing of chemicals for mutagenicity. Committee on Mutagenicity of Chemicals in Food, Consumer Products and the Environment (COM). (Report on Health and Social Security Subjects No. 35.) London, HMSO.

Department of Health. (1991) Guidelines for the evaluation of chemicals for carcinogenicity. Committee on Carcinogenicity of Chemicals in Food, Consumer Products and the Environment (COC). (Report on Health and Social Security Subjects No 42.) London, HMSO.

Department of Health. (2000) Guidance on a strategy for testing of chemicals for mutagenicity. Committee on Mutagenicity of Chemicals in Food, Consumer Products and the Environment (COM). Available at: www.advisorybodies.doh.gov.uk

Doe JE, Boobis AR, Blacker A, *et al.* (2006) A tiered approach to systemic toxicity testing for agricultural chemical safety assessment. *Crit Rev Toxicol* 36(1):37–68.

IGHRC. (2002) Assessment of chemical carcinogens: Background to general principles of a weight of evidence approach. Interdepartmental Group on Health Risks from Chemicals. Institute for Environment and Health, University of Leicester. (IEH is now based at Cranfield University, Silsoe.) Available at: www.silsoe.cranfield.ac.uk

IGHRC. (2003) Uncertainty factors: their use in human health risk assessment by UK Government. Interdepartmental Group on Health Risks from Chemicals. Institute for Environment and Health, University of Leicester. (IEH is now based at Cranfield University , Silsoe.) Available at: www.silsoe.cranfield.ac.uk

IPCS. (1999) Environmental Health Criteria No.210: Principles for the assessment of risks to human health from exposure to chemicals. International Programme on Chemical Safety, World Health Organization, Geneva. Available at: www.inchem.org

IPCS. (2005) Chemical-specific adjustment factors for interspecies differences and human variability: Guidance document for use of data in dose/concentration- response assessment. International Programme on Chemical Safety, World Health Organization, Geneva. Available at: www.who.int

Kimber I, Dearman RJ, Scholes EW, Basketter DA. (1994) The local lymph node assay: development and applications. *Toxicology* 93(1):13–31.

OECD Guidelines for the Testing of Chemicals. Organisation for Economic Co-operation and Development. Available at: www.oecd.org

Scholz G, Genschow E, Pohl I, Bremer S, Paparella M, Raabe H, Southee J, Spielmann H. (1999) Prevalidation of the Embryonic Stem Cell Test (EST) – A new in vitro embryotoxicity test. *Toxicol in vitro* 13(4–5):675–681.

Shelby MD. (1996) Selecting chemicals and assays for assessing mammalian germ cell mutagenicity. *Mutat Res* 352(1–2):159–167.

Tweats DJ, Gatehouse DG. (1988) Further debate on testing strategies. *Mutagenesis* 3(2):95–102.

van den Heuval MJ, Clark DG, Fielder RJ, Koundakjian PP, Oliver GJ, Pelling D, Tomlinson NJ, Walker AP. (1990) The international validation of a fixed dose procedure as an alternative to the classical LD$_{50}$ test. *Food Chem Toxicol* 28(7):469–482.

# Section 1.4

# Introduction to human biomonitoring for public health

Ovnair Sepai

## Learning outcomes

At the end of this chapter and any recommended reading the student should be able to:

1. discuss the application of human biomonitoring in the evaluation of human exposure, uptake and effect of exposure to environmental chemicals;
2. describe the different classes of biomarkers;
3. explain the need for an understanding of the toxicokinetics and toxicodynamics when designing a biomonitoring study;
4. discuss the current knowledge base for the appropriate application of human biomonitoring in the management of both acute and chronic environmental chemical exposures;
5. explain the stages of a biomonitoring study;
6. evaluate the interpretation and utility of human biomonitoring data, and
7. apply their knowledge in the assessment and management of hazardous situations.

## 1    Introduction

Human biomonitoring is a powerful tool used extensively to assess human exposure and uptake of chemicals particularly following occupational exposures. However human biomarkers of environmental exposure are increasingly being used to determine the presence of a chemical(s) in the human body. There are several national human biomonitoring programmes, the most extensive being that of the Centers for Disease Control and Prevention (CDC) in the US. CDC began their National Health and Nutrition Examination Survey (NHANES) in 1971 and published a third extensive report in 2005 (CDC, 2005). The German Environmental Health Survey started in 1985 and since 1995 has focused on childhood exposure (Becker *et al.*, 2006). These surveys are two good examples of the application of human biomonitoring to public health. There are many hundreds of smaller research projects. An internet search reveals more than 500,000 sites related to biomarkers in public health.

The use of biomarkers to assess human exposure and uptake or the effect of the uptake of environmental chemicals is not a simple analytical exercise. There are wider considerations such as the appropriate use and interpretation of the data as well as due consideration of the ethical issues and communication of the results. Advances in analytical technology in the 1980s reduced detection limits and extended the utility of biomarkers from high level occupational exposure to low level environmental exposure. With the more recent advancements in technology, including but not exclusively genomics-based approaches, the field of biomarker development and application has assumed an even greater importance. The advances in technology have overtaken our ability to understand and interpret much of the data that are being produced, thus there is a need for the development of a framework for appropriate application and interpretation of human biomarkers in public health.

Back in 1987 the National Research Council (NRC) in the USA recognised that biomarkers of exposure/uptake and effect may potentially be developed for any of the stages between exposure to the chemical and development of clinical disease (NRC, 1987). This is outlined in Figure 1.

**Figure 1** Human Biomonitoring Continuum.

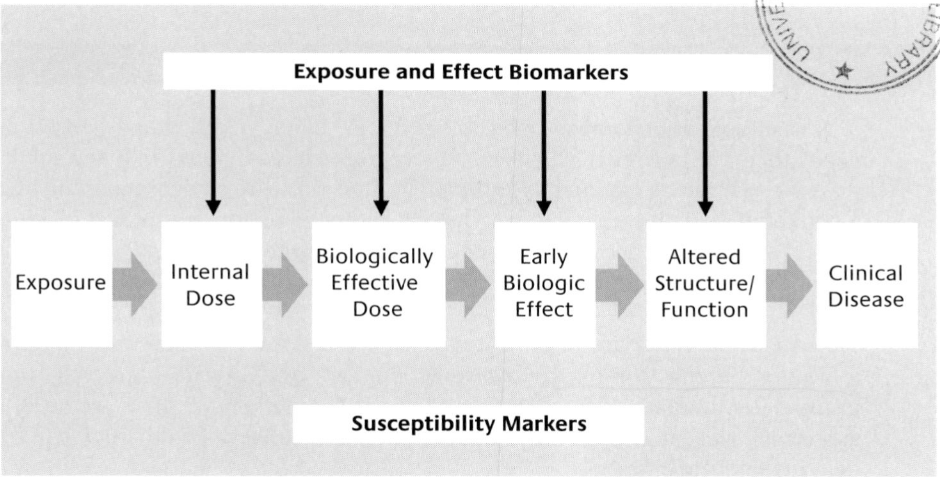

The NRC report established three classes of biomarker, namely, exposure/uptake, effect, and susceptibility. It is clear that the application of biomarkers to public health monitoring is a complicated undertaking but one which represents clear advantages over exposure estimates by measuring uptake and in some cases early effects. This chapter is a primer to human biomonitoring as a tool in public health surveillance and research.

## 2    Defining biomarkers and biomonitoring

A biomarker can be defined for the purposes of environmental exposure as:
*A chemical, biochemical, or functional indicator of exposure to and uptake of (or the effect of exposure to) an environmental chemical, physical or biological agent.*

Biomarkers can be divided into three broad categories (WHO, 2001):

## 2.1    Biomarkers of exposure (and uptake)

Defined as the chemical or its metabolite or the product of an interaction between a chemical and some target molecule or cell that is measured in a biological fluid. Examples include: lead in blood; cadmium in urine; butadiene adducts to haemoglobin; dioxin levels in human breast milk.

Biomarkers of exposure and uptake are measures of internal dose and in some cases biologically effective doses. The internal dose is that which has been absorbed or taken up via all three routes of exposure (See Chapter 1.1 on Toxicology). The advantage of such a biomarker is that it reflects individual exposure from ingestion, skin absorption and inhalation and can be a proxy for population exposure. Biomarkers of exposure are by definition relatively simple to interpret as a measure of exposure and uptake. The challenge here is determining what the health risks, if any, from the internal dose are and, where environmental exposure limits are available, how the internal dose relates to external exposure.

## 2.2    Biomarkers of effect

A measurable biochemical, physiological, or behavioural change resulting from exposure to the chemical which can be recognised as associated with an established or possible adverse health effect. Examples include: 8- hydroxyl deoxyguanine in urine as a marker of oxidative damage; acetyl cholinesterase activity as a marker of exposure to an acetyl cholinesterase inhibitor such as an organophosphate pesticide; chromosomal aberrations or DNA adducts as a marker of exposure to genotoxic agents.

Biomarkers of effect are often not specific for a given chemical exposure and thus are more difficult to interpret. However, markers of effect are potentially important in the determination of mechanisms of effect. Biomarkers of effect are often used in epidemiological studies to relate the occurrence of adverse health effects to exposure to a substance in a study.

## 2.3    Biomarkers of susceptibility

An indicator of an inherent or acquired ability of an organism to respond to the challenge of exposure to a specific chemical. Examples include: genetic polymorphisms in metabolic enzymes; cytochrome P450s, glutathione transferases, N-acetyl transferases, DNA repair genes; excision repair cross-complementing 1 and 2. All these polymorphisms have the potential to affect individual susceptibility, but analysis is often complex and interpretation is difficult.

Variations in absorption, distribution, metabolism, DNA repair, and cell turnover processes can modify the risk for adverse effects and the levels of biomarkers after exposure to toxic agents. Some of these differences are due to heritable variation; individual susceptibility (genetic polymorphisms) as well as gene-environment interactions. Biomarkers of susceptibility are by their nature complex and although they may have a role to play in modulating individual responses to exposure, the interpretation from a health risk point of view is difficult. There are many environmental epidemiological studies that include the measurement of genetic polymorphisms, and metabolic variations could affect the level of biomarkers detected.

In the public health context, biomarkers – markers of susceptibility  – can also be expanded to socio-economic susceptibility, where lifestyle and many other factors may affect population exposure patterns. These aspects are discussed in some detail in Chapter 2.3 on individual susceptibility. Examples include: smoking status, household income.

## 2.4   Biomarkers of clinical disease

A fourth category, biomarkers of clinical disease, is to the right of the continuum in Figure 1. These biomarkers include liver function enzymes, kidney function enzymes or even ECG and lung function tests. Again, although these biomarkers indicate a disease state they are non specific and the contribution of environmental toxicants to the disease state is hard to determine. Biomarkers of disease will not be considered further in this chapter.

## 2.5   Biomonitoring

As applied in this text, biomonitoring is a scientific technique used to sample blood, urine, breast milk and other tissue to assess human exposure uptake or effect of natural and synthetic chemicals.

The use of human biomarkers in environmental epidemiology enables the epidemiologist to determine more accurately population exposure and to associate exposure to adverse health effects.

## 3   Biomarker utility

Our ability to interpret the health significance of any human biomonitoring data lags behind the analytical technology that allows us to measure ever decreasing concentrations of organic and inorganic pollutants. There are an increasing number of studies, subjects and substances determined in human biomonitoring and a parallel increase in awareness of the general public of those chemicals in our bodies. Statements that the presence of an environmental pollutant in a biological sample is not a reflection of risk to health or a cause of disease will not fully address public anxiety (CDC, 2005). There have to be clear guidelines for the appropriate interpretation and use of biomarkers. There have been attempts to develop frameworks for the interpretation and utility of biomarkers (Boogart, 2007).

Four broad categories of activity where biomarkers can be used are 1) scoping, 2) trend analysis, 3) exposure and health research, and 4) risk assessment (Burke *et al.*, 1992). These are considered in turn. Scoping studies are exploratory studies to determine the presence of a pollutant in human tissue and compare this to 'normal values' or background levels if they exist. However, if 'background' levels are not available these preliminary scoping studies can be used to develop reference ranges. Trend analyses assess the concentration of the chemical and whether there are any temporal or spatial trends. Such studies provide valuable information on the effectiveness of control measures aimed at reducing or eliminating exposure. This information also assists in population studies. Biomonitoring studies in health research investigate correlations between health effects in populations. Biological data can be used in risk-based assessments and clinical evaluation to assess individual risks or exposure. Here data are available on the correlation with internal dose (marker of exposure) and effect. Health risk assessment can only be determined with dose-response relationships, ideally in humans (or using animal data with the appropriate uncertainty factors). The classic example of this is blood lead levels and effect.

The interpretation of the significance of biomarker concentration will ultimately depend on the quantum of knowledge about the biomarker. This includes the toxicity, toxicokinetics and individual and population-based variability (genetic susceptibility).

## 4    Study design, conduct and communication

When designing a biomonitoring study it is important to consider in the first instance what the purpose of the study is. Only with this in mind can the appropriate biomarker in the appropriate population be selected. The ethical and communication issues must be considered at the planning or design stage of the project. Biomonitoring study design should also consider in particular the toxicokinetics of the substance under investigation (see Chapter 1.1 on Toxicology) in the selection of appropriate biomarkers.

### 4.1    Selection of the appropriate study population: criteria for taking a human sample

The study population is dependent on the hypothesis to be tested. As a basis for developing a hypothesis it is necessary to use the four categories 1) scoping, 2) trend analysis, 3) exposure and health research, and 4) risk assessment which have been described briefly above. In addition there should be a knowledge of the potential exposure to investigate as well as a knowledge of epidemiology. It may be possible to select a population, a sampling strategy, and where necessary, appropriate controls. An understanding of the intra- and inter-individual sources of variation in exposure is vital when developing a sampling strategy.

Of particular interest to the HPA is the need to consider the place of biomonitoring in investigations of acute incidents and chronic exposure to environmental chemicals. Advice in this area and guidance is being developed by the Laboratory Review and

Liaison Group (LRLG). The Group has also been developing protocols for biomonitoring of the chemicals of most concern associated with acute incidents.

The ideal situation is where the health professional has the luxury of developing a hypothesis and sound study design and is able to include the appropriate biomonitoring protocol following the acute incident. However, there are great pitfalls in taking human samples following an acute incident. Thus there is a need for a set of criteria or an algorithm which would aid the decision as to when and where to take biological samples or when biological samples should not be taken. These criteria have been developed by the LRLG and are summarised in Box 1.

**Box 1**  Criteria for the use of biological samples to investigate a chemical incident

1) *Exposure assessment to guide clinical interventions*
   Testing may be of direct patient benefit where there is the option to use a therapeutic intervention (e.g. antidotes or other medical treatment).

2) *Exposure assessment to monitor clinical effects*
   Testing may be appropriate even where there is no specific treatment to counteract the effect of the chemical (e.g. monitoring the levels of a chemical and/or the specific clinical effects of exposure).

3) *Confirmation of exposure to a known or unknown agent*
   Where there is no specific antidote or other clinical intervention option, testing may still be appropriate in order to confirm exposure to an agent and to quantify the degree of exposure, for a number of reasons:

   A)  Identification of an unknown chemical agent
   B)  Epidemiological follow up
   C)  Reassurance monitoring
   D)  Clinical research
   E)  Medico-legal reasons.

   (Source: Unpublished LRLG)

## 4.2   Selection of the appropriate biomarker

Environmental chemical exposure levels generally are much lower than occupational exposures and therefore there is a need to develop sensitive analytical methods. The analytical procedure must be validated at the exposure levels in question. The exposure may be intermittent and hence the integrated exposure measured at a point in time needs to reflect a known exposure period.

An understanding or estimate of the half life of a chemical or its metabolite (the toxicokinetics) is essential to the design of the study protocol. In a controlled occupational setting where exposures occur over a set working shift it is possible to take biological specimens with the maximum circulating levels in blood or excreted in urine. However, as environmental exposures are not as well defined temporally, it is not possible to take samples at an optimum time.

Metabolites with short half lives reflect exposure over a short period of time often only the previous day (e.g. phthalates and organophosphorus pesticides) where as for persistent compounds (i.e. dioxins, organochlorine pesticides) levels detected in blood, or fat or milk are a reflection of a longer term exposure.

**Table 1** Common Biomonitoring Matrices used in population-based studies

| Sample | Sample type | Exposure Timeframe | Biomarker Category | Example |
|---|---|---|---|---|
| Blood | Invasive | Medium to long term | Exposure, effect | Heavy metals[1], organic compounds |
| Blood fat | Invasive | Longer term – months to years | Exposure uptake | Dioxins, PCBs[2] |
| Urine | Noninvasive | 24–48 hours | Exposure effect | Phthalates[3] |
| Milk | Noninvasive | Reflection of longer term exposure | Exposure | Dioxins, PCBs[4] |
| Exhaled Air | Noninvasive | Short-term – hours | Exposure | Organic solvents (styrene[5]) |
| Hair | Noninvasive | Exposure at a given time – but reflected in the growth of hair | Exposure | Heavy metals (arsenic[6]) organics[7] |
| Nails | Noninvasive | Exposure at a given time – but reflected in the growth of nail | Exposure | Heavy metals (arsenic[8]) |
| Saliva | Noninvasive | Short to medium term | Exposure and effect | Mercury[9] Atrazine[10] |
| Post partum umbilical (cord) blood | Noninvasive | Same as blood | Exposure and effect | Same as blood[11] |

(1. Wilhelm *et al.*, 2004; 2. Schwenk *et al.*, 2002; 3. Koch and Angerer, 2007; 4. Bordajandi *et al.*, 2008; 5. Somorovská *et al.*, 1999; 6. Gebel *et al.*, 1998; 7. Schramm, 1997; 8. Wilhelm *et al.*, 2005; 9. Zimmer *et al.*, 2002; 10. Denovan *et al.*, 2000; 11. Ellwood *et al.*, 1984–5;)

The UK Health and Safety Executive and the German Research Foundation (DFG, Deutsche Forschungsgemeinschaft) produce detailed protocols for the determination of human exposure and uptake markers of occupational exposures. These are a valuable template to consider when developing a study design for environmental exposure. A detailed discussion of the study design is beyond the scope of this chapter.

The specificity of the biomarker also has to be considered, i.e. if the biomarker reflects exposure to one compound only.

## 4.3   Sample collection, storage and analysis

The choice of sample is dependent on the toxicodynamics; which part of the body you would expect to detect the compound or its metabolites. The optimal time at which to take the sample has been discussed above. The appropriate sample collection protocol will include the type of container, the optimum storage and sample processing requirements to meet all quality criteria.

The most frequently used tissues in population-based studies are blood and urine (Table 1, referenced with examples of population-based studies). However, the use of other tissues such as fat, milk etc., have their own advantages and disadvantages. There are many studies that investigate other tissues such as brain, liver and kidney (post-mortem). Such studies are useful to develop the evidence base but of little obvious value to population studies (Chu *et al.*, 2003).

The LRLG are in the process of developing standard protocols for the collection, storage and transport of samples in the context of the investigation of acute incidents. These protocols will be published on the HPA website. The method of analysis is also important when considering how best to collect and process samples.

## 4.4   Confounding factors

There are many confounding factors that may affect the level of biomarker detected as well as the interpretation of the results. These confounding factors include age, gender, ethnic background, socio-economic status and life-style amongst others.

## 4.5   Communication

Communication is a dynamic task and requires the development of tailored material for different groups of stakeholders (Sepai *et al.*, in press). These include the volunteers, the public in general, as well as health professionals. The key aspect to communication is the understanding of our ability to interpret human biomonitoring data and to be able to place the biomarker into one of the categories described in the section on biomarker utility. Whether individual results or population averages are reported will of course depend on the study. However these decisions need to be taken at the design stage of a study and it may be necessary to seek ethical approval.

## 5    Ethical issues

The collection and analysis of human samples for the evaluation of environmental pollutants requires careful consideration of the ethical issues. These issues include the rights of volunteers and data protection issues as well as the need for follow-up and communication of results. The NHS Research Ethics Committees (REC) are generally thought to focus on clinical trials and patient-based studies. However it is unethical to carry out human exposure studies without due consideration of the ethical aspects of the study and, where appropriate, secure REC approval.

## 6    Summary

The use of human biomonitoring in the assessment of environmental exposure is not just an analytical exercise. The continuum from exposure to disease potentially includes biomarkers of exposure and uptake, of effect and of susceptibility. The study design must include consideration of the study population, the sampling regime as well as the current knowledge base with regard to chemical toxicity, toxicokinetics and the analytical sensitivity and specificity. Finally, every population-based human biomonitoring study will have to seek REC approval; this approval includes a description of the communication strategy.

## 7    References

Becker K, Seiwert M, Angerer J, Kolossa-Gehring M, Hoppe H-W, Ball M, Schulz C, Thumulla J, Seifert B. (2006) GerES IV Pilot Study: assessment of the exposure of German children to organophosphorus and pyrethroid pesticides. *Int J Hyg Environ Health* 209: 221–233.

Boogart P (2007) Human biomonitoring activities – programmes by industry. *Int J Hyg Environ Health* 210: 259–261.

Bordajandi L, Abad E, González M (2008) Occurrence of PCBs, PCDD/Fs, PBDEs and DDTs in Spanish breast milk: Enantiomeric fraction of chiral PCBs. *Chemosphere* 70: 567–575.

Burke T, Anderson H, Beach N, Colome S, Drew RT *et al.,* (1992) Role of exposure databases in risk management. *Arch Environ Health* 47(6): 421–429.

CDC Centers for Disease Control and Prevention. (2005) *Third National Report on Human Exposure to Environmental Chemicals.* Atlanta (GA).

Chu S, Covaci A, Schepens P. (2003) Levels and chiral signatures of persistent organo-chlorine pollutants in human tissues from Belgium. *Environ Res* 93(2): 167–176.

Denovan L, Lu C, Hines C, Fenske R. (2000) Saliva biomonitoring of atrazine exposure among herbicide applicators. *Int Arch Occup Environ Health* 73(7): 457–462.

Elwood P, Jones M, James K, Toothill C. (2005) Evidence of a fall in cord blood lead levels in South Wales 1984–85. *Environ Geochem Health* 12: 235–257.

Gebel T, Suchenwirth R, Bolten C, Dunkelberg H. (1998) Human biomonitoring of arsenic and antimony in case of an elevated geogenic exposure. *Environ Health Perspect* 106: 33–39.

Koch H, Angerer J. (2007) Di-iso-nonylphthalate (DINP) metabolites in human urine after a single oral dose of deuterium-labelled DINP. *Int J Hyg Environ Health* 210: 9–19.

NRC National Research Council. (1987) Biologic markers in environmental health research. *Environ Health Perspect* 74: 3–9.

Schramm K. (1997) Hair: a matrix for non-invasive biomonitoring of organic chemicals in mammals. *Bull Environ Contam Toxicol* 59(3): 396–402

Schwenk M, Gabrio T, Päpke O, Wallenhorst T. (2002) Human biomonitoring of polychlorinated biphenyls and polychlorinated dibenzodioxins and dibenzofuranes in teachers working in a PCB-contaminated school. *Chemosphere* 47: 229–233.

Sepai O, Collier C, Van Tongelen B, Casteleyn L. Human biomonitoring data interpretation and ethics, obstacles or surmountable challenges? *Environmental Health* (In Press).

Somorovská M, Jahnová E, Tulinská J, Zámecníková M, Sarmanová J, Terenová A, Vodicková L, Lísková A, Vallová B, Soucek P, Hemminki K, Norppa H, Hirvonen A, Tates AD, Fuortes L, Dusinská M, Vodicka P. (1999) Biomonitoring of occupational exposure to styrene in a plastics lamination plant. *Mutation Research/Fundamental and Molecular Mechanisms of Mutagenesis* 428(1–2): 255–269.

WHO. (2001) Biomarkers in Risk Assessment: Validity and Validation. *Environmental Health Criteria* 222, World Health Organization, Geneva.

Wilhelm M, Ewers U, Schulz C. (2004) Revised and new reference values for some trace elements in blood and urine for human biomonitoring in environmental medicine. *Int J Hyg Environ Health* 207: 69–73.

Wilhelm M, Pesch B, Wittsiepe J, Jakubis P, Miskovic P, Keegan T, Nieuwenhuijsen M, Ranft U. (2005) Comparison of arsenic levels in fingernails with urinary As species as biomarkers of arsenic exposure in residents living close to a coal-burning power plant in Prievidza District, Slovakia. *J Expo Anal Environ Epidemiol* 15(1): 89–98.

Zimmer H, Ludwig H, Bader M, Bailer J, Eickholz P, Staehle H, Triebig G. (2002) Determination of mercury in blood, urine and saliva for the biological monitoring of an exposure from amalgam fillings in a group with self-reported adverse health effects. *Int J Hyg Environ Health* 205: 205–211.

# Section 2
## Applications of Toxicology

# Section 2.1

## Sources of toxicological information

Robie Kamanyire

### Learning outcomes

At the end of this chapter and any recommended reading the student should be able to:

1. explain the importance of the accurate identification of potentially toxic agents and the use of chemical identification numbers;
2. navigate their way though the wide array of available toxicological information sources;
3. take a critical approach to information resources; and
4. apply their knowledge in the analysis and management of hazardous situations.

## 1    Introduction

The environment is increasingly recognised as having an impact on human and ecological health, as well as on specific types of human morbidity, mortality, and disability.

As environmental health concerns continue to increase, it is important for health professionals and other communities to have ready access to information resources. There is a large and diverse potential audience for toxicology and environmental health information, ranging from emergency department physicians to local community advocates attempting to determine the environmental health hazards faced by their communities. Although the user communities in this broad spectrum have diverse information needs it should not be impossible to effectively and efficiently provide relevant information resources.

This chapter aims to provide the tools to direct health professionals through the wide array of information resources that are available for toxicology. Access to the right information at the right time is a crucial ingredient of modern healthcare. The rapid growth of biomedical knowledge and the resulting increase in the number of scientific journals that have inundated health professionals are other factors affecting the need for easily accessible toxicology and environmental health information. Improving access to information is an important factor for all health professionals as well as the public.

Toxicology at its simplest is the study of the nature and mechanism of potential effects of substances on living organisms and other biological systems. The assessment of the health hazards of industrial chemicals, environmental pollutants and other substances represents an important element in the protection of the health of the worker and members of communities.

## 2     Chemical identification

One of the key factors for obtaining good quality toxicology information is to ensure an accurate identification of the chemical or compound of interest. There has been a phenomenal growth in the number of chemical compounds being synthesised (or isolated), and then reported in the scientific literature. In February 2008, the Chemical Abstract Service (CAS) had formally classified over thirty million chemical compounds. The names of many of these compounds are often nontrivial and hence not very easy to remember or cite accurately. Also it is difficult to keep track of them in the literature. Several international organisations like the International Union of Pure and Applied Chemistry (IUPAC) and the Chemical Abstract Service (CAS) have initiated steps to make such tasks easier. CAS provides an abstracting service of the chemical literature, consisting of a numerical identifier, known as a CAS registry number, for each chemical substance that has been reported in the chemical literature. Establishing an accurate identification of a compound of concern allows procession to sources of toxicology information.

Other chemical identification numbers exist such as the EC number: a seven-digit code allocated by the Commission of the European Communities for commercially available chemical substances within the European Union. The "EC number" designation supersedes the older European Inventory of Existing Commercial Chemical Substances Information System (EINECS) and European List of Notified Chemical Substances (ELINCS) designations which were required on the label and the packaging of dangerous substances.

The United Nations Committee of Experts on the Transport of Dangerous Goods assigns four-digit UN numbers that identify hazardous substances, and articles (such as explosives, flammable liquids, toxic substances, etc.) in the framework of international transport. Some hazardous substances have their own UN numbers, while sometimes groups of chemicals or products with similar properties receive a common UN number (e.g. flammable liquids, not otherwise specified, have UN1993). A chemical in its solid state may receive a different UN number than the liquid phase if their hazardous properties differ significantly; substances with different levels of purity (or concentration in solution) may also receive different UN numbers.

## 3     Sources of information

Once a chemical is correctly identified it is then necessary to obtain suitable information on its toxicity. Sources of information can be broadly classified into primary i.e. toxicology journals or secondary i.e. searchable databases or books. It is unlikely for the vast majority of enquiries to use a primary source of information to obtain toxicology information. Secondary sources have a longstanding tradition in toxicology in the form of handbooks or textbooks and more recently databases delivered via the Internet. This chapter will concentrate on a few key textbooks and databases which should be easily accessible from most libraries or via the Internet. This summary is intentionally not an exhaustive list but should provide a basis for initiating a search for information which often leads to further resources.

## 3.1    Text books

*Sax's Dangerous Properties of Industrial Materials* (3 v., 10th ed., 1999) covers over 23,500 toxic, carcinogenic, mutagenic, highly flammable, or potentially explosive substances. Included are health-related and physical property data. There are many pages of synonyms in several languages to assist in using the book and it also includes a CAS Registry Number index. A CD-ROM version is also available.

*Patty's Industrial Hygiene* and *Patty's Toxicology*, now in the 5th edition, collectively cover General Principles, Toxicology, and Theory and Rationale. The focus of the work in recent editions has been extended beyond the industrial workplace to environmental safety and hazard control. The book contains comprehensive toxicological data for industrial compounds from metals to synthetic polymers. Information for each compound includes CAS numbers, Registry of Toxic Effects of Chemicals (RTECS) numbers, physical and chemical properties, threshold limit values (TLV's), permissible exposure limits (PEL's), maximum workplace concentrations (MAK), and biological tolerance values for occupational exposures.

*Ellenhorn's Medical Toxicology: Diagnosis and Treatment of Human Poisoning*, (2nd ed., 1997) Williams and Wilkins. The second edition published posthumously spans 67 chapters with more than 13,000 references. The text, organized into five sections, gives a national and international approach to principles of poison management, individual drugs, intoxicants in the home, chemical poisons, and natural toxins.

*Goldfrank's Toxicologic Emergencies*. This book uses a case-study approach to medical toxicology. This comprehensive reference is comprised of 117 chapters covering toxicological emergencies, related environmental problems, and issues affecting emergency departments, the poison centres and the poisoned patient. In addition, an accompanying study guide provides several case studies as well as a questions and answer section.

Textbooks, including some of the texts listed above, have evolved from print-based materials to electronic Internet-based resources.

## 3.2    Internet resources

However, when accessing toxicology resources on the Internet care must be taken as there are numerous sites and it is important to access sources which can be considered to be reputable or 'accredited'.

Individuals have varying skill in their abilities to conduct Internet searches for reliable information. When using Internet resources it is important to ensure the results of searches have been critically appraised, especially ensuring that any information has been subjected to independent peer review. A small selection of such sites is presented below.

### 3.2.1  Compendia of Chemical Hazards, HPA

The Health Protection Agency's Chemical Hazards and Poisons Division produces as part of its information resource a series entitled the **Compendium of Chemical Hazards**. The aim is to produce an online information resource for the public and all professionals who may be involved in advising and responding to chemical incidents, mainly public health professionals and emergency services. Each Compendium entry is split into three sections:

- *General Information* which provides background information on the compound, including its uses and 'frequently asked questions'.
- *Incident Management* focusing on information that may be needed during chemical incidents, such as physicochemical properties, health effects and decontamination.
- *Toxicological Overview* provides more in-depth toxicology of the compound.

### 3.2.2  INCHEM, IPCS

The International Programme on Chemical Safety (IPCS) produces **INCHEM** as a co-operative programme and is an invaluable tool for those concerned with chemical safety and the proper management of chemicals. IPCS INCHEM directly responds to one of the Intergovernmental Forum on Chemical Safety (IFCS) priority actions to consolidate current, internationally peer-reviewed chemical safety-related publications and database records from international bodies, for public access. IPCS INCHEM offers rapid access to internationally peer-reviewed information on chemicals commonly used throughout the world, which may also occur as contaminants in the environment and food. The site provides quick and easy electronic access to thousands of searchable full-text documents on chemical risks and the sound management of chemicals:

- Concise International Chemical Assessment Documents (CICADS)
- Environmental Health Criteria Monographs (EHC)
- Joint Expert Committee on Food Additives – Monographs and Evaluations (JECFA)
- Health and Safety Guides (HSG)
- International Agency for Research on Cancer – Summaries and Evaluations (IARC)
- International Chemical Safety Cards (ICSC)
- Joint Meeting on Pesticide Residues – Monographs and Evaluations (JMPR)
- Pesticide Data Sheets and Documents (PDS)
- Screening Information Data Set for High Production Volume Chemicals (SIDS)

### 3.2.3   TOXNET, NLM

The US National Library of Medicine (NLM) toxicology data service **TOXNET** is a free service with access to a range of free toxicology databases. Included are:

- Toxicology Data Search for factual information in the databases HSDB (see below), Gene-Tox, CCRIS (carcinogenesis), IRIS (the US Environmental Protection Agency's (EPA) risk assessment database) and the Registry of Toxic Effects of Chemical Substances (RTECS).
- Toxicology Literature Search for bibliographic records from TOXLINE and the genotoxic/reproductive database DART/ETIC.
- TRI (Toxic Release Inventory) Search, reporting EPA's annual estimate of releases of toxic substances into the environment.
- Chemical Information Search for identification of substances by name, structure, etc. (ChemIDplus contains >367,000 records and >182,000 structures; HSDB: >4,500 records; and NCI-3D: >213,000 substances).

### 3.2.4   HSDB

The **Hazardous Substances Data Bank** (HSDB, available through TOXNET) contains around 5,000 chemical records, each of which can have as many as 150 or so fields of data, covering human health effects, emergency medical treatment, animal toxicity studies, metabolism/pharmacokinetics, pharmacology, environmental fate and exposure, environmental standards and regulations, chemical/physical properties, chemical safety and handling, occupational exposure standards and more. HSDB is peer-reviewed by a committee of experts, the Scientific Review Panel (SRP).

### 3.2.5   IRIS, EPA

The **Integrated Risk Information System** (IRIS) is prepared and maintained by the U.S. Environmental Protection Agency (U.S. EPA), and is an electronic database containing information on human health effects that may result from exposure to various chemicals in the environment. The information in IRIS is intended for those without extensive training in toxicology, but with some knowledge of health sciences. The dataset contains descriptive and quantitative information in the following categories:

- oral reference doses and inhalation reference concentrations (RfDs and RfCs, respectively) for chronic noncarcinogenic health effects;
- hazard identification, oral and inhalation unit risks for carcinogenic effects.

### 3.2.6   Pocket Guide to Chemical Hazards, NIOSH

The **NIOSH Pocket Guide to Chemical Hazards** is intended as a source of general industrial hygiene information for workers, employers, and occupational health professionals. The Pocket Guide presents key information and data in abbreviated tabular form for 677 chemicals or substance groupings (e.g., manganese compounds, tellurium compounds, inorganic tin compounds, etc.) that are found in the work environment. The industrial hygiene information found in the Pocket Guide should help users recognise and control occupational chemical hazards. The chemicals or substances contained in this revision include all substances for which the National Institute for Occupational Safety and Health (NIOSH) has recommended exposure limits (RELs)

### 3.2.7   ATSDR

**Agency for Toxic Substances and Disease Registry (ATSDR)** is the principal federal public health agency charged with the responsibility of evaluating the human health effects of exposure to hazardous substances. The United States Congress requires ATSDR to provide toxicological profiles to state health and environmental agencies and to make them available to other interested parties. The toxicological profiles are summaries of ATSDR's evaluations concerning whether and at what levels of exposure adverse health effects occur and levels at which no adverse effects occur. The profiles include information about exposure and environmental fate that may help readers determine the significance of levels found in the environment. Toxicological profiles provide interpretations of data, which distinguishes them from ordinary reviews. Interpretations are useful for those health professionals who may not have the resources to gather and consider all the toxicological data themselves.

### 3.2.8   ECETOC

**European Centre for Ecotoxicology and Toxicology of Chemicals (ECETOC)** was established in 1978 as a scientific, non-profit, non-commercial association. It is financed by 51 of the leading companies with interests in the manufacture and use of chemicals. A stand-alone organisation, it was established to provide a scientific forum through which the extensive specialist expertise in the European chemical industry could be harnessed to research, review, assess and publish studies on the ecotoxicology and toxicology of chemicals. ECETOC produces a range of peer-reviewed technical reports and monographs reviewing generic topics or issues fundamental to the application of sound science in evaluating the hazards and risks of chemicals to human health and the environment.

## 3.3   UK Independent Advisory Committees

### 3.3.1   CoC and CoM

**Committee of Carcinogenicity and Committee on Mutagenicity (CoC and CoM)** are independent advisory committees that provide advice to UK government departments and agencies on matters concerning the potential carcinogenicity or mutagenicity of chemicals ranging from natural products to new synthetic chemicals used in pesticides or pharmaceuticals. The committees consist of a panel of independent doctors and scientists recruited for their individual expertise from universities and research institutes and, in some cases, industry. The committees are tasked with providing advice on a range of issues related to the carcinogenicity or mutagenicity of chemicals.

### 3.3.2   Committee on Medical Effects of Air Pollution (COMEAP)

COMEAP is an Advisory Committee of independent experts that provides advice to UK Government Departments and Agencies on all matters concerning the potential toxicity and effects upon health of air pollutants.

## 3.4   UK Agency Guidance

### 3.4.1   Environment Agency: Contaminated Land Exposure Assessment (CLEA)

The Department for Environment, Food and Rural Affairs (Defra) and the Environment Agency published a series of reports that provide a scientifically-based framework for the assessment of risks to human health from land contamination. The health criteria values and the soil guideline values (SGVs) published through the CLEA programme are developed through an extensive period of consultation between independent experts, peer reviewers and regulatory authorities. Authoritative health criteria values for each contaminant are established through a review of scientific literature. The health criteria values are protective of human health and are used in the derivation of SGVs and can be used for site-specific risk assessment.

### 3.4.2   Health and Safety Executive

The UK's Health and Safety Commission's advisory committee on toxic substances (ACTS) advise the Health and Safety Commission on matters relating to the prevention, control and management of hazards and risks to the health and safety of persons arising from the supply or use of toxic substances at work, with due regard to any related risks to consumers, the public and the environment. ACTS is sub-divided into a number of sub committees to cover issues such as workplace exposure limits or packaging hazards.

## 3.5   World Health Organization

### 3.5.1   Air Quality

The *WHO Air Quality Guidelines for Europe* aim to provide a basis to protect public health from the adverse effects of air pollutants, and to eliminate, or reduce to a minimum, pollutants that are known or are likely to be hazardous to human health and well-being. In providing pollutant levels below which lifetime exposure or exposure for a given averaging time does not constitute a health risk, they form a basis for setting national standards for air pollution.

### 3.5.2   Water Quality

The WHO Guidelines for Drinking-Water Quality include fact sheets and comprehensive review documents for many individual chemicals. The guidelines are addressed primarily to water and health regulators, policymakers and their advisors, to assist in the development of national standards. The guidelines and associated documents are also used by many others as a source of information on water quality and health and on effective management approaches.

## 4    Summary

This chapter summarises a few key resources in the field of toxicology which should enable anyone involved in health protection to access information they would require to answer questions relating to the exposure of a population to noxious chemicals.

## 5    Further reading

Advisory Committee on Toxic Substances (ACTS), UK Health and Safety Commission. www.hse.gov.uk

Agency for Toxic Substances and Disease Registry (ATSDR), US Centers for Disease Control and Prevention. www.atsdr.cdc.gov

Chemical Abstract Service (CAS), American Chemical Society. www.cas.org

Chemical Hazards and Poisons Division (CHaPD) Chemical Compendium, UK Health Protection Agency. www.hpa.org.uk

Committee on Carcinogenicity of Chemicals in Food, Consumer Products and the Environment (COC), UK Department of Health www.advisorybodies.doh.gov.uk

Committee on the Medical Effects of Air Pollutants (COMEAP), UK Department of Health. www.advisorybodies.doh.gov.uk

Contaminated Land Exposure Assessment (CLEA), UK Environment Agency. www.environment-agency.gov.uk

European Centre for Ecotoxicology and Toxicology of Chemicals (ECETOC). www.ecetoc.org

Hazardous Substances Database Network (HSDN), Toxicology Data Network (TOXNET). www.toxnet.nlm.nih.gov

INCHEM, International Programme on Chemical Safety. www.inchem.org

Integrated Risk Information System (IRIS), US Environmental Protection Agency. www.epa.gov

National Institute for Occupational Safety and Health (NIOSH) *Pocket Guide to Chemical Hazards*, US Centers for Disease Control and Prevention. www.cdc.gov/niosh

Toxicology Data Network (TOXNET). www.toxnet.nlm.nih.gov

United Nations Committee of Experts on the Transport of Dangerous Goods, UN Economic Commission for Europe (UNECE). www.unece.org/trans

WHO air quality guidelines for Europe 2000. 2nd Edition, World Health Organization. www.euro.who.int

WHO Guidelines for drinking-water quality. World Health Organization.  www.who.int

# Section 2.2

# Medical management of chemical incidents

Simon FJ Clarke

## Learning outcomes

At the end of this chapter and any recommended reading the student should be able to:

1. explain how the state of the patient is assessed following toxic exposure;
2. describe and discuss the supportive and symptomatic management of poisoned patients;
3. describe and discuss decontamination techniques, methods used to reduce absorption of toxic substances, antidotes, and the enhancement of the elimination of toxic substances;
4. explain the roles of the various agencies involved, including the accident and emergency services and hospital emergency departments;
5. critically discuss the protocols used in the management of the poisoned patient e.g. in the prevention of secondary contamination, and
6. apply their knowledge in the analysis and management of hazardous situations.

## 1    Introduction

Toxicology has been defined as the study of the adverse effects of xenobiotics (extraneous chemicals) on biological systems. If this definition is applied to human medicine, it can be seen that it incorporates a number of scenarios involving pharmaceuticals (adverse drug reactions, interactions, and overdose) and exposure to non-pharmaceuticals (domestic and industrial chemicals, and chemical warfare agents). Although poisoning by pharmaceuticals is more commonly encountered in clinical medicine, exposure to non-pharmaceutical chemicals during chemical incidents is more important from the health protection perspective. This is due to the potential for spread of contamination to other individuals (both members of the public and healthcare staff) and the environment, as well as disruption to infrastructure.

Toxins can be absorbed via the gastrointestinal tract (ingested), absorbed across the lungs (inhaled), or absorbed across the skin or eyes.

This chapter will focus on the medical management of chemical incidents. The issues that will be discussed include:

- the risk of *secondary contamination* of healthcare staff and facilities and systems used to reduce that risk (*containment*);
- the diagnostic challenges presented by exposure to chemicals;
- the treatment strategies available, such as:
  - *reducing absorption* of chemical (*decontamination*),
  - *promoting elimination* of any toxin that has been absorbed,
  - specific therapies for individual chemicals (*antidotes*), and
  - the *symptomatic and supportive* approach, which is the mainstay of clinical toxicology;
- sources of expert help for both clinicians and public health practitioners.

## 2    Secondary contamination

The main feature that sets chemical incidents apart from other causes of presentation to Emergency Departments (EDs) is the fact that there is a risk that healthcare staff and facilities may themselves become affected by the chemicals. There are many reported cases where casualties have caused significant disruption to EDs, Operating Theatres and Intensive Care Units (Burgess, 1999; Geller *et al.*, 2001; Davey *et al.*, 2004; Harrison *et al.*, 2002; Stewart *et al.*, 2003; Stacey *et al.*, 2004). Even single patients have caused significant disruption; however, the most widely reported incident was the sarin attack on the Tokyo subway in 1996 where 10–20% of emergency responders and healthcare staff developed clinical features of sarin poisoning (Nozaki *et al.*, 1997; Okumura *et al.*, 1996; Ohbu *et al.*, 1997), many of whom required medical treatment, and some of whom suffered from persistent symptoms for at least seven years after the incident (Miyaki *et al.*, 2005).

Secondary contamination can occur from a number of sources:

- Residues can be brought in on the patients' clothes and skin. This can be transferred to other individuals either by direct splashing onto their skin or in their eyes or by inhalation in the case of volatile chemicals and particulates.
- Volatile agents may be found in significant concentrations in the casualty's expired air (*respiratory off-gassing*). These can be inhaled by other individuals nearby, particularly those who are managing the patient's breathing.
- Chemicals may be present in body fluids; in particular, ingested toxins can be present in high concentrations in vomitus. Again, these pose a risk of skin or eye contamination for members of staff treating the patient, or an inhalational risk if the body fluids contain volatile agents.

The risk of secondary contamination depends upon a number of chemical properties (Horton *et al.*, 2003; Cox, 1994; Brennan *et al.*, 1999; Moles *et al.*, 1999; Baker, 1999):

- *Volatility:* this indicates how rapidly an agent evaporates. Such agents may present an immediate risk of inhalation injury but they disperse rapidly; external decontamination does not eliminate the risk of secondary contamination because the patients may continue to "off-gas" (continuing evaporation of chemical after external decontamination) with their expired breath, but the risk is relatively short-lived in a well-ventilated environment.

- *Persistence:* this is the inverse of volatility. These agents pose more of a risk from direct contact, although the risk can be eliminated by efficient external decontamination.
- *Toxicity:* this is the potential for a chemical to cause harm to biological systems. Chemical warfare agents have been specifically designed to have a particularly high degree of toxicity, which means that small doses can cause harm.
- *Latency:* this is the period of time between exposure and the onset of symptoms; it is of particular concern if there is a delay in symptoms becoming apparent as the casualties may not realise that they are being exposed and therefore do not seek to escape from the area and minimise contamination.
- *Corrosiveness:* strong acids and alkalis produce tissue damage by a variety of mechanisms; in addition, some chemicals, such as certain elemental metals, react violently with moisture on the skin and can produce thermal burns. Agents such as phosgene react with metals in a moist environment which can damage equipment such as metal valves in breathing systems; strong acids can degrade plastic material.

The risk of secondary contamination can be minimised by early recognition that a chemical incident has occurred, appropriate use of personal protective equipment, and adequate decontamination of the patient. It is important for each healthcare facility to have a single, generic, well-rehearsed protocol for dealing with such incidents (Burgess *et al.*, 1999; Tan *et al.*, 2002; Timm *et al.*, 2007) using the following principles:

- Recognition
- Containment
- Decontamination with life support measures
- Definitive care

These will be discussed in the following section.

# 3    Management of a chemical incident

## 3.1    Recognition

Chemical substances can be released overtly or covertly. In many cases it is obvious that a chemical incident has occurred. Ideally the Emergency Department (ED) will receive a formal warning from the emergency services or directly from an industrial site. Patients may allege that they have been involved in a chemical incident, arrive obviously contaminated, or attend complaining of feeling ill after smelling a "funny" or "chemical" odour. It should be noted that the ability to smell certain chemicals is genetically determined and not everyone has the ability to detect them; in addition, odour may only be detected at a level that exceeds the toxic threshold, which is important when staff members notice the smell.

Unfortunately, recognition that a chemical incident has occurred may not be so obvious and a degree of vigilance is necessary by emergency services or healthcare staff. Multiple patients may arrive unannounced with similar symptoms (e.g. respiratory or neurological symptoms) from the same geographical location. This is the basis of the STEP 1-2-3 protocol used by the emergency services (see Box 1).

Individual or multiple patients may arrive with certain toxidromes, which are clusters of symptoms and signs suggestive of exposure to chemicals (see Table 1). Interestingly, clinicians who had treated patients from the Matsumoto sarin release were amongst the first to recognise the features of sarin poisoning whilst watching news footage of the Tokyo attack (Murakami, 2003).

A number of protocols have been devised to reduce the risk of secondary contamination.

**Box 1** STEP 1-2-3 System

**Step 1. One casualty:** approach using normal procedures

**Step 2. Two casualties:** approach with caution, consider all options
Report on arrival and update Control

**Step 3. Three or more casualties:**
Do NOT approach
Withdraw
Contain
Report
Isolate yourself and SEND for SPECIALIST HELP

## 3.2    Containment

- The hospital needs to be 'locked down' which means that all of the entrances are secured except the one where patients enter the ED and a separate access point for staff.
- The air conditioning must be isolated to prevent spread of volatile agents to other parts of the hospital.
- Patients who present to the waiting room following a chemical incident should be asked to go outside where they should be assessed by a senior clinician. A rapid risk assessment will need to be undertaken as to whether the waiting room should be evacuated and ventilated. In most instances the risk of secondary contamination from a single, ambulant casualty is minimal.

Not every chemical presents a risk of secondary contamination; for example, patients exposed to gases may be free of residual contamination. Although both fire and ambulance services have the capability to detect and identify the chemicals at the scene of release, precise information about the nature of the chemical is unlikely to be rapidly available. Also the current generation of detection and identification monitors available to EDs are based on military models which were designed for battlefield identification of Chemical Warfare Agents (CWAs); unfortunately, they do not identify most Toxic Industrial Chemicals (TICs) and provide false positive readings in the presence of ethanol, alcohol hand gel and some perfumes. Therefore, the safest default option is to assume that all patients presenting from the scene of an incident pose a risk until definite information is available.

## 3.3  Decontamination

### 3.3.1  External decontamination

***The process***

Decontamination is the process of removing chemical from the patient before it is absorbed. External decontamination describes the method of removing chemical from the patient's skin, hair, eyes and any wounds.

The aims of decontamination are:
- to stop ongoing exposure for the patient and reduce their absorbed toxic dose, and
- to reduce the risk of secondary contamination of healthcare facilities and staff.

There are a number of different possible methods of undertaking decontamination: firstly, physically removing the chemical by washing with soap and water (or brushing for dry powders); secondly, inactivating the chemical such as using hypochlorite solution to inactivate organophosphorous compounds (Duirk and Colette, 2006); thirdly, using adsorbents such as Fuller's Earth (Taysse *et al.*, 2007); lastly, chelating agents such as diphoterine (Nehles *et al.*, 2006) have been recently advocated to bind chemicals. Wet decontamination using soap and water is currently recommended in the UK (Heptonstall and Gent, 2007; Morgan *et al.*, 2007) primarily for logistical reasons, since water is universally available. It should be remembered that external decontamination does not reduce the damage that is caused by chemicals that have already been absorbed (Hall *et al.*, 2006), therefore it is imperative that it must be undertaken as soon as possible after exposure has occurred. Resources have recently been allocated to the blue light services to allow rapid deployment of decontamination equipment to the scene of the incident (Communities and Local Government, 2008).

The patients disrobe and are then decontaminated following the 'Rinse-Wipe-Rinse' system:

- *Rinse 1*. The patient is drenched under the shower. This removes particulate matter and water-soluble substances.

- *Wipe.* Detergent solution (10ml in a bucket of water) is applied with a soft brush/sponge. This removes organic chemicals.
- *Rinse 2.* The patient is drenched again under the shower. This removes the detergent and chemicals.

Particular attention should be paid to the patient's face and the process should be repeated if there is any visible, residual contamination. In addition, wounds should be thoroughly irrigated. Water should be lukewarm; there is a known risk of inducing hypothermia in the patients (Black, 2003) if it is too cold, while water that is too warm may promote transcutaneous absorption of chemical (Renshaw *et al.*, 2006; Moody *et al.*, 2006). Eyes should be thoroughly irrigated with 1–2 litres of normal saline or Hartmann's solution (two common forms of intravenous rehydration therapy). Contact lenses should be removed. In the case of mustard gas, irrigation should continue for at least 30 minutes (Department of Health, 2003). If an acid or alkali has contaminated the patient's eyes, irrigation should continue until a neutral pH has been achieved.

### Limitations of decontamination
It must be remembered that the process described above only removes most of the chemical from the patient's exterior (Lavoie *et al.*, 1992; Schultz and Wabeke, 1995; Al-Damouk and Bleetman, 2005). Some chemicals may be present in significant concentrations in the patient's expired air. Thus if advanced life support techniques need to be performed, it must be assumed that staff are still at risk of exposure to chemical agent (Davey *et al.*, 2004; Harrison *et al.*, 2002). The Tokyo subway attack (Okumura *et al.*, 1996) showed that these risks can be reduced by regularly rotating staff out of the area, keeping the resuscitation room well ventilated (i.e. keep the external doors open) and sending ventilated patients to an area which has a scavenging system (i.e. theatres/recovery rather than ICU).

Similarly, bodily secretions, such as vomitus, may contain ingested chemical (Stacey *et al.*, 2004) and should be cleared up and disposed of rapidly. Lastly, blisters should be kept intact until the responsible agent is formally identified because those caused by Lewisite contain active chemical (Chilcott, 2007), unlike those due to mustard gas or TICs with a blistering action.

Ambulance Services and Fire Brigades both have equipment that can cope with decontaminating large numbers of casualties. On the other hand, there are concerns about limitations in capacity of the current decontamination equipment supplied to hospitals (Malpass and Blunden, 2003); although plans are in place to upgrade their facilities, there is currently a possible gap in resilience which needs to be addressed locally at the planning stage (e.g. developing agreements with the local fire service to provide tenders to the hospital to rapidly wash large numbers of self-presenting casualties) (Clarke *et al.*, 2008).

### Treatment prior to decontamination
Personal protective equipment (PPE) limits dexterity and restricts patient assessment to visual clues, so before decontamination is undertaken, only basic life saving techniques should be performed (simple airway opening manoeuvres, bag-valve-mask ventilation, pressure on wounds, and external cardiac massage). In addition,

**Table 1** Toxidromes of Chemical Warfare Agents (please refer also to Chapter 4.5 on Chemical Warfare Agents)

| Agents | Odour | Onset | Symptoms | Signs | Differential Diagnosis |
|---|---|---|---|---|---|
| Nerve Agents | Fruity | Rapid | Weakness, dyspnoea, runny nose, blurred vision, painful eyes | Muscle fasciculations, miosis, wheeze, copious secretions, altered mental state, collapse | Organo-phosphate/carbamate pesticides; cyanide; myasthenia gravis |
| Blister Agents | Mustard/Garlic/Horseradish | *Mustard:* hours *Lewisite:* minutes | Burning/itchy skin, sore throat/painful eyes | Erythema/blisters, haemoptysis/pulmonary oedema | Contact with caustics, sodium hydroxide, and ammonia |
| Choking Agents | *Chlorine:* characteristic *Phosgene:* hay/mown grass | *Chlorine:* rapid onset, mild to more severe over hours *Phosgene:* 1–24 hours | Sore throat/painful eyes; throat/chest tightness; dyspnoea; wheeze | Laryngeal oedema/inflamed throat; pulmonary oedema | Upper airway sepsis |
| Cyanide | Bitter almonds | Rapid | Painful eyes; dizziness/headache; dyspnoea; collapse | Convulsions; hypotension; rapid, deep respirations; metabolic acidosis and high venous oxygen content | Nerve agents; carbon monoxide; hydrogen sulphide |
| Ricin | None | 18–24 hours (ingestion); 8–36 hours (inhalation) | *Ingestion:* Diarrhoea/vomiting/abdominal pain. *Inhalation:* cough/tight chest; fever; nausea; weakness. | Combined acute pulmonary and gastrointestinal signs | Atypical infections/biological weapons (tularaemia, plague, Q-fever) Phosgene |

it will be possible to administer treatments, where available, by the intramuscular or subcutaneous routes. Until recently, it was accepted practice for medical care to be started only once the casualties have been removed from the contaminated area (the 'hot zone'); this has recently been questioned and it is becoming recognised that earlier medical intervention in the hot zone may be life saving (personal communication DJ Baker; Byers *et al.*, 2008).

### 3.3.2    Gastrointestinal decontamination

There are a number of techniques available to try to prevent absorption of ingested drug. However, these techniques are limited because to be effective they need to be administered before a significant amount of drug has been absorbed. Although the evidence base for these techniques is limited, expert consensus has agreed that it must be given within one hour of ingestion in most situations.

*Activated Charcoal (AC)* (American Academy of Clinical Toxicology, 2005): binds drug in the bowel lumen which prevents it from being absorbed. Unfortunately, AC is not palatable and it is often difficult to persuade the patient to take it. It may be given via a wide-bore nasogastric tube but this can precipitate vomiting in the conscious patient. The airway must be secured in those with reduced conscious levels to prevent aspiration. Certain agents are not adsorbed onto AC:

- metals (e.g. iron, lithium, mercury)
- acids and alkalis
- hydrocarbons.

*Whole Bowel Irrigation (WBI)* (American Academy of Clinical Toxicology, 2004b): the aim of this treatment is to flush the bowel lumen so that the drug passes through without being absorbed. The patient is required to drink 1.5–2 litres of polyethylene glycol per hour, or it can be administered via a nasogastric tube. This is continued until the rectal effluent is clear. It is particularly useful for substances not adsorbed onto AC, for slow-release formulations of medicines, or for well-wrapped packets of illicit drugs swallowed for the purposes of smuggling.

*Induced Emesis and Gastric Lavage* (American Academy of Clinical Toxicology, 2004a, 2004c): neither of these techniques is recommended because of lack of evidence of efficacy and the unacceptable risk of serious complications, such as injury to the patient's oesophagus, or aspiration of stomach contents.

### 3.4    Definitive care

### 3.4.1    Symptomatic and supportive therapy

There are 33 million organic and inorganic substances registered with the Chemical Abstract Service (CAS, 2008); clearly it is not possible to have individual treatments for each chemical.

Once the patients have been decontaminated, they should be managed using a standard approach which ensures that the most rapidly dangerous clinical problems are identified first. As a physiological abnormality is identified, appropriate treatment measures are implemented to try to reverse the problem, before moving on with the assessment. In reality, these patients are likely to be looked after by a clinical team, individual members of which will be responsible for each of the areas outlined below, so a number of assessments will continue concurrently.

- *Airway:* ensure that the airway is clear and that a gag reflex is present (taking care not to stimulate vomiting). There are a number of techniques that can be used to open a patient's airway, but the definitive method is to insert a tube into the patient's trachea (endotracheal intubation), usually assisted by the administration of anaesthetic drugs.

- *Breathing:* look for central cyanosis (blue discolouration of the lips, tongue, and finger nails due to lack of oxygen), count the respiratory rate, look at the pattern of respiration and attempt to assess depth of breathing. Monitor the patient's oxygen saturations using a pulse oximeter. The simplest treatment of inadequate respiration is the administration of supplemental oxygen. More profound ventilatory failure may require the patient to be intubated and artificial ventilation to be instituted.

- *Circulation:* measure pulse rate and blood pressure. Hypotension often responds to intravenous administration of fluids. Rarely, drug therapy to support the circulation may be necessary, but this should be undertaken with advice from the National Poisons Information Service (NPIS) and once invasive monitoring (arterial and central venous pressures) has been set up. Slow heart rates are often well tolerated by patients but some casualties may need atropine or even application of temporary pacemakers to maintain a satisfactory heart rate. Fast heart rates (tachyarrhythmias) may need drug therapy but again this should only be started after advice from the NPIS because in some cases of poisoning these drugs may exacerbate the arrhythmia.

- *Disability:* assess the conscious level of the patient; there are two standard methods:
    - AVPU (**A**lert, responds to **V**oice, responds to **P**ainful stimulus, **U**nresponsive)
    - Glasgow Coma Scale (GCS – see Box 2) (Teasdale and Jennett, 1974).
Although neither of these assessment tools has been formally validated for toxicological causes of impaired consciousness, there are currently no other systems available and it seems reasonable to continue to use them. In addition to meticulous attention to the airway, breathing and circulation, the patient's blood glucose level should be monitored closely.

- *Exposure:* this involves removing the patient's clothes and undertaking a 'top-to-toe' examination. Again, problems that are identified should be treated as necessary.

The importance of this approach cannot be overemphasised; during the Moscow theatre siege in 2002 (BBC, 2002) patients died as a result of inadequate basic airway management, not due to delays in identifying the chemical agents involved or administering specialised treatments.

**Box 2** Glasgow Coma Scale

**Eye Opening**
    Spontaneously – 4
    To verbal command – 3
    To painful stimulus – 2
    Not opening – 1

**Verbal Response**
    Orientated – 5
    Disorientated but converses – 4
    Inappropriate words – 3
    Incomprehensible words – 2
    No response – 1

**Motor Response**
    Obeys commands – 6
    Localises pain – 5
    Flexion (withdraws from pain) – 4
    Abnormal flexion – 3
    Abnormal extension – 2
    No response  – 1

Agent-specific therapies (antidotes) are available for only a small number of toxins. They should be given if there is strong clinical suspicion (from the presence of toxidromes – see Table 1) as to the identity of the causative agent or after chemical analysis from the scene.

### 3.4.2   Enhanced elimination techniques

In some circumstances, the elimination of absorbed toxins can be encouraged. The simplest method is to ensure that the patient is well hydrated, which increases the glomerular filtration rate (the volume of blood that is filtered by the kidneys per unit time). This promotes elimination of renally excreted drugs or metabolites of drugs. In a limited number of cases, more specialised techniques are available to increase the rate of elimination of certain drugs. To be successfully eliminated, substances must have a low volume of distribution (they are located primarily in the blood stream) and be poorly bound to plasma proteins.

*Urinary Alkalinisation* (Morgan and Polak, 1971; Prescott *et al.*, 1982): administration of bicarbonate promotes excretion of weakly acidic drugs; they form the ionised form in the kidney which prevents reabsorption back into the bloodstream and hence promotes excretion in the urine. This technique may be useful for poisoning by the herbicide 2,4-dichlorophenoxyacetic acid.

*Extracorporeal Techniques*: haemoperfusion, haemofiltration and haemodialysis may be useful for eliminating a small number of substances. They require specialised equipment and are usually only available on critical care units (haemofiltration) or renal units (haemoperfusion and dialysis). Filtration and dialysis may also be used to support failing kidneys.

*Artificial Ventilation*: some volatile chemicals are excreted via the lungs. In theory, by intubating and artificially ventilating the patient, the depth and rate of respiration can be intentionally increased to speed up the elimination of the chemical.

### 3.4.3  Antidotes

Antidotes are treatments that are specific to individual toxins. There are relatively few, some of which are held in regional centres so are not readily available to EDs. Therefore, the emphasis on acute treatment is based on the symptomatic, supportive approach described above.

The non-pharmaceutical chemicals which have known antidotes include:

- *Cyanide* – there are a number of antidotes which bind cyanide and form non-toxic compounds. These include dicobalt edetate, sodium nitrite, sodium thiosulphate, and hydroxocobalamin. All of these have significant side-effects if given in the absence of cyanide exposure, with the possible exception of hydroxocobalamin. However, there is little data for the use of hydroxocobalamin with hydrogen cyanide and large volumes have to be given, so currently, dicobalt edentate is recommended as the first line treatment and has been stockpiled by the Department of Health (Department of Health, 2003).
- *Organophosphate compounds (including nerve agents)* – atropine is used to counteract the cholinergic effects of these compounds. Pralidoxime is used to reactivate the inhibited enzyme, cholinesterase. Both of these agents have been stockpiled by the Department of Health.
- *Heavy metals* – there are a number of antidotes, including sodium calcium edetate and succimer (DMSA), both particularly useful for lead poisoning. Unithiol (DMPS) and dimercaprol are used for mercury poisoning. These are relatively rare conditions and use of the antidotes should be supervised by a clinical toxicologist and advice sought from the National Poisons Information Service (NPIS).
- *Thallium* – the antidote is Prussian Blue, and again, this should be used under the supervision of a clinical toxicologist and advice sought from the NPIS.

A full list of all antidotes available in the UK can be found on the web-site of the British Association of Emergency Medicine (College of Emergency Medicine, 2006).

## 4    Sources of information – role of the NPIS and Chemical Hazards and Poisons Division (CHaPD) of the Health Protection Agency

There are a number of sources of information for clinicians, when faced with poisoned patients. Toxbase is an on-line information resource developed by the National Poisons Information Service (NPIS) and is widely used as the first source of information for acute clinicians. It is found at www.toxbase.org and an institutional password is needed to access this site.

The NPIS, a service commissioned by the HPA, runs a telephone advice service and is able to give advice about the clinical treatment of individual patients and other aspects of management when the chemical has been identified. Some of the individual poisons units that comprise the NPIS hold regional stocks of some antidotes and also have laboratories that can undertake certain toxicological analyses. Lists of accredited toxicological laboratories can also be found on the web-site www.assayfinder.com.

During an acute chemical incident, the Chemical Hazards and Poisons Division (CHaPD) of the Health Protection Agency can provide information about the toxic effects of chemicals, but will also liaise with the local Health Protection Unit, assist the emergency services in identifying the chemical(s), and advise other agencies, such as the utilities and local authority. CHaPD undertakes surveillance of acute chemical incidents and therefore should be informed of all such events. Both CHaPD and the NPIS provide a 24 hour service. Chapter 2.1 contains more details of sources of toxicological information.

## 5    Planning and preparation

All EDs should have developed a Chemical Incident Plan which should be separate from, but dovetails into, their Major Incident Plan. This should use the above system but be adapted to their specific facilities and geography. An assessment of the risks in the catchment area of the hospital should be made which should include local industry, including Control of Major Accident Hazards (COMAH) sites (Control of Major Accident Hazards Regulations, 2005), transport systems (motorways, railways and airports), and possible terrorist targets.

The plan should include contact details of sources of information, which should include:
- NPIS
- CHaPD
- local HPU
- institutional password for Toxbase.

It is helpful if an individual or group of members of staff have responsibility for updating the plan and organising appropriate training. It is useful if that group establishes links with those responsible for Chemical Response in the blue light services and with the local Health Emergency Planning Advisors. The plan should be tested and specific aspects, such as setting up the decontamination equipment and donning the PPE should be practised regularly. In particular, each hospital should determine in advance who will be undertaking decontamination; there are pros and cons to using clinical and non-clinical staff.

## 6    Summary

Treatment of all types of poisoning is primarily symptomatic and supportive, with gut decontamination, enhanced elimination techniques, and antidotes only being suitable for relatively few cases.

In chemical incidents, risk of secondary contamination can be reduced by external decontamination of casualties and appropriate use of PPE by staff that come into contact with patients before and during decontamination.

Advice should be sought from the NPIS and CHaPD should be informed.

Chemical incident plans should be developed by all EDs and these should be thoroughly tested and practised.

## 7    References

Al-Damouk M, Bleetman A. (2005) Impact of the Department of Health initiative to equip and train acute trusts to manage chemically contaminated casualties. *Emerg Med J.* 22: 347–350.

American Academy of Clinical Toxicology. (2004a) European Association of Poisons Centres and Clinical Toxicologists. Position paper: ipecac syrup. *J Toxicol Clin Toxicol* 42: 133–143.

American Academy of Clinical Toxicology. (2004b) European Association of Poisons Centres and Clinical Toxicologists. Position paper: whole-bowel irrigation. *J Toxicol Clin Toxicol* 42: 843-854.

American Academy of Clinical Toxicology. (2004c) European Association of Poisons Centres and Clinical Toxicologists. Position paper: gastric lavage. *J Toxicol Clin Toxicol* 42: 933–943.

American Academy of Clinical Toxicology. (2005) European Association of Poisons Centres and Clinical Toxicologists. Position paper: single-dose activated charcoal. *J Toxicol Clin Toxicol* 43: 61–87.

Baker D. (1999) Management of respiratory failure in toxic disasters. *Resuscitation* 42: 125–131.

BBC (25 October 2002) *Moscow theatre siege.* British Broadcasting Corporation. www.news.bbc.co.uk

Black J. (2003) Exercise Alex. *Chemical Incident Response* 28: 16–19.

Brennan R, Waerckerle J, Sharp T, Lillibridge S. (1999) Chemical warfare agents: emergency medical and emergency public health issues. *Ann Emerg Med* 34: 191–204.

Burgess J, Kirk M, Borron S, Cisek J. (1999) Emergency department hazardous materials protocol for contaminated patients. *Ann Emerg Med* 34: 205–212.

Burgess J. (1999) Hospital evacuations due to hazardous materials incidents. *Am J Emerg Med.* 17: 50–52.

Byers M, Russell M, Lockey D. (2008) Clinical care in the 'Hot Zone'. *Emerg Med J* 25: 108–112.

CAS (accessed February 2008) Chemical Abstract Service Registry. www.cas.org

Chilcott R. (2007) Dermal effects of chemical warfare agents. In: Marrs TC, Maynard RL and Sidell FR. *Chemical warfare agents: toxicology and treatment.* (2nd Ed.) J Wiley & Sons; Chichester.

Clarke SFJ, Chilcott RP, Wilson JC, Kamanyire R, Baker DJ, Hallett A. 2008 Decontamination of multiple casualties who are chemically contaminated: a challenge for acute hospitals. Prehosp and Disas Med: 23: 175–181.

College of Emergency Medicine. The antidotes guidelines can now be found at the following site: www.collemergencymed.ac.uk/CEM

Communities and Local Government (Accessed February 2008) *New Dimensions mass decontamination programme.* Available at: www.communities.gov.uk

The Control of Major Accident Hazards (Amendment) Regulations 2005. Statutory Instrument No. 1088. London, HMSO.

Cox R. (1994) Decontamination and management of hazardous materials exposure victims in the Emergency Department. *Ann Emerg Med* 23: 761–770.

Davey A, Moppett I. (2004) Postoperative complications after CS spray exposure. *Anaesthesia* 59: 1219–1220.

Department of Health. (2003) Expert Group on the Management of Chemical Casualties Caused by Terrorist Activity. First report. Treatment of poisoning by selected chemical compounds.

Duirk S, Collette T. (2006) Degradation of chlorpyrifos in aqueous chlorine solutions: pathways, kinetics, and modeling. *Environ Sci Tech* 40: 546–51.

Geller R, Singleton K, Tarantino M, Drenzel C, Toomey K. (2001) Nosocomial poisoning associated with Emergency Department treatment of organophosphate toxicity – Georgia, 2000. *J Toxicol Clin Toxicol* 39: 109–111.

Hall A, Maibach H. (2006) Water decontamination of chemical skin/eye splashes: a critical review. *Cutaneous Ocular Toxicol* 25: 67–83.

Harrison H, Clarke S, Wilson A, Murray V. (2002) Chemical contamination of healthcare facilities and staff. *Chemical Incident Report* 25: 2–5.

Heptonstall J, Gent N. (2007) Generic Incident Management. CBRN incidents: clinical management and health protection. Version 2. Health Protection Agency. Available at: www.hpa.org.uk

Horton D, Berkowitz Z, Kaye W. (2003) Secondary contamination of ED personnel from hazardous materials events, 1995-2001. *Am J Emerg Med* 21: 199–204.

Lavoie F, Coomes T, Cisek, J, Fulkerson L. (1992) Emergency Department external decontamination for hazardous chemical exposures. *Vet Hum Toxicol* 34: 61–64.

Malpass T, Blunden M. (2003) Deployment of PPE in the event of a chemical incident. The importance of pre-planning and estimating capacity. Chemical Hazards and Poisons Report 1: 23–24.

Miyaki K, Nishiwaki Y, Maekawa K, Ogawa Y, Asukai N, Yoshimura K, Etoh N, Matsumoto Y, Kikuchi Y, Kumagai N, Omae K. (2005) Effects of sarin on the nervous system of subway workers seven years after the Tokyo subway sarin attack. *J Occup Health* 47: 299–304.

Moles T, Baker D. (1999) Clinical analogies for the management of toxic trauma. *Resuscitation* 42: 117–124.

Moody R, Maibach H. (2006) Skin decontamination: Importance of the wash-in effect. *Food Chem Toxicol* 44: 1783–1788.

Morgan A, Polak A. (1971) The excretion of salicylate in salicylate poisoning. *Clin Sci* 41: 475–484.

Morgan D, Said B, Walsh A, Murray V, Clarke S, Lloyd D, Gent N. (2007) Initial investigation and management of outbreaks and incidents of unusual illnesses: A guide for health professionals. Health Protection Agency. Available at: www.hpa.org.uk

Murakami H. (2003) *Underground. The Tokyo gas attack and the Japanese psyche.* Vintage Books, New York.

Nehles J, Hall A, Blomet J, Mathieu L. (2006) Diphoterine for emergent decontamination of skin/eye chemical splashes: 24 cases. *Cutaneous Ocular Toxicol* 2006: 25; 249–58.

Nozaki H, Hori S, Shinozawa Y, Fujishima S, Takuma K, Sagoh M, Kimura H, Ohki T, Suzuki M, Aikawa N. (1995) Secondary exposure of medical staff to sarin vapor in the emergency room. *Intes Care Med* 21: 1032–1035.

Ohbu S, Yamashina A, Takasu N, Yamaguchi T, Murai T, Nakano K, Matsui Y, Mikami R, Sakurai K, Hinohara S. (1997) Sarin poisoning on Tokyo subway. *South Med J* 90: 587–593.

Okumura T, Takasu N, Ishimatsu S, Miyanoki S, Mitsuhashi A, Kumada K, Tanaka K, Hinohara S. (1996) Report on 640 victims of the Tokyo subway sarin attack. *Ann Emerg Med* 28: 129–135.

Prescott L, Balali-Mood M, Critchley J, Johnstone A. (1982) Diuresis or urinary alkalinisation for salicylate poisoning? *BMJ* 285: 1383–1386.

Renshaw B. (1947) Observations on the role of water in the susceptibility of human skin to injury by vesicants. *J Invest Dermatol* 9: 75–85.

Schultz M, Cisek J, Wabeke R. (1995) Simulated exposure of hospital emergency personnel to solvent vapors and respirable dust during decontamination of chemically exposed patients. *Ann Emerg Med* 26: 324–329.

Stacey R, Morfey D, Payne S. (2004) Secondary contamination in organophosphate poisoning: analysis of an incident. *QJM* 97: 75–80.

Stewart A, Whiteside C, Tyler-Jones V, Ghebrehewet S, Reid J, McDonald P, Kennedy C, Pennycock A, Gent N, Seddon D. (2003) Phosphine suicide. *Chemical Incident Report* 27: 23–25.

Tan G *et al.* (2002) Chemical-Biological-Radiological (CBR) response: a template for hospital Emergency Departments. *Med J Australia* 177: 196–199.

Taysse L, Daulon S, Delamanche S, Bellier B, Breton P. (2007) Skin decontamination of mustards and organophosphates: comparative efficiency of RSDL and Fuller's earth in domestic swine. *Hum Exp Toxicol* 26: 135–141.

Teasdale G, Jennett B. (1974) Assessment of coma and impaired consciousness. A practical scale. *Lancet* 2: 81–84.

Timm N, Reeves S. (2007) A mass casualty incident involving children and chemical decontamination. *Disaster Management & Response* 5: 49–55.

# Section 2.3

# Concept of susceptibility to environmental hazards

Charlotte NB Aus

## Learning outcomes

At the end of this chapter and any recommended reading the student should be able to:

1. discuss how risks to human health from chemicals are assessed;
2. identify susceptible or vulnerable population groups, and explain why they are more susceptible;
3. explain how a hazardous chemical affects human health using a source-pathway-receptor model;
4. discuss aspects of susceptibility/vulnerability using examples, and
5. apply their knowledge in the analysis and management of hazardous situations.

## 1   Introduction

When the risk to human health from exposure to potentially hazardous environmental chemicals is assessed, this is on the basis of the best available data. There are rarely adequate toxicology data for exposure to environmental chemicals available from human populations, therefore, risk assessments will largely use experimental animal data with added uncertainty factors to allow inter-species variability (between animals and humans) and for intra-species variability (between different groups within the same species).

With better understanding of the factors resulting in human disease and of the variation in human susceptibility to disease induced by chemicals, together with extremes of variability in exposure, there has been some proposal that risk assessments should be directed towards specific groups, such as children, as well as the general public. An example of where this has happened is in the USA, where the 1996 Food Quality Protection Act (FQPA) mandated the use of an additional safety (or uncertainty) factor to account for differences between adults and children when risk assessing pesticides, to account for developmental risks and incomplete data when considering a pesticide's effect on infants and children, and any special sensitivity and exposure to pesticide chemicals that infants and children may have. More recently, the UK Committee on the Toxicity of Chemicals in Food, Consumer Products and the Environment (COT) published a report on variability and uncertainty in the toxicology of chemicals which gives detailed consideration of vulnerable subgroups including children (COT, 2007). The working group were specifically asked to consider the appropriateness of the uncertainty factors customarily used to extrapolate toxicological data from animals to humans and for variability in the human population, including children. They found that results suggest that the current approaches and uncertainty factors in use are adequate in the case of interspecies extrapolation and generally appropriate in the case of variability in the human population, but recommended that the area be kept under review.

## 2    Understanding susceptibility

Specific subgroups of the population who might be particularly vulnerable to exposure to some chemicals due to some deviation from the 'normal' exposed person, can be considered in the following three ways:

**a. A sub-group of a population is considered to be more susceptible than the population as a whole to a chemical hazard assuming that there are no other confounders or biasing factors.** i.e. exposure to a chemical at a particular dose will elucidate a harmful effect in the susceptible person, where no effect would be noticed in a 'normal' person.

**b. The level of exposure (dose) to a hazard that is needed to elucidate an adverse response in the susceptible group compared to the population as a whole.** i.e. the susceptible person will require a smaller exposure compared to a 'normal' person, for an adverse response to occur.

**c. The time period before the adverse effect manifests in different equally exposed groups.** i.e. the adverse effect will occur much earlier in time in the susceptible person, compared to the 'normal' person.

Population subgroups may be innately more susceptible to the effects of exposure to pollutants than others due to genetic predisposition or to incomplete development of normal (adult) physiological functions. Individuals who have specific genetic or immunological variations from the 'normal' are likely to be vulnerable throughout their lives. On the other hand, some population groups may be particularly vulnerable at specific times during their lives, such as during pregnancy, childhood, or old age (Risk Assessment and Toxicology Steering Committee, 1999). Also important are those who become more susceptible as a result of environmental or social factors, or personal behaviour (acquired susceptibility) and those who are simply exposed to unusually large amounts of pollutants. Members of the last group are vulnerable by virtue of the magnitude of exposure rather than as a result of individual susceptibility, for example by living near a busy road.

Susceptible subgroups of the population can be split into three main groups based on biological, socio-cultural or ethnic characteristics that may affect their vulnerability to adverse effects resulting from environmental exposure to a particular hazardous chemical, shown in Table 1. However, it is important to remember that susceptibility will vary with different chemicals.

**Table 1** Factors affecting vulnerability to an environmental hazard (adapted from Risk Assessment and Toxicology Steering Committee 1999)

| Biological | Sociocultural | Ethnic |
|---|---|---|
| Age group (e.g. infant, elderly)<br>Sex<br>Disease state/medication<br>Genetic susceptibility<br>Pregnancy (e.g. foetal development)<br>Physiological variation (e.g. height, weight) | Diet<br>Smoking status<br>Alcohol, drugs<br>Socioeconomic position<br>Religion<br>Housing quality<br>Housing location<br>Occupation | Genetic<br>Social (e.g. diet) |

For the purposes of this chapter, these following four broad groups are considered in further detail in the following sections:

1. Developing foetuses, infants and very young children;
2. The elderly;
3. Groups of people with genetic polymorphisms;
4. Those who are socially and economically deprived.

## 3    Source-Pathway-Receptor Model

In order for a hazardous chemical present in the environment to pose a risk to human health, three factors need to be present. A source of the chemical of concern; pathways by which it can come into contact with the public, which include air, water, land and food; and a receptor – in this case the person, or group of people.

Other factors that need to be considered are:
- Age at time of exposure, e.g. infancy, childhood;
- Duration of exposure: brief, intermittently, or over a long period of time;
- Level of exposure: a high or low dose.

This is simplified into the Source-Pathway-Receptor Model (Figure 1).

## 4    Increased susceptibility of developing foetuses, infants and very young children

The Third Ministerial Conference on Health and the Environment 1999 stated that children are not 'little adults'. Children are considered to be particularly susceptible to environmental chemicals compared to the general population of adults because of their fundamental differences to adults, which may lead to an unusual pattern of exposure (see Table 2). Young children also spend the majority of their time within the home, with one estimate of an average of 19.3 hours per day in the UK (Farrow and Golding, 1997). The home environment is a unique environment known to accumulate

**Figure 1** Illustrating the Source-Pathway-Receptor Model.

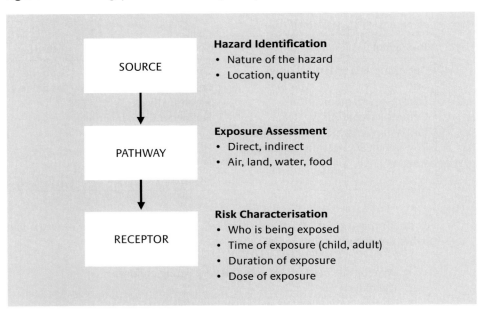

air pollutants at a higher concentration than outdoors (Whitmore *et al.*, 1994). Children also have a longer expected length of life left which all lead to a potentially greater exposure to toxic chemicals.

## 4.1   Physical differences

Children are physically very different to adults. They are much smaller, which means that they tend to be in much closer contact with the ground. Proportionally they have a larger surface area of skin compared to their body size, which increases the potential for exposure and the absorption of chemicals through their skin. Proportional to body weight, children breathe more air, drink more water and eat more food than adults do. The amount of air breathed in by a child while resting, per unit time on a weight-by-weight basis, may be nearly three times that of an adult.

## 4.2   Time windows

Children are both growing and developing rapidly, with their internal structures constantly being developed and matured, and important internal connections made. This is vital for the correct functioning of their bodies, for example their ability to produce specific hormones. During critical 'time windows' during development, damage may be caused which is irreparable and renders the body unable to function properly. The organs that are particularly sensitive to chemical damage during development include the brain and central nervous system, the immune system and the reproductive system.

## 4.3    Metabolic pathways

Many of the internal functions of infants and young children may differ from adults, making children more vulnerable to exposure. Their mechanisms for detoxifying and excreting environmental chemicals are immature and less efficient. Metabolic pathways may not yet include the same enzymes, or the same amount of a particular enzyme, which an adult would use to metabolise and detoxify the chemicals that have entered their bodies (Eskenazi *et al.*, 1999). This means that a dose of a specific

**Table 2** Differences between children and adults

| Factor | How children differ from adults |
|---|---|
| **Exposure to hazard** | Sources of exposure (e.g. industry, use in gardens) |
| | Pathways of exposure (e.g. dust, water, soil) |
| | Routes of exposure (e.g. dermal, inhalation, ingestion) |
| | Greater intake of air/food/water per unit body |
| | Increased surface area to weight ratio |
| **Physiological factors** | Greater rate of circulation |
| | Higher cell growth in many organs |
| | Shorter height |
| | Lighter weight |
| | Faster rate of respiration |
| **Pharmacokinetics** | Greater intake through the gut in the very young |
| | Higher rate of intake through the lungs |
| | Reduced ability to breakdown harmful chemicals in the very young |
| | Higher membrane permeability affecting oral absorption of chemicals in the very young |
| | Undeveloped ability to bind and store chemicals |
| | Increased bioavailability in body |
| | Decreased excretion from the body in the very young |
| **Pharmacodynamics** | Immature immune system |
| | Different extent of effect and response to toxic substances in the very young (may be increased or decreased sensitivity depending on substance) |
| | Increased sensitivity of particular organs |

chemical, which an adult body could quickly get rid of before damage was caused, does have the potential to cause harm to a child.

## 4.4    Behavioural patterns

Younger children have age-specific behaviours that may increase their exposure to hazardous chemicals. Their unique behavioural patterns, such as playing close to the ground and crawling, can increase their potential exposure through the skin. Younger children routinely explore their environment by putting fingers, toys and other objects into their mouths; hand contact with floors, carpets, lawns and other surfaces during crawling may lead to enhanced exposure via hand-to-mouth and object-to-mouth transfer. Some children exhibit pica behaviour, which is the deliberate ingestion of non-food items. Skin contact with surfaces during crawling or play may also contribute to exposure. Children have a higher ratio of skin surface area to body weight, compared to adults. In general, children will experience more intensive contact with their surroundings in the home than adults, all of which would lead to an increased potential for exposure.

## 5    Increased susceptibility in the elderly

This susceptibility is most often the result of disease states that are frequent in the older age groups compromising their physiological reserves and the ability to withstand stress and other disorders or dysfunctions due to chemicals interfering with cellular function. Disease states such as heart disease or high blood pressure would considerably reduce the ability to compensate for the changes in blood volume or falls in blood pressure or the risk of disturbances of heart rhythm that may follow toxic exposures.

The alteration in the structure of blood vessels such as thickening of the walls of the arteries with age-related arteriosclerosis, will prevent compensatory increases in blood flow that may be necessary (due to loss of elasticity) to prevent ill-health following toxic exposures. Similarly, chest or respiratory diseases such as emphysema or chronic bronchial asthma would prevent compensatory respiratory mechanisms coming into effect during times of respiratory compromise following toxic exposures.

The elderly and those who have been exposed previously or concurrently to relatively high levels of other xenobiotics such as therapeutic drugs may have compromised functions of vital organs which would prevent the normal body compensatory mechanisms coming into effect following toxic exposures. An example is an individual who is treated with a drug to slow the heart rate. The presence of such a drug will diminish the ability of the heart to increase the rate as a compensatory response.

## 6    Increased susceptibility due to genetic polymorphisms

Genetic polymorphisms often affect the qualitative and quantitative functions of metabolising enzymes which are necessary for the inactivation or detoxification of toxic chemicals. One of the better known examples is the absence of the enzyme to metabolise alcohol in some population groups. This enzyme – alcohol dehydrogenase – is absent for example in nearly 20% of the Japanese population and such individuals develop adverse effects after even minimal doses of alcohol. Similarly the genetic polymorphism associated with metabolising enzymes, the cytochrome P450 enzymes in the liver and gut, produces variations in the ability to inactivate many xenobiotics – often drugs. Such polymorphisms, in certain instances, have resulted in grouping individuals as fast metabolisers and slow metabolisers.

## 7     Increased susceptibility due to socio-economic deprivation

Socially and economically deprived populations can be more at risk of overcrowding, poor nutrition and poor sanitation, which may lead to disease states such as anaemia, diarrhoea and infections of the chest and skin. Such socio-economic factors invariably lead to a greater vulnerability to communicable diseases as well as greater vulnerability to toxic insults from chemicals.

These groups may react more strongly to a given exposure, either as a result of increased responsiveness to a specific dose and/or as a result of a larger internal dose of some pollutants than those of a higher socio-economic status exposed to the same concentration.

## 8     Examples of susceptibility and exposure to chemicals

When responding to an incident that involves a potentially harmful chemical, it is important to consider whether there are any susceptible sub-groups of the population that may be at greater risk from exposure and adverse health effects compared to the general population. Public health personnel need to be particularly concerned about these groups and to identify them quickly in order to ensure that they can be removed from the exposure if they are at an increased risk, and treated if they are displaying health effects from the exposure.

### 8.1     Case study of lead exposure

A three-year-old child was referred to hospital by their General Practitioner who had noticed the child looked pale. A full blood count revealed iron deficiency, microcytic, hypochromic anaemia and a haemoglobin of 6.6 g/dl. Blood lead levels were found to be 404 µg/l (1.95 µM/l) [a normal result is <100 µg/l]. His parents said that he often ate soil from the garden and paint chips from the walls of the house and his usual diet was not thought to be very good.

The child was started on oral iron therapy and the family advised that he should be prevented from eating soil and paint. Community follow up was arranged through the local health visitors to help improve his diet. One week later his lead level had reduced to 318 µg/l (a sample from his younger sibling at that time was 46 µg/l). Within two months his lead level had reduced to 229 µg/l and haemoglobin increased to 11.7g/dL.

An Environmental Health Officer (EHO) from the Local Authority visited the house a week after the initial diagnosis and took a water sample from the kitchen tap, where the results indicated that the lead levels were within permitted bounds at 5 µg/L. A second visit to the house was undertaken by a senior EHO and Consultant in Communicable Disease Control (CCDC) a week later and samples were taken for analysis from the house paint and soil from the garden. The house was built in the 1930s which meant the most likely source of lead was paint. The parents were strongly advised to make sure that the child did not eat any more paint from the walls.

**Figure 2** Old paintwork containing high levels of lead that is flaking can lead to oral exposure in children.

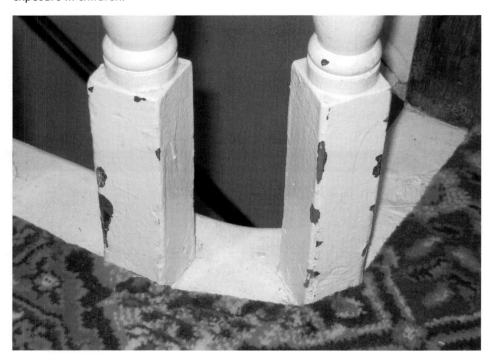

The lead analysis results were insignificant for most samples, except the paintwork from the stairs, which indicated high lead levels (6.2%) which would pose a problem if eaten over a long period of time.

The case study illustrates an example of a child receiving high oral exposure to lead-based paint in the home environment and developing symptoms of adverse health effects, because of biological sensitivity to lead toxicity, as well as a particular behaviour (in this case pica) causing higher potential for exposure.

## 8.2    Air pollution episodes involving sulphur dioxide

Sulphur dioxide ($SO_2$) is produced when a material or fuel containing sulphur is burned. Globally, much of the sulphur dioxide in the atmosphere comes from natural sources, but in the UK the predominant sources are power stations burning fossil fuels, principally coal and heavy oils. Widespread domestic use of coal can also lead to high local concentrations of $SO_2$.

According to the UK's Advisory Group on the Medical Aspects of Air Pollution Episodes in 1992 (Department of Health, 1992), during episodes of elevated sulphur dioxide concentrations in the air, those suffering from pre-existing respiratory diseases (particularly asthma) may need to take steps to reduce their exposure. The evidence they reviewed indicated that although individuals not suffering from respiratory disease should not be affected by the kind of air pollution episodes of elevated concentrations of sulphur dioxide typically found in the UK, asthmatic patients were found to be more sensitive to exposure to sulphur dioxide. Sulphur dioxide pollution is also considered more harmful when particulate and other pollution concentrations are high (UK Air Quality Archive, 2007). In parts of the UK, levels of sulphur dioxide can regularly exceed those at which effects of clinical significance, including tightness of the chest, coughing and wheezing, have been demonstrated in these susceptible individuals, with the effects being acute and reversible, but where medical attention may be needed (Department of Health, 1992), or indeed some form of public health intervention, such as an alerting system when such an episode is occurring, so that these susceptible groups can limit their exposure by adapting their behaviour (such as staying indoors).

## 9    References

COT. (2007) Variability and Uncertainty in the Toxicology of Chemicals in Food, Consumer Products and the Environment. Committee on the Toxicity of Chemicals in Food, Consumer Products and the Environment. Available at: www.food.gov.uk

Department of Health. (1992) Advisory Group on the Medical Aspects of Air Pollution Episodes. Second Report. Sulphur Dioxide, Acid Aerosols and Particulates. London: HMSO.

Eskenazi B *et al.* (1999) Exposures of children to organophosphate pesticides and their potential adverse health effects. *Env Health Pers* 107(s.3): 409–419.

Farrow A, Golding J. (1997) Time spent in the home by different family members. *Environ Technol* 18: 605–614.

Risk Assessment and Toxicology Steering Committee. (1999) Risk Assessment Strategies in Relation to Population Subgroups (cr3)

UK Air Quality Archive. (2007) www.airquality.co.uk

Whitmore R, Immerman F, Camann D, Bond A, Lewis R, Schaum J. (1994) Non-occupational exposures to pesticides for residents of two US cities. *Arch Env Health* 26: 47–59.

## 10    Further reading

WHO. (2005). Chapter 5: determinants of susceptibility. In: *Air quality guidelines. Global update 2005. Particulate matter, ozone, nitrogen dioxide and sulfur dioxide.* World Health Organization, Geneva.

# Section 2.4

# Exposure assessment using environmental monitoring and modelling

Richard Mohan, Giovanni Leonardi

### Learning outcomes

At the end of this chapter and any recommended reading the student should be able to:

1. explain how exposure assessment is crucial for understanding the impact of the environment on human health;
2. understand the limitations of using simple methods of exposure assessment;
3. understand the complexities involved with pollutant dispersal in the environment and with population movement, and their impact on exposure assessment;
4. evaluate the strengths and weakness of different approaches to exposure assessment;
5. explain how the use of Geographical Information Systems (GIS) and environmental monitoring and modelling facilitates improved estimates of exposure, and
6. apply their knowledge in the analysis and management of hazardous situations.

## 1 Introduction to exposure assessment

This chapter provides a general overview of exposure assessment. For a more detailed description of exposure assessment readers should refer to Nieuwenhuijsen (2003) or the Interdepartmental Group on the Health Risks of Chemicals guide for assessing exposure (IGHRC, 2004; Nieuwenhuijsen, 2003). Exposure in health studies is usually defined as any contact between a substance and the surface of the human body. Exposure assessment is the study of the distribution and determinants of substances or factors affecting human health. It is usually carried out to try and establish the nature of the relationship between any exposure and its possible health effects. Exposure assessment can be used for epidemiological studies, risk assessments or health surveillance. In developed countries, the health risks associated with environmental exposure to chemical hazards would generally be expected to be relatively low, which means that, in order to detect risks when and where they exist, exposure assessments need to be very refined to accurately determine differences in exposure (Nieuwenhuijsen, 2003).

**Figure 1** Routes of exposure used in the CLEA model.

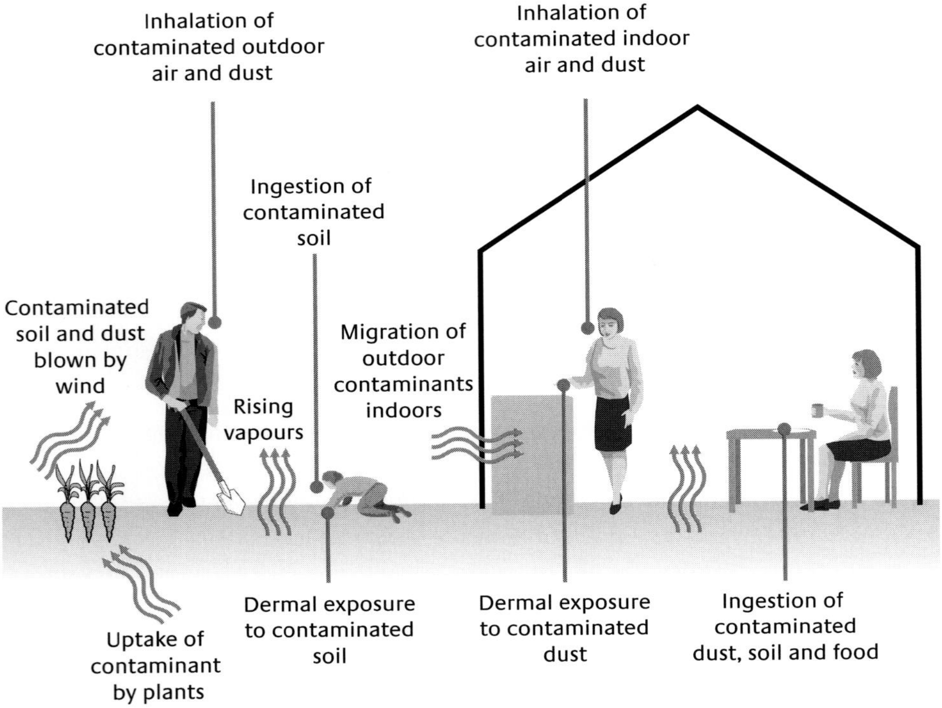

In order for an individual to be exposed to a substance, there must be a pathway linking the source to the person. This is sometimes known as the source-pathway-receptor model. This relationship is often described by a conceptual model, describing all the exposure pathway(s) between the source(s) and the receptor(s) (people). Figure 1 shows an example of the pathways that are included in the Contaminated Land Exposure Assessment (CLEA) model (Defra and Environment Agency, 2002). These describe the potential exposure pathways between the sources of pollution and individuals. For more information on contaminated land, see Chapter 3.3.

It is not only the concentration of the pollutant in the environment that determines the exposure. For example, with a contaminated garden, the exposure will depend on the concentration of pollutants in the soil, the number of relevant exposure pathways (for example, whether people eat vegetables from their garden), the frequency of exposure and the duration of each exposure event, for example how often do they use their garden.

## 2    Estimating exposure at an individual level

Ideally, exposure should be measured at an individual level with quantified estimates of the pollution levels that people are exposed to over time (Nieuwenhuijsen, 2003). Perhaps the most obvious way of measuring exposure to atmospheric pollutants is to ask individuals to wear personal monitors. A study by Gulliver and Briggs is a good example – this measured individual exposures to particulate matter of 10 micrometers or less ($PM_{10}$) during walking and car journeys in Northampton (Gulliver & Briggs, 2004). Particle measurements were made using a small monitor that was worn by the individual that was participating in the study. This approach allowed accurate estimate of the individual's exposure to $PM_{10}$ matter over time. The study found that the concentrations of $PM_{10}$ to which people were exposed were higher inside cars than those walking. This approach to exposure assessment should estimate an individual's exposure quite accurately. However, it is quite expensive and labour intensive and may therefore not always be practical.

Another technique that can be used to measure uptake of a chemical at an individual level is using biological markers or biomarkers. These analyse the concentration of a specific marker of exposure in human tissue or fluid (WHO, 2000). Potential problems associated with estimating exposure and uptake in this way include the fact that there are difficulties in differentiating between sources and the fact that obtaining biomarkers may prove to be invasive. For more information on biomarkers see Chapter 1.4.

| 3 | Estimating exposure at a group level using simple approaches |

Due to the limitations discussed, the level of detailed information about personal exposure gained by measurements using either personal monitors or biological markers is rarely available. In health studies, it is more common to attribute individuals to different exposure groups based on either environmental monitoring or modelling. Although this method of exposure assessment may not be as representative as personal monitoring, it has the advantage of being relatively cheaper and more practical. This means that it is possible to study a greater number of individuals, which may decrease problems associated with having insufficient variability in the exposure estimates (Nieuwenhuijsen, 2003). Theoretically, it also enables study of the effects of different sources and pathways. One of the simplest ways of estimating exposure is to use the distance that someone lives from a source of pollution as a proxy for exposure.

An example of such an approach to exposure assessment was the EUROHAZCON study which investigated risks of congenital anomalies around hazardous waste sites in Europe (Dolk *et al.*, 1998). This study assumed that persons living less than 3 km from a landfill were exposed, while those living 3 to 7 km away from a landfill site were unexposed. The study found an increased risk of congenital anomalies among individuals who were classified as exposed compared to those who were unexposed, with the risks increasing with decreasing distance from the site.

However, exposure assessment using this approach which provides no information regarding actual exposures to chemical substances is very different from data obtained from personal exposure monitoring. It is also very difficult to determine within-group variation. For example, given what is known from tracer studies about the dispersion of potential atmospheric pollutants from landfill sites, it would be reasonable to expect that those who live within 100 m of the landfill sites studied in the EUROHAZCON study would be exposed to much higher concentrations of potential atmospheric pollutants than those who lived 900 m from the site, and yet they were all classified within the

**Figure 2** The relationship between modelled concentrations of atmospheric pollutants from a landfill and distance from the centre of the landfill (Mohan, 2006).

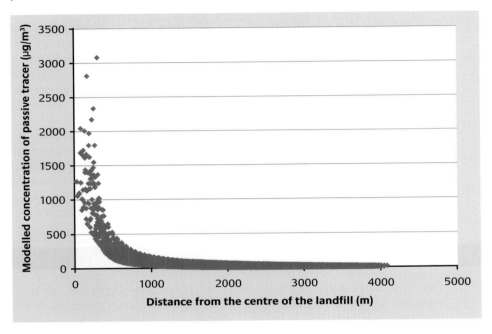

same exposure group. It also ignores environmental factors such as wind direction, topography and ground water flow which are all known to affect pollutant dispersion and therefore exposure. An example is given in Figure 2 of the relationship between modelled concentrations of atmospheric pollutants from a landfill site and distance, which shows that the relationship is not linear (Mohan, 2006).

## 4    Use of Geographical Information Systems (GIS) for exposure assessment

A GIS is essentially a database that allows large quantities of information to be analysed and viewed within a geographical context (Vine *et al.*, 1997). This enables data to be manipulated, integrated and graphically displayed on maps. Essentially, GIS has the ability to integrate data as illustrated in Figure 3, which makes it useful for exposure assessment. GIS allows for the source – pathway – receptor model to be represented in both space and in time, meaning that the two spatial patterns of interest in exposure assessment – the distribution of pollutants and the distribution of people – can be linked together. As such it represents an extremely useful tool for exposure assessment.

## 5    Using GIS to integrate dispersion modelling results with population data to estimate exposure.

There are numerous software models available for estimating the distribution of pollutants in the environment (James *et al.*, 2004; Carruthers *et al.*, 1992). Models are

**Figure 3** How GIS enables information to be integrated both in space and time to assess exposure. Courtesy of Briggs, 1992.

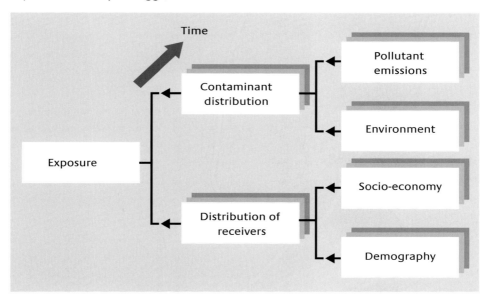

used because adequate environmental monitoring data are rarely available for the entire area and time period of interest. These models are widely used for regulatory purposes; however, by using GIS and considering other variables that may affect exposure, they can also be applied for exposure assessment. One of the most widely used types of modelling for exposure assessment is air dispersion modelling.

In a case control study of stillbirths, Ihrig *et al.* (1998) investigated adverse reproductive outcomes around an industrial plant in Texas, USA, which released arsenic into the atmosphere. Information was collected on 119 cases and 267 controls between 1983 and 1993, with exposure being estimated using a dispersion model called the fugitive dust model that was developed by the United States Environmental Protection Agency. The model took account of the amount of arsenic emitted from the plant, the prevailing wind direction and other atmospheric conditions, the velocity of the emissions, the height of the stack and the size of the particles emitted. The model was used to predict arsenic concentrations for a 16-year period from 1973 to 1989. Exposure levels were estimated for residential addresses of study subjects at the time of delivery of their babies. Maternal age, race/ethnicity and marital status were obtained from medical records and socio-economic status was calculated from census data. The results of this study revealed a higher rate of stillbirths among mothers who were exposed to higher concentrations of arsenic. This study is superior to some other studies regarding exposure assessment because estimating exposure using predicted levels of specific pollutants is better than using a simple proxy measure such as distance from place of residence to source.

During a fire in Paignton, Devon, UK, a decision was made to evacuate some nearby residents to a local leisure centre (Kinra *et al.*, 2005). During fires, health professionals

**Figure 4** Estimated relative 48 hour exposure from a fire in a plastics factory (Kinra *et al.*, 2005).

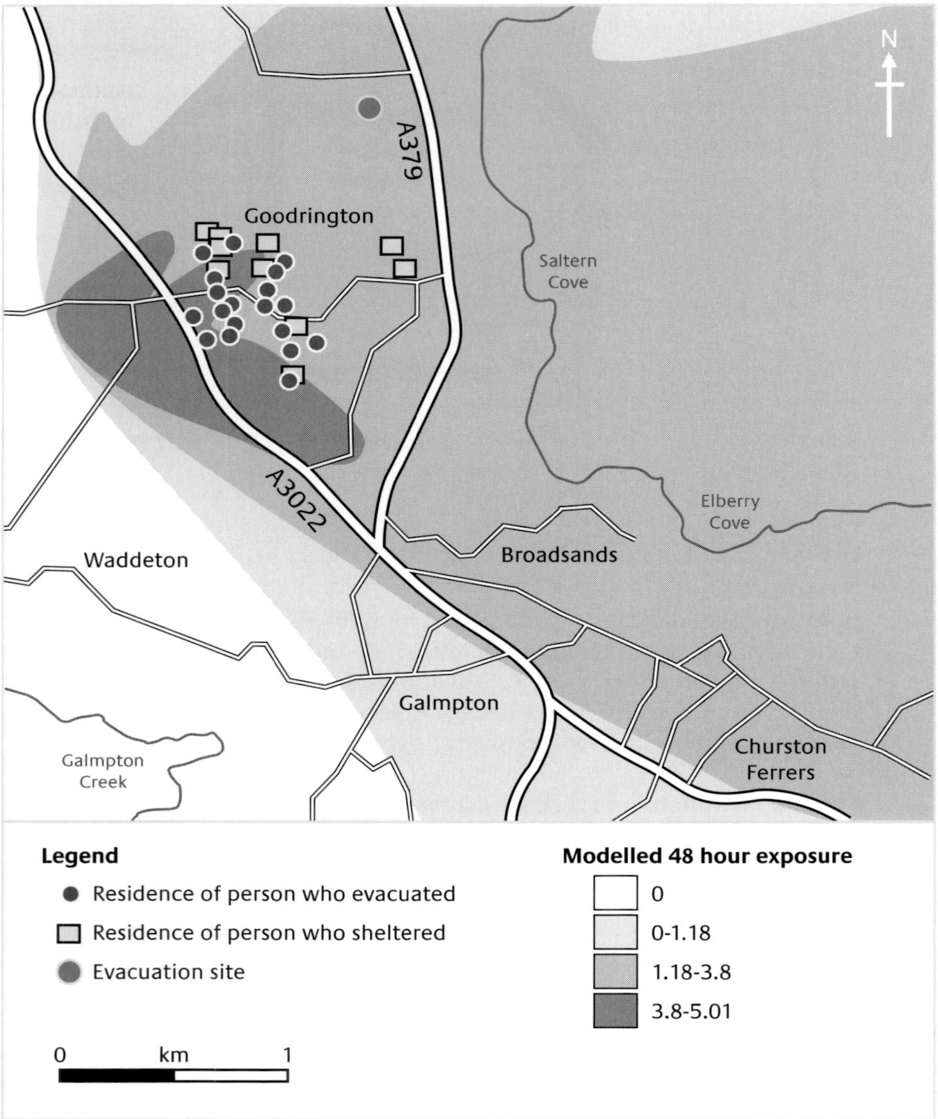

generally advise that residents should stay indoors and close windows and doors instead of evacuating, which may lead to exposure to higher concentrations of smoke. After the Paignton fire, an epidemiological study was carried out to determine whether evacuation was the correct decision by comparing adverse health effects between the residents who were evacuated and those who sheltered in their own homes.

Atmospheric dispersion modelling was used to provide exposure estimates for the epidemiological study. The Numerical Atmospheric dispersion Modelling Environment

(NAME III) was used to model atmospheric emissions from the fire (Jones *et al.*, 2006). This modelling used real time meteorological data from the nearby meteorological station to predict relative concentrations of pollutants over the 48-hour duration of the incident as well as a six hour run for the period before the evacuation took place (Figure 4). GIS software was used to link the relative concentrations of pollutants to postcoded population data to estimate exposure. Using this exposure assessment, the epidemiological study suggested that evacuation conferred no protective advantage over sheltering and that there was some evidence of adverse health effects associated with evacuation.

## 6    Using GIS to interpolate monitoring data to estimate exposure

The ability of GIS to integrate data means that it is possible to assess exposure using either modelled or monitored concentrations of pollutants. It is especially useful with environmental monitoring data as it is not possible to monitor at all locations. Therefore, interpolation techniques can be used to estimate pollutant concentrations at unmeasured locations.

Pikhart *et al.* (2001) used kriging (a form of data interpolation) to interpolate the concentrations of sulphur dioxide from 50 sites in Prague, Czech Republic, and 80 sites in Poznan, Poland (Pikhart *et al.*, 2001). A GIS package was then used to link these data to pollution data, with the exposure assessment used for a cross-sectional epidemiological study. The results showed an association between long-term concentration of pollution and wheezing and asthma in children.

Despite the fact that interpolation is relatively straightforward to carry out using GIS, there are few published health studies that have used interpolation solely to determine exposure (Briggs, 2005). The chief reason for this is that the main method of interpolating data, kriging, is not effective at accurately predicting pollution values, because pollution generally has very complex spatial patterns. For example, air pollution from ground level sources has extremely steep gradients which could only be properly interpolated with a very dense network of monitors. This means that on many occasions it is simply not practical to interpolate monitoring data or that the interpolation methods must be matched to the physical processes and their consequences.

## 7    Interpolating concentrations of pollutants using intelligent interpolation models

A better way of estimating pollution values is to use what Briggs describes as '*intelligent interpolation models*', which make use of information on not only monitored pollution values but also other variables which affect pollution concentrations (Briggs, 2005). These variables include any factors that are related to pollution and which have a geographical attribute, for example, traffic volumes on a road or housing density. Techniques such as co-kriging which involve the use of covariates to estimate pollution values have been successfully applied in several studies (Briggs, 2005; Cyrys *et al.*, 2005; Hoek *et al.*, 2002).

Cyrys *et al.* (2005) applied a form of stochastic modelling using monitored levels of nitrogen dioxide and $PM_{2.5}$ (particulate matter less than 2.5 micrometers) pollutant levels for 40 locations along with information on traffic intensity and population density. This study involved the use of a regression model to predict exposures at unmonitored locations, which were then linked to population data to estimate exposure. In addition, atmospheric dispersion modelling from sources of pollution was carried out using a Gaussian model and the results were linked to population data. To compare the two measures of exposure, the modelled concentrations were classified into three categories: high, medium and low, based on tertiles so that there were equal distributions in each category. The two exposure assessments showed good agreement, with 70% of the study subjects classified into the same exposure category in both studies.

Exposure is not merely the concentration of pollutants present in a particular media. It is also influenced by a number of factors, including the length of time an individual spends in a particular microenvironment. This means that when studying population exposure, it is important to consider population movement, as people constantly move from one location to another, thus changing the degrees/extents of exposure. This type of study is not carried out often, due to the complexities involved. Therefore, many health studies make the unrealistic assumption that individuals spend all their time at their place of residence. There have been attempts at modelling exposure considering population movement, using what Briggs describes as integrated exposure assessment (Briggs, 1992). These intersect geographical models of the distribution of pollution with population movement and are likely to become an important part of exposure assessment for health studies in the future.

## 8    Conclusions

This chapter has given a brief background to exposure assessment and showed how exposure assessment can be carried out using numerous approaches. Although exposure assessment is conceptually easy to understand, the fact that it involves environmental science and human behaviour means that in practice it is normally extremely difficult to carry out. GIS has been used to help study this complicated relationship. GIS is simply a tool for manipulating, integrating, interrogating and displaying geographical data and cannot on its own provide answers to questions about the effects of the environment upon human health. Even the most elaborate GISs still require accurate input data! A lack of accurate data remains one of the main reasons why the effects of the environment on human health are not better understood and exposure assessment remains a major challenge to those investigating the effects of the environment upon human health.

## 9    References

Briggs D. (1992) Mapping environmental exposure. In: Elliott P. *et al.* (eds) *Geographical and Environmental Epidemiology: Methods for Small Area Studies.* 2nd edition. Oxford University Press, Oxford. pp158–176.

Briggs DJ. (2005) The role of GIS: coping with space (and time) in air pollution exposure assessment. *Journal of Toxicology and Environmental Health, Part A*, 68:1243–1261.

Carruthers DJ, Holroyd RJ, Hunt JCR, Weng WS, Robins AG, Apsley DD, Thomson DJ, Smith J. (1994) UK-ADMS: A new approach to modelling dispersion in the earth's atmospheric layer. *Journal of Wind Engineering and Industrial Aerodynamics* 52: 139–153.

Cyrys J, Hochadel M, Gehring U, Hoek G, Diegmann V, Brunekreef B, Heinrich J. (2005). GIS based estimation of exposure to particulate matter and $NO_2$ in an urban area: Stochastic versus dispersion modelling. *Environmental Health Perspectives* 113(8): 879–992.

Department for Environment Food and Rural Affairs (Defra) & Environment Agency. (2002) *The contaminated land exposure assessment model (CLEA): Technical basis and algorithms*. Environment Agency R&D Publication, CLR 10.

Dolk H, Armstrong B, Abramsky L, Bianchi F, Garne E, Nelen V, Robert E, Scott JES, Stone D, Tenconi R. (1998) Risk of congenital anomalies near hazardous-waste landfill sites in Europe: The EUROHAZCON Study. *The Lancet* 352: 423–427.

Gulliver J, Briggs DJ. (2004) Personal exposure to particulate air pollution in transport microenvironments. *Atmospheric Environment* 38(1):1–8.

Hoek G, Brunekereef B, Goldbohm S, Fischer P, Van Den Brant P. (2002) Association between mortality and indicators of traffic-related air pollution in the Netherlands: a cohort study. *Lancet* 360: 1203–1209.

Ihrig MM, Shalat SL, Baynes C. (1998) A hospital based case control study of stillbirths and environmental exposure to arsenic using an atmospheric dispersion model linked to a Geographical Information System. *Epidemiology* 9(3): 290–294.

IGHRC. (2004) Guidelines for good exposure assessment practice for human health effects of chemicals. Interdepartmental Group on Health Risks from Chemicals. Institute for Environment and Health, University of Leicester. Available at: www.silsoe.cranfield.ac.uk

James L, Matthews I, Nix B. (2004) Spatial contouring of risk, a tool for environmental epidemiology. *Epidemiology* 15(3): 287–292.

Jones A, Thomson D, Hort M, Devenish BJ. *The UK Met Office's next generation atmospheric dispersion model*, NAME III, Kluwer (in press).

Kinra S, Lewendon G, Nelder R, Herriott N, Mohan R, Hort M, Harrison S, Murray V. (2005) Evacuation decisions in a chemical air pollution incident: Cross-sectional survey. *British Medical Journal* 330: 1471–1475.

Mohan R. (2006) *Public health perspectives on municipal waste management.* Engineering Doctorate Thesis, University of Surrey.

Nieuwenhuijsen M. (2003) *Exposure assessment in occupational and environmental epidemiology.* Oxford Medical Publication, Oxford.

Pikhart H, Bobah M, Gorynski P, Wojtyniak B, Danova J, Celko MA, Kriz B, Briggs DJ, Elliot P. (2001) Outdoor sulphur dioxide and respiratory symptoms in Czech and Polish school children: a small-area study (SAVIAH). *International Archives of Occupational and Environmental Health* 74: 574–578.

Vine MF, Degnan D, Hanchette C. (1997) Geographical Information Systems: Their use in environmental epidemiological research. *Environmental Health Perspectives* 105(6): 598–605.

WHO. (2000) *Human Exposure Assessment.* World Health Organization, Geneva.

# Section 3

Environmental Toxicology

# Section 3.1

# Occupational toxicology

Virginia Murray, Norman Parkinson, Sarah McCrea

## Learning outcomes

At the end of this chapter and any recommended reading the student should be able to:

1. understand the importance of occupational toxicology in relation to health protection activities;
2. be aware of important sources of information about toxic agents in the workplace;
3. discuss the methods by which occupational exposure to toxic substances may affect health during manufacture, transport, storage and use;
4. critically discuss incidents that have resulted from occupational exposures to toxic chemicals, and understand how they are investigated;
5. evaluate the guidelines and protocols that are used to prevent or minimise ill health due to occupational exposures, and
6. apply their knowledge in the analysis and management of hazardous situations.

## 1    Introduction

Occupational toxicology is concerned with the investigation, management and prevention of diseases arising from chemicals in the workplace. While it is primarily concerned with the health of workers exposed to toxic agents, it recognises that their families and the general public may also be affected. There may also be concurrent environmental impacts.

Occupational toxicology is a sub-set of environmental public health that requires the close co-operation of many professional groups, including: occupational physicians; occupational hygienists; environmental health practitioners; government inspectors; safety officers; toxicologists; chemists and chemical engineers; design engineers; managers; trades union representatives; information scientists, and the workers themselves (Figure 1). Occupational toxicologists provide the other professionals with vital understanding of the nature of toxic agents and hazards, to enable the assessment and management of risks, and appropriate responses to chemical incidents.

**Figure 1** Occupational toxicology is a sub-set of environmental public health that requires the close co-operation of many professional groups and the workers themselves. Adapted from the University of New South Wales, Australia.

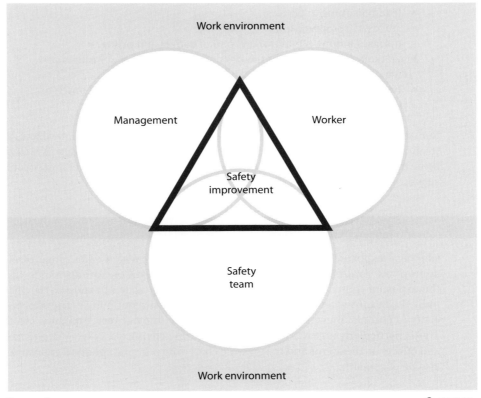

Government

Technology

Work environment

Management

Worker

Safety improvement

Safety team

Work environment

Economics

Customer

The UK's Health and Safety at Work (etc.) Act 1974 (HASAWA) is the primary piece of legislation covering health and safety in the UK. The Act established the Health and Safety Commission (HSC) and its operating arm the Health and Safety Executive (HSE). The HASAWA and related legislation is enforced by the HSE or, in certain cases, mainly relating to distribution, retail, leisure and catering sectors, by Local Authorities. The Act recognises the pluralistic approach and places general duties regarding health and safety on all people at work (except domestic servants), including employers, the self employed and employees, as well as the HSE and HSC itself.

## 2    History of occupational diseases

Occupational toxicology is not new. The Romans recognised that certain occupations were associated with particular diseases. The first such textbook is attributed to Bernardino Ramazzini (1633–1714), who worked as a physician and professor in Padua and Modena, Italy. In 1713 he published *De morbis artificum diatriba* (An account of the diseases of work), in which he described over 50 occupational disorders, along with an account of working conditions at the time:

- occupational asthma in grain workers;
- pneumoconiosis and other diseases of miners;
- lead poisoning in potters;
- silicosis in stonemasons;
- diseases among metal workers and of gilders and printers;
- workers that cleaned out the city cesspits developed eye infections which led to sight loss or total blindness;
- breast cancer occurred more often in nuns than in other women of similar age.

Ramazzini methodically collected data relating to diseases of manual workers and the relation to their occupations. In the same way, today, when a disease is shown to be more prevalent in a particular group of workers than it is in the general population, it is suggestive of an occupational disease.

## 3    Types of adverse effects

Chemical exposure in the occupational setting can cause a wide range of effects if appropriate controls are not in place. These will depend on various issues, including the exposure route, duration and dose and the frequency of exposure as well as the individual exposed and any pre-existing diseases or susceptibilities. The effects may be acute or chronic or even delayed with a long lead time between exposure and disease. This is particularly important with cancer-causing chemicals. Issues relating to fertility and effects on the foetus and the growing child from parental chemical exposure should also be of concern.

In this chapter, two examples of adverse effects from occupational use of chemicals are provided. The first describes the acute effects of chlorine, and the second describes the acute but more importantly the chronic effects of vinyl chloride monomer.

### 3.1    Chlorine: health effects of acute / single exposure

In a properly managed safe system of work, acute exposure to chlorine will not occur. However, should there be a release, the immediate symptoms following inhalation of chlorine include a burning sensation in the eyes and pain or burning of the lungs during respiration. Sufficient exposure may induce reflex cholinergic bronchoconstriction with associated signs of coughing, wheezing and dyspnoea (HPA, 2007). Exposure to a sufficiently high dose may result in pulmonary oedema and respiratory failure, the onset of which may be delayed by up to 36 hours. In extreme cases, pulmonary haemorrhage may also occur (NPIS, 2002). There is some evidence to suggest that exposure to chlorine may be associated with long-term neuropsychological changes (Dilks and Matzenbacher, 2003), although further studies are required to confirm this

**Table 2** Summary of acute toxic effects in relation to approximate (air) concentration of chlorine (IPCS, 1996). Concentration (mg/m³) are approximate conversions from the corresponding ppm value.

| Concentration | | Signs and symptoms |
| --- | --- | --- |
| ppm | mg/m³ | |
| 1–3 | 3–10 | Mild mucous membrane irritation. |
| 5–15 | 15–45 | Moderate irritation of upper respiratory tract. |
| 30 | 90 | Immediate chest pain, vomiting, coughing. |
| 40–60 | 115–175 | Toxic pneumonitis and pulmonary oedema. |
| 430 | 1250 | Lethal after 30 minutes exposure. |
| 1000 | 2900 | Lethal in minutes. |

hypothesis. A summary of the acute effects of chlorine exposure by concentration are given in Table 2.

### 3.1.1   Delayed effects following an acute exposure

Most studies of survivors of World War I gassing incidents have reported a high incidence of acute respiratory damage and a lower incidence of chronic sequelae following acute exposure (Ayres and Baxter, 2004). Similar sequelae have also been reported for individuals following acute exposure to the accidental release of chlorine gas, with the most consistently reported chronic effect being a reduction in the forced expiratory volume (FEV) (IPCS, 1999a). A relatively recent report relating to accidental exposure to chlorine gas suggests that chronic sequelae following acute exposure may be more frequent than previously anticipated: a follow-up study in July 1999 on twenty individuals (previously exposed in 1995) indicated that 75% had residual lung volumes below 80% of their predicted value and nearly half the subjects tested for airway reactivity to methacholine had a greater than 15% decline in FEV (Schwartz *et al.*, 1990). There is some evidence to suggest that a single, acute exposure to chlorine gas may cause reactive airways dysfunction syndrome (RADS), also known as irritant-induced asthma (Ayres and Baxter, 2004; Winder, 2001).

### 3.2   Vinyl Chloride: Exposure and Health Effects

Vinyl chloride (Figure 2) is toxic by all routes of exposure. It is metabolised to the active metabolites chloroethylene oxide and chloracetaldehyde which are responsible for its toxicity. In the absence of proper controls, acute exposure will produce immediate signs and symptoms such as respiratory irritation, producing coughing, wheezing and breathlessness following inhalation and also systemic effects including headache, ataxia, drowsiness and coma. In addition, some halogenated hydrocarbons can cause cardiac arrhythmias (NPIS, 2004; IPCS, 1999b).

**Figure 2** Vinyl chloride monomer

H\           /Cl
  \C = C
H/           \H

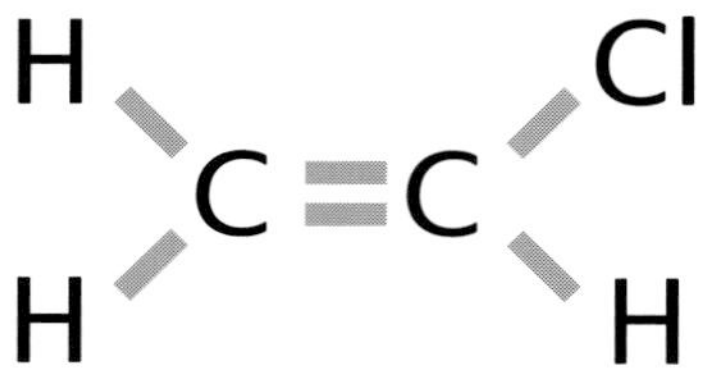

Where there are inadequate controls, long-term exposure may cause impotence, blood disorders, liver problems (angiosarcoma) and the pathopneumonic disease of acroosteolysis following adult exposure to vinyl chloride. Bone loss in the finger-tips due to exposure to vinyl chloride monomer has been observed among polyvinyl chloride (PVC) reactor workers (NIOSH, 2001). The term acroosteolysis was used to name the condition (the word acroosteolysis is derived from Greek words *Akron* = extremity, *Osteon* = bone, *Lysis*= dissolution), and has been defined as a shortening of the terminal digits.

The Department for Work and Pensions (2005) review concluded that there was consistent evidence that the inhalation of vinyl chloride monomer (VCM) in PVC production workers causes a characteristic clinical triad of osteolysis of the terminal phalanges, scleroderma and Raynaud's phenomenon, but not all three are invariably present together (DWP, 2005). These effects occurred in workers who had been exposed to levels of VCM very much higher than the current control limits. Surveys of factory workforces have shown that among those exposed to VCM who do not have radiological evidence of osteolysis, the prevalence of Raynaud's phenomenon and scleroderma is greater than in the general population (by two fold).

The mechanisms of toxicity for non-cancer VCM effects are not completely elucidated. VCM disease exhibits many characteristics of autoimmune diseases (e.g. Raynaud's phenomenon and scleroderma). B-cell proliferation, hyperimmunoglobulinemia, and complement activation, with increased circulating immune complexes or cryoglobulinaemia indicating stimulation of immune response have been observed.

Postulated mechanisms for the non-cancer effects include:

1. Immunological
   • a reactive vinyl chloride intermediate metabolite, such as 2-chloroethylene oxide or 2-chloroacetaldehyde, binds to a protein such as IgG;
   • altered protein initiates an immune response, with deposition of immune products along vascular endothelium;

- circulating immune complexes are proposed to precipitate in response to exposure to the cold, and these precipitates are proposed to produce blockage of the small vessels.

2. Resorptive bone changes in the fingers may be due to activation of osteoclast secondary to vascular insufficiency in the finger tips (ATSDR, 2006).

However, the International Agency for Research on Cancer has classified vinyl chloride as a known human carcinogen, based upon evidence of carcinogenicity in both humans and animals (IARC, 1987). It is mutagenic and its carcinogenic action is believed to occur via a genotoxic mechanism. VCM is covered by the Carcinogens Directive, and the current Workplace Exposure Limit of 3 ppm is based on its recognised carcinogenicity rather than non-cancer endpoints.

## 4  Assessing occupational disease and hazardous chemicals

It is important to recognise that occupational diseases are preventable by adopting appropriate control measures, yet they can be responsible for temporary and permanent disablement, discomfort and distress, as well as lost productivity. The risks extend to co-workers, the worker's family, and the environment. Occupational hygienists stress the importance of *anticipation* and *prevention* before a system of work is introduced.

Occupational diseases can be difficult to recognise (Figure 3). Occupational illnesses may resemble non-occupational illnesses, and a very long latency period can sometimes exist between exposure and the emergence of signs and symptoms. There are thousands of jobs, chemicals, and diseases, and an association may not be readily apparent. In addition, medical students and most other health professionals are not trained in occupational toxicology!

**Figure 3** Ways of identifying occupational toxicity related diseases.

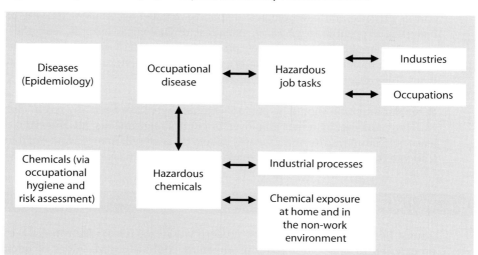

Occupational disease can be identified by consideration of *health data*, i.e. epidemiological studies, health assessments, the incidence of particular diseases in a workforce, or the appearance of signs and symptoms in individual workers or their families, together with *knowledge of the chemicals* in the workplace, the available data on their toxicity, risk assessment and monitoring. In most cases, risk assessment will be based on the available toxicology data (largely from experimental studies in animals) together with estimates of exposure.

An investigation into suspected ill-health from workplace exposure to a hazardous chemical will start with an analysis of the system of work, to identify which chemicals are used in which locations by which workers and consideration of the data on their toxicity. The *source-pathway-receptor* model is a useful starting point. The exact activities, times and durations should be recorded. Existing risk assessment documentation and inventories *should* provide information to identify critical control points, but they must be assessed critically.

Investigations may involve biological/clinical sampling to detect and measure the presence of the toxic agent or its metabolic products in body tissue or excreta – typically blood, urine or exhalation samples. In some cases it may be necessary for medical examination of the exposed workers and function tests. Clearly there are practical and ethical issues here, including consent and confidentiality, not to mention the possibility of personal distress, and industrial relations problems. These will need careful handling and good communications.

Environmental sampling may be carried out to provide data for an exposure assessment. This may involve air and dust sampling. In some hazardous situations there may already be continuous monitoring data. The sampling strategy should be appropriate to the pattern of work and activities of individual workers, and their locus and exposure to the particular hazardous chemicals.

Environmental and/or biological sampling data must be complemented by taking the work history, present and past, of the affected individuals including the type of work and its physical and psychological demands; detailed accounts of working practices including exposures to physical, chemical or biological hazards, and the control measures employed (e.g. personal protective equipment) should be recorded. This should not be confined to the worker's current work activity and employer, but should if possible cover their entire working lives.

Particular attention should be paid to whether there have been any recent changes in working practices, materials employed or control mechanisms. Absenteeism, sickness leave, and employee turnover records should be analysed. Analysis and evaluation will lead to recommendations for risk management control measures (see section 5).

## 4.1    Multi-exposure to hazardous chemicals

It must be remembered that in the modern workplace it is unlikely that a worker will be exposed to only one hazardous chemical. Multi-exposure issues of interactions between substances include:

- **independent** – no cross reaction between the compounds, e.g., carbon monoxide and cadmium;
- **antagonistic** – exposure protects against the production of toxicity, e.g., antidotes;
- **potentiative** – the single compound has no effect unless another is present, e.g., carbon tetrachloride and 2-propanol;
- **additive** – effect is additive in nature, e.g., solvents;
- **synergistic** – effect is exponential, e.g., asbestos and smoking.

## 5    Risk management

The exposure of workers to hazardous chemicals must be prevented or adequately controlled. The Control of Substances Hazardous to Health Regulations (COSHH) (see section 6 below) make risk assessment and risk management mandatory.

A **Hierarchy of Control Measures** is given below. *Elimination* and *Substitution* should **always** be considered first, whether as long term or short term solutions, before the use of engineering controls. It should be noted that the use of personal protective equipment is a last resort after all other controls have been implemented.

- Elimination of hazardous chemical
- Substitution with less hazardous materials or forms of the material (e.g. pellets instead of powder), or processes
- Minimisation of inventories or stocks or amounts of available hazards
- Engineering controls at source, such as automation or process enclosure
- Engineering controls to reduce exposure, such as segregation, partial enclosure, mechanical handling, suppression methods or ventilation
- Administrative controls, such as safe working procedures, job rotation, good housekeeping
- Reduction of the number of workers exposed
- Personnel procedures, such as adequate supervision, information dissemination and training
- Health surveillance
- Personal protective equipment

COSHH impose special controls over carcinogens. The concept of substitution is encouraged which is the second most effective measure in the hierarchy of control measures. Table 3 provides recommendations for substitution of materials.

## 6    Legal controls and standards

The Control of Substances Hazardous to Health Regulations (COSHH) made under HASAWA, apply to substances or mixtures of substances classified as dangerous to health under the Chemicals (Hazard Information and Packing for Supply) Regulations. These regulations impose labelling requirements and, significantly, require suppliers to provide a **safety data sheet**. COSHH require a risk assessment to be carried out, and

**Table 3** Substitution: some examples

| Old product | New product | Industry |
|---|---|---|
| Flammable solvents | Less flammable or non-flammable materials | Many processes |
| White phosphorus | Sespui-Sulfide | Matches |
| Cleaning solvents | Detergents | Cleaning |
| Trichloroethylene | 1,1,1-Trichloroethane | Degreasing |
| Asbestos | Synthetic mineral fibres | Insulation |
| Leaded glazes | Leadless glazes | Pottery |
| Toluene di-isocyanate | Less volatile isocyanates or pre-polymers | Polyurethane and paints |
| Solvent based paints | Water based paints | Paint industry |
| Organochlorine pesticides | Organophosphorus pesticides | Agriculture and pest control |

Source: University of New South Wales, Australia

control measures to be implemented to prevent or control exposure. Control measures may include the monitoring of the exposure of workers and appropriate health surveillance. Workers must be properly trained and supervised, and control measures must be properly maintained and implemented. Occupational exposure limits have been set (see section 7 below) and these are found in the Health and Safety Executive's (HSE) publication EH40.

In 2005, existing requirements to follow good practice were brought together by the introduction of eight principles in the Control of Substances Hazardous to Health (Amendment) Regulations 2004 (Box 1).

Basic advice on the implementation of the COSHH regulations is also provided on the HSE website *COSHH Essentials.*

# 7    Occupational Exposure Limits

## 7.1    Workplace Exposure Limits

Workplace Exposure Limits (WELs) have now replaced Maximum Exposure Limits (MELs) and Occupational Exposure Standards (OESs). Many of the old MELs and OESs have

**Box 1** Principles of Good Practice for the Control of Substances Hazardous to Health

- Design and operate processes and activities to minimise emission, release and spread of substances hazardous to health.

- Take into account all relevant routes of exposure – inhalation, skin absorption and ingestion – when developing control measures.

- Control exposure by measures that are proportionate to the health risk.

- Choose the most effective and reliable control options which minimise the escape and spread of substances hazardous to health.

- Where adequate control of exposure cannot be achieved by other means, provide, in combination with other control measures, suitable personal protective equipment.

- Check and review regularly all elements of control measures for their continuing effectiveness.

- Inform and train all employees on the hazards and risks from the substances with which they work and the use of control measures developed to minimise the risks.

- Ensure that the introduction of control measures does not increase the overall risk to health and safety.

Source: The Control of Substances Hazardous to Health (Amendment) Regulations 2004

been converted to WELs, apart from about 100 OESs that have been deleted. There are no WELs for asbestos and lead and other substances that have specific legislative controls.

The list of exposure limits is known as **EH40** and is available from the HSE Direct website. Readers are advised to familiarise themselves with HSE COSHH guidance publications including EH40.

The Health and Safety Commission's Advisory Committee on Toxic Substances (ACTS) recommends new WELs or revisions to current WELs on the advice of the Working Group on Action to Control Chemicals (WATCH). They take into account all the available toxicity data including carcinogenicity, reproduction toxicity, and irritation and sensitisation potential.

All UK WELs are air limit values. They are expressed in both ppm (parts per million) and mg.m$^{-3}$ (milligrams per cubic metre of air) and are given as **Long-term Exposure Limits** (LTELs) – 8-hour time weighted average reference period (TWA) and **Short-term Exposure limit** (STELs) – 15-minute time weighted average reference period. The TWA calculation methods are explained in EH40. Some potent substances are only given a STEL.

A 'Comments' column in EH40 gives further advice – for example 'skin' indicates that substance's ability to penetrate human skin.

There are some WELs for multi-substance exposure, prescribing process emissions such as welding fumes.

Biological monitoring results may be used as indicators of exposure, although they do not have legal status. **Biological Monitoring Guidance Values** (BMGV) are also provided in EH40.

Employers are now legally obliged to:

- apply the principles of good practice (above) for the control of substances hazardous to health;
- ensure that the WEL is not exceeded, and
- ensure that exposure to substances that can cause occupational asthma, cancer, or damage to genes that can be passed from one generation to another is reduced *__as low as is reasonably practicable__*.

## 7.2    As Low As is Reasonably Practicable 'ALARP'

The duty to control and reduce risks to *as low as is reasonably practicable* has its legal foundations in the case of *Edwards v. The National Coal Board* (1949) which addressed the adequacy of safety precautions in a mine. The Court of Appeal held that:

> "the risk… has to be weighed against the measures necessary to eliminate the risk. The greater the risk, no doubt, the less will be the weight to be given to the factor of cost."

The Court decided that 'reasonably practicable' is a narrower term than 'physically possible'. There must be an assessment of the risk on one side, and this must be compared with, on the other side, the 'sacrifice' in terms of the time, trouble and money necessary for averting the risk. The sacrifice should not be *grossly disproportionate* to the risk. Inherent in the use of the word *grossly*, is a bias on the side of health and safety. Nevertheless, it must be accepted that even when ALARP is adopted there will still be some risk.

Consideration of the balance between risk and cost should be revisited when there is new scientific evidence about the risk (whether higher or lower), or when new control technologies become available.

Complex ALARP decisions involving high risks usually include the consideration of formal Cost-Benefit Analysis (CBA), but ALARP decisions are never based on CBA alone. The inclusion of CBA means that when considering chemicals with no threshold, e.g. genotoxic carcinogens, their use in, say, cosmetics would be prohibited, but industrial exposures, under very strict controls, might still be tolerated.

## 8    Surveillance systems and sources of information

### 8.1    THOR

THOR is an example of a UK system for occupational disease surveillance. The Health and Occupational Reporting activity (THOR) at the Centre of Occupational and Environmental Health, University of Manchester, has a range of surveillance programmes. It includes Surveillance of Work-Related & Occupational Respiratory Disease (SWORD) and in particular occupational asthma, benign and malignant pleural disease, mesothelioma, lung cancer and pneumoconiosis surveillance. The most common cause of occupational asthma in the UK consists of the di-isocyanates (used in various industries such as in 'twin-pack' spray painting). Other important asthma hazards include colophony fume (from soldering flux). The SWORD scheme successfully picked up trends such as an increase in asthma associated with exposure to latex, and thus helped in raising awareness and reducing the risks.

### 8.2    International resources in occupational toxicology

A new European Community regulation on chemicals and their safe use, 'REACH', deals with the **R**egistration, **E**valuation, **A**uthorisation and **R**estriction of **Ch**emical substances (EC, 2006). The new law came into force on 1 June 2007. The REACH agency will manage a European database of chemical hazards information to which the public will have access (EC, 2006).

The American College of Occupational and Environmental Medicine (ACOEM) was founded in 1916. The College periodically issues position papers and committee reports that set practice guidelines for a variety of workplace/environmental settings. These position papers/committee reports cover topics such as spirometry, mould, environmental tobacco smoke, noise-induced hearing loss, multiple chemical sensitivities, workplace drug screening, confidentiality of medical information, depression screening, and reproductive hazards. In their 2005 position paper on toxicology, it was identified as a core content of occupational and environmental medicine.

### 8.3    Haz-Map

Haz-map is an occupational toxicology database designed to link jobs to hazardous job tasks which are linked to occupational diseases and their symptoms. It has been published on the website of the National Library of Medicine since 2002. It is a relational database of chemicals, jobs and diseases. Haz-Map was designed to be a decision-support computer application for occupational safety and health professionals. Its aim is to assist physicians, physician assistants, occupational health nurses, and industrial hygienists in the recognition of diseases caused by toxic chemicals and infectious agents in the workplace.

For more on other toxicology databases such as **TOXNET,** please see Chapter 2.1.

## 9    References

ATSDR. (2006) Toxicological Profile for Vinyl Chloride. US Department of Health and Human Services, Agency for Toxic Substances Disease Registry.

Ayres J, Baxter P. (2004) Irritant Induced Asthma and RADS. EPAQS short report.

The Control of Substances Hazardous to Health (Amendment) Regulations 2004. Statutory Instrument 2004 No. 3386. HMSO, London.

EC. (2006) European Community Regulation on Chemicals and their Safe Use No. 1907/2006. *Official Journal of the European Union* L396:2–849.

DWP. (2005) Vinyl Chloride Monomer-Related Diseases. (cm6645) Department for Work and Pensions. HMSO, London.

Dilks LS, Matzenbacher DL. (2003) Residual neuropsychological sequelae of chlorine gas exposure. *Neurotoxicol Teratolol* 25: 391.

*Edwards v National Coal Board* (1949) All ER 743 (CA).

HPA. (2007) Chlorine. *Compendium of Chemical Hazards* Version 2. Health Protection Agency.

IARC. (1987) Vinyl Chloride. International Agency for Research on Cancer – Summaries & Evaluations. Supplement 7, p.373.

IPCS. (1996) Chlorine. International Programme on Chemical Safety. *Poisons Information Monograph* PIM 947.

IPCS. (1999a) Disinfectants and disinfectant by-products. International Programme On Chemical Safety Monograph. *Environmental Health Criteria* 216.

IPCS. (1999b) Vinyl chloride. International Programme on Chemical Safety Monograph. *Environmental Health Criteria* 215.

NIOSH. (2001) Occupational Dermatoses Program for Physicians: Index of Occupational Dermatoses slides. National Institute for Occupational Safety and Health. Available at: www.cdc.gov

NPIS. (2002) Chlorine. *TOXBASE®*, National Poisons Information Service. Last updated 05/2002. Available at: www.toxbase.org

NPIS. (2004) Vinyl chloride. *TOXBASE®*. National Poisons Information Service. Last updated 09/2004. Available at: www.toxbase.org

Ramazzini B. (1713) *De Morbis Artificum Bernardini Ramazzini Diatriba* [Diseases of Workers: The Latin Text of 1713 Revised]. Wright WC, trans-ed. Chicago, Ill: University of Chicago Press; 1940.

Schwartz DA, Smith DD, Lakshminarayan S. (1990) The pulmonary sequelae associated with accidental inhalation of chlorine gas. *Chest* 97: 820–825.

Winder C. (2001) The toxicology of chlorine. *Environ Res* 85: 105–114.

## 10   Further reading

ACOEM (American College of Occupational and Environmental Medicine). Available at: www.acoem.org

Gardiner K & Harrington JM. (2005) *Occupational Hygiene*. Blackwell Publishing, Oxford.

HAZ-MAP. Occupational Exposure to Hazardous Chemicals, National Library of Medicine. Available at: hazmap.nlm.nih.gov

HSE (Health and Safety Executive) documentation including COSHH Guidance and EH40. Available at: www.hse.gov.uk

HSE (Health and Safety Executive) COSHH Essentials. Available at: www.coshh-essentials.org.uk

REACH (**R**egistration, **E**valuation, **A**uthorisation and Restriction of **C**hemical) information. Available at: ec.europa.eu/environment/chemicals

Stacey N H & Winder C. (2004) *Occupational Toxicology*. Taylor and Francis, London.

THOR (The Health and Occupational Reporting Network), University of Manchester. Available at: www.medicine.manchester.ac.uk/coeh

University of New South Wales, School of Safety Science. Available at: www.safesci.unsw.edu.au

# Section 3.2

# Air pollution and health in the UK

Robert L Maynard

## Learning outcomes

At the end of this chapter and any recommended reading the student should be able to:

1. outline the history of air pollution, and discuss the evolution of concerns about air pollution;
2. explain and discuss the effects of common air pollutants, including ozone, sulphur dioxide, nitrogen dioxide, carbon monoxide and particulate matter;
3. explain the consequences of exposure to organic chemicals, particularly carcinogenic outdoor air pollutants;
4. discuss the problem of indoor air pollution, and its relationship with outdoor air pollution;
5. understand the setting of air quality standards, and;
6. explain the role of international organisations such as the European Union and the WHO in air pollution control.

## 1    Introduction

Concern about air pollution in the UK has a long history. Smoke from burning sea coal was recognised as a nuisance in the 17th century and the rising industrialisation of the 18th and 19th centuries led to many towns and cities becoming densely polluted. London experienced particularly dense smogs (smog = smoke + fog) and in December 1952 an episode of London smog claimed at least 4000 lives. Such an impact had been predicted before 1940. The 1952 London smog was characterised by record levels of particulate air pollution: Black Smoke monitors overloaded at about 6 mg/m$^3$ and 24 hour average concentrations of sulphur dioxide reached 4 mg/m$^3$. These are extraordinary concentrations by modern standards. Deaths from cardio-respiratory causes were increased and the older and very young age groups were particularly vulnerable. Public reaction to the smog was sharp and in 1956 the Clean Air Act, the first of its kind in the world, was passed. This paved the way for cleaning up UK cities and towns and funds were provided for replacing open hearths burning house coal with grates that burnt smokeless fuel. At the same time, the use of gas and electricity for domestic space heating was increasing rapidly and by the early 1970s the great London smogs were a thing of the past. Research into the effects on health of air pollutants undertaken by the Medical Research Council's Air Pollution Research Unit at St Bartholomew's Hospital led to the development of early time-series techniques which showed an association between daily levels of pollution and the health status of patients suffering from chronic bronchitis. This association, so clear in the late 1950s and early 1960s, had all but disappeared by the 1970s. These studies led to the concept of thresholds of effect of air pollutants, but more recent work (see below), has called these into question. It is accepted today that levels of air pollution which would have been regarded as harmless in the 1960s, are capable of causing significant damage to health. Chronic bronchitis was very much the English Disease when these early studies were being done: it has declined as a result of encouraging people to give up smoking; reductions in levels of air pollutants may have played a part in its decline.

In countries and regions warmer than the UK, the rapid increase in the use of motor vehicles led to another form of smog being recognised in the early 1950s. This was photochemical smog, characterised by high concentrations of ozone and nitrogen oxides. Los Angeles experienced particularly dense smogs of this kind. This oxidant smog was very different from the chemically reducing coal smoke smogs of London. In more recent years photochemical pollution has been recognised as a problem in the UK. In 1976, record concentrations of ozone were recorded in London and across Southern England. Concentrations peaked at about 250 ppb (500 µg/m³) but, at the time, effects on health were not noted. Later studies suggested an increase in deaths of almost 10% though it was difficult to separate the possible effects of exposure to ozone from those of temperature.

In the past twenty years, developments in epidemiological techniques have shown that even low concentrations of air pollutants can damage health. More worrying still is the evidence that long-term exposure to air pollutants can reduce life expectancy. Current levels of particulate air pollution in the UK (measured as $PM_{2.5}$, see below) of about 13 µg/m³, on average, may be associated with, on average, a reduction in life expectancy of about 8 months. This is a very significant effect and as outlined below seems to be due largely to an effect on diseases of the heart and circulation. Such an effect was not even thought of as little as fifteen years ago. Though air pollution levels in the UK have fallen dramatically in the last 50 years much more remains to be discovered about this apparently universal risk to health.

## 2    Particulate air pollution

The air we all breathe can be thought of as an aerosol: a fairly stable suspension of particles and liquid droplets of varying size and composition. Particles found in the air come from a variety of sources. In urban areas of the UK three main sources can be identified: particles produced locally by motor vehicles (primary particles), particles produced by the oxidation of gases including the oxides of sulphur and nitrogen, often far from towns, and carried into towns by air movements (secondary particles) and particles thrown up from the earth's surface by attrition by vehicles and the wind. The latter particles are rather larger in size than the former two groups and are thought to have less significant effects on health. Particle concentrations may be measured by a number of methods but measurement of the mass concentration of particles falling within specified size ranges are the methods in most general use today. Thus particulate matter (PM) may be monitored as $PM_{10}$: the mass of particles of, generally, less than 10 μm diameter, per cubic meter of air. $PM_{2.5}$ is similarly defined. $PM_{10}$ corresponds closely to the mass concentration of particles defined by inhalation toxicologists as the thoracic fraction of the ambient aerosol. This specifies those particles likely to pass through the upper airways of the nose, mouth and throat and which may be deposited, with varying efficiency depending on their diameter, in the airways and air spaces of the lung. $PM_{2.5}$ reflects those particles with a higher probability of being deposited deep in the lung, in the air spaces involved in gas exchange.

Particles defined as $PM_{10}$ vary, of course, in size and composition. Metal species such as iron, nickel and vanadium are present, as are large amounts of organic and inorganic carbon. Organic compounds such as polycyclic aromatic hydrocarbons are adsorbed onto the surfaces of the particles. Particles deposit in the airways by impaction, sedimentation and diffusion. Impaction and sedimentation depend on the square of the diameter of the particle; diffusion depends on the reciprocal of the particle diameter. Small particles thus deposit effectively by diffusion whilst larger particles impact in the airways. Deposition by sedimentation depends on settling under the influence of gravity and is thus increased by slow deep breathing. The efficiency of deposition of particles reaches a minimum at about 0.5 μm diameter. Particles deposited in the lung are cleared by a variety of processes: in the airways cilia sweep particles upwards, in the alveoli macrophages ingest particles and carry them to the ciliary escalator for removal. Some particles pass through alveolar walls and enter the interstitial tissues, the lymphatic system and the blood. Clearance from the airways is rapid; clearance from the alveolar spaces is slow. Reaction of particles with the thin film of fluid lining the airways and alveoli leads to the formation of oxidative free radicals. These react with anti-oxidants including reduced glutathione, ascorbic acid and uric acid and are effectively neutralised. However, failure to deal with these radicals may lead to local inflammatory responses that can trigger further changes in the walls of blood vessels nearby. Very small particles can enter the blood stream and may interact with clotting factors: an increase in clotting factors has been described in animals exposed to such particles. This may lead to effects on atherosclerotic plaques in the coronary arteries: a link may thus exist between inhalation of particles and the triggering of heart disease. Additionally, it has been argued that particles may react with receptors in the airways and trigger subtle reflex changes in the heart rate. This is a new and unexpected finding which may prove important in explaining why patients susceptible to cardiac arrhythmias may be at increased risk when concentrations of particles are raised.

Epidemiological studies have revealed associations between mass concentrations of particles ($PM_{10}$ and $PM_{2.5}$) and a range of effects on health. These include daily death rates, admissions to hospital for treatment of cardio-respiratory disorders, visits to General Practitioners and increases in symptoms. Those with pre-existing cardio-respiratory disease and diabetes seem to be at increased risk of such effects. These associations have been debated at length but are now accepted as likely to be causal in nature. Interestingly, no thresholds of effect have been identified: this may be because of the wide distribution of exposure and of sensitivity within the population. Recent work has focused on two epidemiological techniques: time series studies and cohort studies. The former probe the link between daily variations in levels of air pollution and daily counts of health end-points; the latter study the effects of long-term exposure to air pollutants on the risk of death at all ages. Cohort studies have shown a major effect of particles on heart disease but little on respiratory disease. This is surprising, but recent experimental work using rabbits that are genetically susceptible to heart disease has shown that exposure to particles accelerates the development of atherosclerotic disease in the coronary arteries. Again this is a startling finding. These findings and others relating to effects on cardiovascular disease have recently been reviewed in detail: see reading list.

Much emphasis has been placed on the possible role of very small particles. These are referred to as ultrafine particles if their diameter is less than 100 nm (0.1µm). Such particles can also be described as nano-particles and findings from the air pollution field have been central to the increasing level of concern about the possible effects on health of exposure to engineered nano-particles. This is a rapidly expanding field and many advances in nano-toxicology are expected in the coming decade.

## 3     Air pollutant gases

Ambient air contains a number of pollutant gases in addition to the usual constituents: oxygen, nitrogen, carbon dioxide and the inert gases. Some, such as sulphur dioxide and nitrogen dioxide are emitted by combustion processes, others, including again nitrogen dioxide, and ozone are produced from precursors in the atmosphere. Carbon monoxide is produced by the incomplete combustion of carbon: complete combustion produces carbon dioxide. Carbon monoxide production by poorly ventilated gas, oil and solid fuel heating devices is a major problem indoors. Ozone is produced by the photochemical breakdown of nitrogen dioxide which yields nitric oxide and an oxygen free radical. The latter reacts with oxygen to form ozone. This process takes place in polluted air drifting away from cities and towns and ozone levels tend to be higher in rural and semi-urban areas than close to traffic – the major source of the precursor pollutants. Organic species are important in facilitating the production of ozone.

### 3.1     Ozone

Ozone is a rather insoluble gas which, in high concentrations, causes brisk inflammation of the airways. It is poorly absorbed in the upper airways: peak tissue concentrations of absorbed ozone occur in the terminal bronchioles. Concentrations rise on warm sunny days and exposure occurs outdoors. Ozone levels indoors tend to be low because of the lack of primary indoor sources and as a result of the rapid reaction of ozone with furnishings and fittings. Exposure to ozone is associated with significant effects on indices of lung function and an increase in admissions to hospital for the treatment of respiratory disorders. The effects of ozone on lung function are increased by exercise and thus those most likely to suffer effects are those exercising outdoors on warm days in summer. High concentrations limit the capacity for full inspiration, perhaps due to pain produced presumably as a result of airway inflammation. Effects on lung function can be detected on exposure to concentrations as low as 80 ppb (160 µg/m$^3$) in subjects exercising in exposure chambers. To produce these effects exposure has to be prolonged for about 6 hours: shorter periods of exposure require higher concentrations to produce the same effects. Epidemiological studies, unlike experimental studies with volunteers, have not shown thresholds of effect: effects have been detected at concentrations of only 40 ppb. This may be because sensitive subjects such as those with asthma tend not to be studied experimentally, but it is interesting to note that by no means all asthma sufferers are unusually sensitive to ozone. Recent work has suggested that one of the genes that may play a part in the causation of asthma may also confer increased sensitivity to ozone: more work is needed on this. Exposure to concentrations of ozone of over 100 ppb (200 µg/m³) may cause eye irritation but whether this is due to ozone *per se* or to associated photochemical pollutants is uncertain.

## 3.2   Sulphur dioxide

Sulphur dioxide is a water-soluble gas that is absorbed well in the upper airways and acts as an airway irritant as a result of interaction with airway receptors. This leads to broncho-constriction and asthmatic subjects are particularly sensitive. Epidemiological studies have shown associations between 24 hour average concentrations of sulphur dioxide and the number of deaths occurring each day from cardio-respiratory causes; hospital admissions are also increased. Effects on the airways appear rapidly after exposure begins: this is not the case with ozone. The rapidity of onset of the effects of sulphur dioxide has led to air pollution standards being defined with very short averaging times: 10 or 15 minutes in addition to the more usual averaging time of 24 hours.

## 3.3   Nitrogen dioxide

The major source of oxides of nitrogen in urban areas is traffic: exhaust gases contain high concentrations of nitric oxide and some nitrogen dioxide. The nitric oxide is oxidised to nitrogen dioxide in the ambient air. The combination of nitric oxide (NO) and nitrogen dioxide ($NO_2$) is sometimes referred to as NOx. Nitrogen dioxide causes inflammation of the airways and, as in the case of sulphur dioxide, those suffering from asthma are at increased risk though the effect of nitrogen dioxide on these subjects is less marked than that of sulphur dioxide. Long-term exposure to nitrogen dioxide is associated with an increased prevalence of symptoms of respiratory disease in children and perhaps with an increase in the prevalence of asthma. Nitric oxide is an important transmitter substance in the body: it plays a part in relaxing the walls of blood vessels. Exposure to ambient levels of nitric oxide has not been regarded as likely to cause harm to health but recent work has shed doubt on this. The effects of nitrogen dioxide are difficult to distinguish from those of fine particles emitted by motor vehicles. The close association between concentrations of nitrogen dioxide and those of fine particles make distinguishing their effects by epidemiological means very difficult. Some experts believe that many of the effects attributed to nitrogen dioxide are actually caused by exposure to fine and perhaps ultrafine particles.

## 3.4 Carbon monoxide

Carbon monoxide competes with oxygen for binding to haemoglobin and thus reduces the capacity of the blood to transport oxygen. In addition, the bi      o ur carbon monoxide to haemoglobin inhibits the release of such oxygen as is transported from haemoglobin. These effects are particularly dangerous to the heart and brain where a high percentage of the transported oxygen is usually given up by the blood. Concentrations of carbon monoxide outdoors are generally too low to cause serious effects on health but indoor concentrations can be high and each year many deaths and hospital admissions are caused by accidental exposure to this gas. Damage to the brain may be due to the direct effect of the reduced supply of oxygen but further injury after exposure to carbon monoxide has stopped may also occur. This is an example of re-perfusion injury and is due in part to the formation of oxidative free radicals. Long-term exposure to levels of carbon monoxide that cause only modest symptoms (headaches, tiredness) may be associated with damage to the brain: this is not yet accepted by all experts in the field and more work on this potentially very important effect is needed. Epidemiological studies have shown associations between peak daily outdoor concentrations of carbon monoxide and effects on the heart. As in the case of nitrogen dioxide, it is difficult to be sure that these effects are due to carbon monoxide *per se*: they may be due to fine particles. For more details on carbon monoxide poisoning see Chapter 4.1

## 3.5 Carcinogenic outdoor air pollutants

In addition to those pollutants described above, ambient air contains organic chemical species including benzene, 1,3-butadiene and polycyclic aromatic hydrocarbon (PAH) species. These are all known to be carcinogenic though at the concentrations found in ambient air it is difficult to predict their impact on health. That some risk occurs is likely. Recent epidemiological work using cohort study methods has shown that long-term exposure to fine particles ($PM_{2.5}$) is associated with an increased risk of lung cancer. This may be due to PAH compounds adsorbed onto the surfaces of particles.

## 3.6 Indoor air pollutants

Much more emphasis has been placed on the study of the effects of outdoor exposure to air pollutants than on those of indoor exposure. This is paradoxical as we all spend more than 80% of our lives indoors and indoor concentrations of pollutants such as nitrogen dioxide and carbon monoxide often exceed those found outdoors. One reason for this disproportionate study of outdoor air pollution is that the means of controlling outdoor levels of air pollutants are more easily adopted by governments. Standards for outdoor concentrations of air pollutants are also more easily enforced than standards set for indoor concentrations. The indoor environment is, of course, connected to the outdoor environment and pollutants generated outdoors infiltrate into buildings. Much of our daily exposure to particles generated outdoors must occur indoors. This means that studies which link outdoor concentrations of pollutants with effects on health should not be regarded solely as studies of outdoor exposure.

The indoor environment presents special problems: direct sources of pollutants such as cookers and fires may vent into the limited indoor space. This can lead to high indoor concentrations of pollutants especially in houses with a low air exchange rate. Modern trends in building design which reduce the need for space heating by insulation exacerbate this problem. Some pollutants including organic species released by carpets and adhesives reach effective concentrations only indoors; formaldehyde, released from composition boards, is also a special indoor air problem. The dangers of indoor exposure to carbon monoxide have been discussed above. Tobacco smoke is also a special indoor air problem: high concentrations of carbon monoxide and nitrogen dioxide are found in tobacco smoke.

## 4 · Air quality standards

### 4.1 UK standards

It is often assumed that policies to reduce levels of air pollutants must be based on air quality standards. This is quite untrue. In the 1950s and 60s air pollution levels in the UK fell dramatically without any standards being set. Much more important than standards is the recognition that air pollution damages health and the political will to address this problem. This is comparatively easy to sustain during periods of high air pollution when the effect on health or the pollution itself is easily seen. When pollution levels are low, maintaining pressure for further reductions is more difficult. Standards allow the effectiveness of policies to be judged and provide targets for further action.

Standards for air pollutants tend to be defined in terms of concentrations and averaging times. Sulphur dioxide is an acute irritant of the airways and controlling short term peak concentrations is important. Thus the standard for sulphur dioxide is set in terms of a 15 minute averaging time. Carcinogens such as PAH compounds exert their effects by causing damage that accumulates over time: thus an annual average concentration is defined as the standard. Often the form of air quality standards is dictated by the type of study that has led to effects on health being recognised. Time series studies employ 24 hour average concentrations and thus this averaging period is widely used in standard settings. Details of air pollution standards currently in use in the UK can be found on the Defra website. It is, of course, necessary to specify more than a concentration and an averaging period when defining a standard. The method to be used, the location of the monitoring sites and how the data will be checked and reported should also be set out in detail.

Setting standards when it is believed that there is no discernible threshold of effect is clearly likely to be difficult. In these cases it must be assumed that all reductions in pollutant concentrations will be associated with some benefit to health. In the UK, the National Air Quality Strategy is based on balancing the costs of policies against the benefits to health which they are predicted to deliver. Expressing benefits to health in monetary terms presents formidable difficulties but this can be done. Progressive, cost-benefit tested, reduction in concentrations of air pollutants has to some extent replaced an emphasis on standards.

## 4.2   International dimensions

For many countries, including the UK, the solution to air pollution problems is impossible without international cooperation. Ozone concentrations in the UK are, in part, dictated by the background hemispheric concentrations of this pollutant. Furthermore, the production of volatile organic compounds across Europe affects the photochemical processes that lead to ozone and this too affects the UK. International organisations such as the European Union rightly take a strong interest in air pollution and EC policies are set out in a series of Air Quality Directives. Some specify levels of performances for vehicle engines, others deal with the composition of fuel and some set Limit Values for air pollutants. These are binding on Member States.

In recent years EC Directive Limit Values have been increasingly based on recommendations from the World Health Organization. These recommendations are summarised in the WHO Air Quality Guidelines. WHO guidelines are set without regard for cost, but cost and feasibility must be taken into account by the EC and dates for achievement of Limit Values and allowed levels of exceedence of these values reflect these considerations.

## 5   Conclusion

Air pollution continues to be a problem in both developed and developing countries. Our knowledge of the effects of air pollutants on health continues to expand rapidly but much remains to be learnt. Levels of air pollution in many developing countries are not falling, in some cases they are rising, and this presents a challenge. In the UK, levels of air pollutants are, in historical terms, low but further reductions are desirable. The use of cost-benefit tested policies is accepted by many but it should be recalled that such policies will not be possible unless research to underpin our understanding of the effects of air pollutants on health is pursued.

## 6   Further reading

Department for Environment, Food and Rural Affairs. (2006) Air pollution in the UK: 2005.

Department of Health Committee on the Medical Effects of Air Pollutants. (2006) Cardiovascular Disease and Air Pollution. Available at: www.advisorybodies.doh.gov.uk

Holgate ST, Samet JM, Koren HS, Maynard RL. (1999) *Air Pollution and Health.* Academic Press, London.

World Health Organization. (2000) *Air Quality Guidelines for Europe*, second edition. WHO Regional Publications, European Series Number 91.

# Section 3.3

# Contaminated land assessment

James Wilson

## Learning outcomes

At the end of this chapter and any recommended reading the student should be able to:

1. describe and discuss the nature of land contamination, and the UK's approach to regulation;
2. describe the methods used for assessing land contamination;
3. explain how toxicological information is used in the UK to assess public health risks posed by land contamination;
4. explain the exposure assessment tools available for managing risks to health posed by land contamination; and
5. apply their knowledge in the analysis and management of land contamination cases.

# 1 Introduction

## 1.1 Aims

The aim of this chapter is to provide environmental and public health practitioners in the UK with a broad overview of what 'contaminated land' is, how contaminated land is investigated and how the risks it poses to human health are assessed. Contaminated land assessment involves comparing the contaminant concentrations present on a site (especially in soil) to 'assessment criteria' such as the UK Soil Guideline Values. Assessment criteria are generated using toxicological information and exposure assessment models. Therefore, in order for environmental/public health practitioners to contribute to the design or evaluation of a risk assessment strategy or to appreciate the implications of a risk assessment, it is necessary for them to be aware of the rudiments of site investigation procedures (such as soil sampling and analysis), the statistical treatment of analytical data, the use of exposure assessment models and the application of toxicological information. The skills required to produce contaminated land assessments are clearly varied and may draw on a number of disciplines. Specialist contractors are often commissioned to produce risk assessments, often on the behalf of regulators, which for the majority of potentially contaminated sites in the UK are local authorities. Regulators may in turn seek advice from public health professionals on managing incidents of land contamination.

## 1.2    Definition of 'contaminated land'

The legal definition of 'contaminated land' is given in Part IIA of the Environmental Protection Act (1990). Sites that are undergoing assessment, or might not necessarily fulfil the legal criteria, are generally referred to as having 'land contamination' (Box 1).

**Box 1** 'Contaminated Land' and Part IIA of the Environmental Protection Act (1990)

Section 57 of the Environment Act 1995 created a new legal framework for managing contaminated sites that are considered to present a hazard or potential hazard to human health and/or the environment. These new provisions were inserted into the Environmental Protection Act 1990 under Part IIA and came into force on 1 April 2000. 'Contaminated Land' for the purposes of Part IIA of the Environmental Protection Act (1990) can be defined as:

> "any land which appears to the LOCAL AUTHORITY in whose area it is situated to be in such a condition, by reason of substances in, on or under the land, that –
> (a) SIGNIFICANT HARM is being caused or there is a SIGNIFICANT POSSIBILITY of such harm being caused; or
> (b) POLLUTION OF CONTROLLED WATERS is being, or is likely to be, caused" (Defra Circular 01/06)."

'Harm' is defined as: 'death, disease, serious injury, birth defects and the impairment of reproductive functions'. 'Disease' is taken to mean: 'an unhealthy condition of the body or a part of it and can include, for example, cancer, liver dysfunction, or extensive skin ailments. Mental dysfunction is only included insofar as it is attributable to the effects of a pollutant on the body of the person concerned' (Defra Circular 01/06).

## 1.3    The nature of land contamination

A wide range of industries may be associated with land contamination, a few examples include: gas/coke works, chemical works, metal works, asbestos works, engineering works, manufacturing plants, oil refineries, textile and dye works, sewage works, timber treatment works, waste recycling works, garages and filling stations, landfills and electrical manufacturing works. Each type of industry may have one or a series of processes (and waste streams) associated with it. In addition to industrial activities, the underlying geology of an area may lead to 'naturally occurring' concentrations of potentially harmful substances which are deemed to be elevated (in areas with significant heavy metal mineralisation for example). Prior to conducting site investigations of a potentially contaminated area, a desk-based study of the land use history of a site along with its underlying geology is therefore recommended to identify what hazardous substances/man-made structures may still be present, and can be useful in deciding on sampling and analytical strategies for site investigations. In the UK, the former Department of the Environment 'Industry Profiles' provide useful technical background information on the processes, materials and wastes associated with individual industries (these are available from the Environment Agency website).

## 2    Site investigation

### 2.1    Background

Site investigation is an essential part of assessing the health risks associated with land contamination. Site investigations usually include soil sampling, groundwater sampling (in order to determine whether 'controlled waters' are being affected) and may include soil vapour/gas sampling. In most cases, soil is the environmental media that is primarily of interest for assessing health-related risks related to land contamination. Guidance on site investigation for regulators has been published by government departments/agencies such as the Department for Environment, Food and Rural Affairs (Defra) and the Environment Agency (e.g. CLR 4, Department of the Environment, 1994; Environment Agency, 2000a,b and references therein) and others (e.g. Petts *et al.*, 1997; Nathanail *et al.*, 2002).

### 2.2    Environmental sampling

The primary aim of any environmental sampling for human health risk assessment is to identify what substances are present on a site to which the public may be exposed and to measure their concentrations. Samples may be taken from topsoil (by using a hand trowel or auger for example) or deeper soil horizons (by excavating trenches). Boreholes may also be drilled which can be used for water and/or vapour extraction. Factors to consider when designing or evaluating a sampling strategy include: depth of sampling, spatial arrangement and density of sample along with procedures for taking and storing/preserving samples. Sampling at various depths may be useful in order to characterise the distribution of contamination on a site. However, members of the public are more likely to be exposed to surface or near-surface soil during their daily activities and it is samples of this material which are most likely to be of use for assessing risks to health.

In general, soil sampling strategies fall into two broad categories: 'targeted' and 'non-targeted' (Petts *et al.*, 1997). 'Targeted sampling' involves using some degree of judgement in order to focus sampling on a particular area where there is a known or suspected discrete point source of a pollutant (around a leaking tank for example).

The non-targeted approach involves taking samples on a grid arrangement in order to characterise the overall spatial distribution of contaminant concentrations, and to identify the presence of 'hotspots', i.e. localised patches of especially elevated contaminant concentrations (Petts *et al.*, 1997; Nathanail *et al.*, 2002).

There are many types of soil sampling grid that may be used (Figure 1), of which the 'herringbone' has been identified as being the most efficient at detecting hotspots (Ferguson, 1992).

For some sites, it may not be viable to take soil samples using a regular grid pattern, (for example, on a housing estate with irregularly spaced areas of hard and soft cover). For other sites, it may be the case that more than one set of samples has been taken in order to characterise a potential hotspot, resulting in samples being unevenly spaced. In such cases, the clustering of sample points may have implications for the validity of statistical tests commonly used for human health risk assessments (see Nathanail, 2004 for details).

The density of points on sampling grids requires careful consideration, in order to ensure that there are enough data to ascertain with some degree of confidence, the distribution of contaminant concentrations to which 'receptors' (such as members of the public) may be exposed. The density of sampling points may also affect the effectiveness with which a soil sampling strategy can detect 'hotspots' (CLR 4, Department of the

**Figure 1** Examples of soil sampling grids.

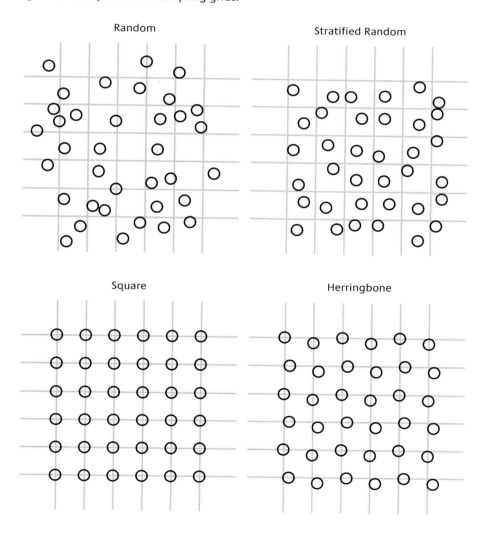

Environment, 1994). The statistical methods chosen to assess typical concentrations to which receptors may be exposed may also influence sampling strategy design.

The design of a soil sampling strategy also requires the methods of sample collection and storage to be carefully chosen to minimise the potential for sample degradation (such as the loss of volatile substances) or cross-contamination to occur.

## 2.3    Chemical analysis

Once samples have been collected, analytes will need to be chosen. The choice of analytes may be influenced by factors such as land use history and the availability of guidelines or standards to assess risks to human health and the environment. In addition, evidence may be observed during site surveys/soil sampling (odours or visual observations) that may suggest the presence of certain substances which are subsequently included in soil analyses (gas works waste and asbestos – containing materials, for example).

Chemical analysis of soils (and other environmental media) for regulatory purposes should be conducted by an accredited laboratory. In the UK, accreditation is given by the United Kingdom Accreditation Service (UKAS). The use of accredited services should ensure that appropriate analytical methods are used which have sufficient quality assurance/control measures in place that the data obtained are reliable.

Risk assessors should be aware that the form in which the contaminants are present in soil will not necessarily be identified during analysis. This is an important consideration, as the different forms of a given contaminant will have different physico-chemical (and therefore toxicological) properties. Contaminants may be present as discrete particles (e.g. loose asbestos fibres), as constituents of organic or inorganic soil particles, as part of organic and inorganic complexes sorbed to soil particles or they may be present as complex mixtures (such as the hydrocarbon compounds present in petroleum and tar).

A good example of where contaminant form affects toxicity is given by the cyanide compounds which are often associated with sites where town gas has been manufactured. The most prevalent forms of cyanide at such sites are likely to be the relatively less toxic, iron-complexed forms, such as ferric ferrocyanide, rather than the highly toxic 'free' cyanide forms (Shifrin *et al.*, 1996). The methods available for cyanide analysis can measure for 'total' cyanide, readily soluble or 'free' cyanide and cyanide that is present in complexed forms (such as 'weak acid dissociable' cyanide and cyanide that is 'amenable to chlorination') (Rayment *et al.*, 2003).

## 2.4    Bioaccessibility testing

Heavy metal contamination and the risks it may pose to health are often of concern on potentially contaminated sites. Analytical results for metals (such as lead) and metalloids (such as arsenic) are generally reported as total mass of element per unit mass of soil, although they may be present in different compounds that may have different oral bioavailabilities (i.e. the ability to be absorbed, generally across the gastrointestinal tract). *In-vitro* methods have been developed in order to measure soil contaminant bioaccessibility, as an indication of bioavailability. Bioaccessibility methods generally involve laboratory tests that extract metals/metalloids (such as lead and arsenic) from soil by simulating the action of fluids present in the stomach and small intestine (e.g. Environment Agency and British Geological Survey, 2002a, 2002b; Oomen *et al.*, 2002, 2003; Ruby *et al.*, 1996).

**Box 2** Health Criteria Values
(CLR7, CLR 9, Defra/Environment Agency, 2002).

For substances that exhibit threshold effects, Health Criteria Values (HCVs) take the form of tolerable daily soil intakes (TDSIs) which may be better described as tolerable daily intakes *from* soil. The approach taken for a given substance is to initially identify a Tolerable Daily Intake (TDI) which is expressed as mass of substance per unit mass body weight, per day. This is typically extrapolated from a 'No Observable Adverse Effect Level' (NOAEL) often identified from animal experiments. Once this is identified, a number of uncertainty factors may be applied to account for variability in response, due to factors such as inter- and intra-species variation. If a NOAEL is not available for a given substance, the 'Lowest Observable Adverse Effect Level' (LOAEL) may be adopted with the application of an additional uncertainty factor. Once a TDI has been identified, the mean daily intake (MDI) of substances from sources other than soil is identified (drinking water and food products for example). The TDSI is equal to the TDI minus the MDI, except in cases where the MDI ≥ 80% of the TDI. In those cases, the TDSI is equal to 20% of the TDI (in order to ensure that resources are not devoted to inappropriately reducing exposure to substances from soil sources). The approach taken for lead is somewhat different. The lead HCV is a target blood lead level and assessment criteria are based on a model of the relationship between concentrations of lead in soil/dust and those in blood (Tox Report 6 and lead SGV Report, Defra/Environment Agency 2002).

For non-threshold substances, HCVs are in the form of 'index doses' which are daily intakes (also expressed as mass of substance per unit mass receptor body weight per day) that have a corresponding 'minimal' risk of causing adverse health outcomes, typically cancer. Although intakes can be identified which correspond to a minimal risk, there is an additional exhortation that exposure to non-threshold substances should be kept 'as low as reasonably practicable' or 'ALARP', because no 'safe' level of exposure can be identified. It is also assumed that exposures to non-threshold substances from sources other than soil will also be reduced to levels that are 'as low as reasonably practicable' and as such, intakes of non-threshold substances from sources other than soil are not considered.

It should be remembered that HCV values identified in the Tox Reports essentially represent daily intakes that are *unlikely* to result in widespread manifestation of adverse health effects within a population, whereas 'contaminated land' is defined in terms of 'significant harm' (Box 1).

However, issues have been identified regarding the robustness of the data produced by such methods and the degree to which they correlate with *in vivo* bioavailability (Saikat, 2006). The regulatory guidance in the UK states that although such methods may be potentially useful, their applicability at present is limited (Environment Agency, 2005b). However, work on validating *in vitro* bioaccessibility tests is ongoing (for example Drexler and Brattin, 2007) and they could play a more prominent role in contaminated land risk assessments in the future.

## 2.5    Data quality

An important aspect of any risk assessment is the quality of the data upon which it relies. All chemical analyses will have some degree of random and systematic error associated with them (Gill and Ramsey, 1997). Sampling may also have random error associated with it, the magnitude of which generally reflects soil heterogeneity. Techniques have been developed that allow random errors from sampling and analysis to be estimated, thereby indicating the degree to which samples taken from a site represent the true distribution of contaminant concentrations (Ramsey *et al.*, 1992, 2002; Ramsey, 1993, 1994). In addition to error estimation, the limit of detection for an analytical technique should be considered, as it will clearly need to be lower than a given assessment criterion to ensure that the data obtained can be reliably used for risk assessment purposes.

## 3    Toxicological information

In constructing human heath risk assessments for land contamination, toxicological information has to be carefully evaluated in order to determine the possible effects that soil pollutants may have on health and to choose toxicological information to use in the generation of assessment criteria such as Soil Guideline Values (SGVs). Considerations have to be given to the toxicological properties of a contaminant/pollutant related to acute as well as chronic exposures (including, for example, carcinogenicity, genotoxicity, reproductive toxicity and teratogenicity). It should be noted that toxicological data are often only available from animal studies and that the form (and therefore bioaccessibility) of the substance used in the experiments may not be the same as that present in the environment.

In the UK, compilations of toxicological information of commonly occurring soil pollutants have been published by Defra/Environment Agency, as a series of 'tox' reports (CLR 9, and associated Tox Reports, Defra/Environment Agency, 2002). These documents aim to summarise the published views of authoritative expert bodies in order to choose the most appropriate Health Criteria Values (HCVs) to use with exposure models to generate contaminated land assessment criteria.

## 4    Exposure assessment models

Exposure models are used in order to generate assessment criteria such as Soil Guideline Values (SGVs). An assessment criterion is the concentration of a substance present in soil that may result in a daily intake which is equal to, or less than a Health Criteria Value.

The exposure pathways present on a given site are identified by constructing a 'conceptual model'. In order for a hazardous substance to pose a risk to human health, there has to be a source of that substance, viable exposure pathway(s), as well as receptors that can be exposed. If a source, pathway(s) and receptors are present, there may be a complete 'pollution linkage' (Figure 2) which will have some degree of risk associated with it.

In 2002, the Environment Agency released the Contaminated Land Exposure Assessment (CLEA) model (CLR10, Defra/Environment Agency, 2002) which was subsequently updated to CLEA UK (released in 2005). The model has been used to generate SGVs for three generic land use scenarios: residential (both with and without plant uptakes), allotments, and commercial/industrial. The CLEA model includes a number of potential exposure pathways (Figure 3). In addition to those included in the CLEA model, risk assessors may also wish to consider the potential for organic chemicals to permeate drinking water pipes made of plastic (Goodfellow *et al.*, 2002). The approach used is to identify 'a critical receptor' which for a given exposure is likely to receive the greatest dose and therefore, potentially be most at risk. For a typical residential site, the critical receptor is taken to be a young female child. The CLEA model can also be used to generate site-specific assessment criteria (SSAC) where generic exposure parameters are altered to reflect more closely the conditions present on the site of interest.

**Figure 2** Source-pathway-receptor model.

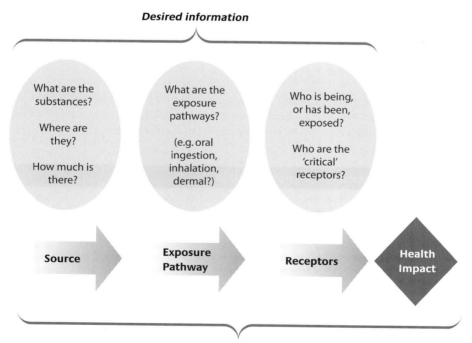

**Figure 3** Routes of exposure used in the CLEA model.

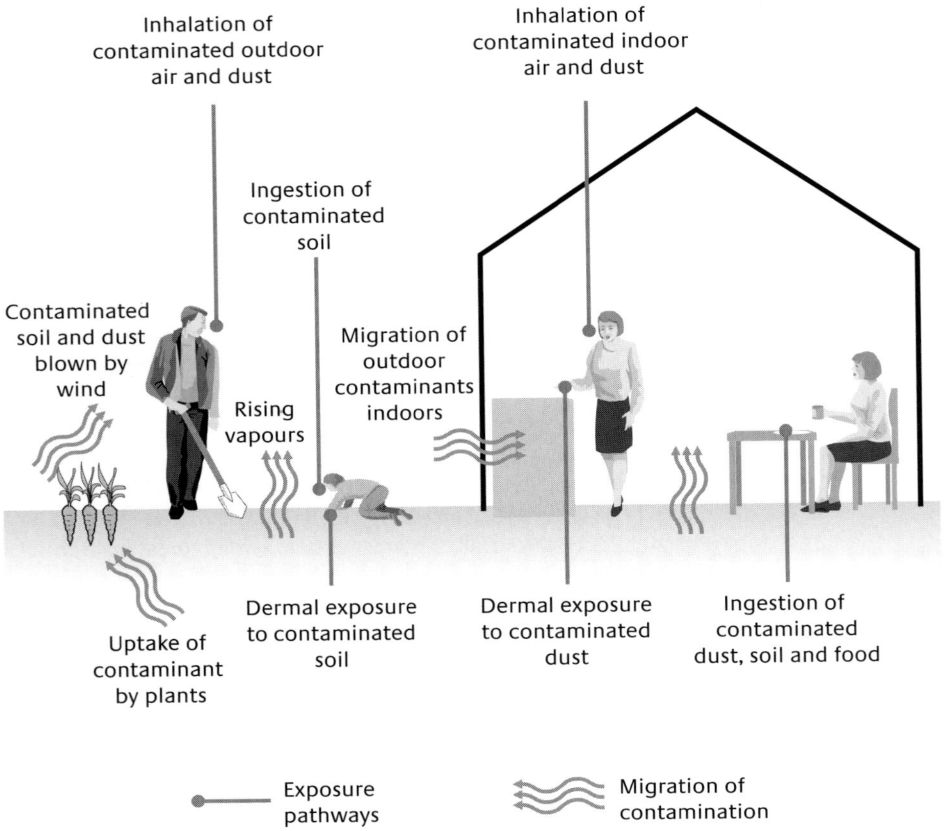

A number of other exposure assessment models have also been developed (such as SNIFFER and RBCA). The Environment Agency has a produced a series of fact-sheets on these models that can be downloaded from their website.

## 5    Statistical treatment of analytical data

Once a site investigation is complete, contaminant concentrations are compared to generic criteria (such as SGVs) or site specific criteria (SSACs). The approach recommended by the Environment Agency (CLR 7, 2002) is to split sites into a number of 'averaging areas' and to apply statistical tests to the data taken from samples within each area, which should be representative of exposure potential. The designation of averaging areas may be influenced by factors such as the geography of the site (type and/ or sources of contamination), soil type as well as land use patterns. For each averaging area, statistical tests can be applied to measured soil contaminant concentrations in order to identify 'outliers' that could correspond to contaminant 'hotspots' and to estimate average contaminant concentrations to which receptors may be exposed. The approach recommended in CLR 7 (Defra/Environment Agency, 2002) is to apply the 'maximum value test' to identify outliers and to estimate mean contaminant concentrations within each averaging area (CLR 7, Defra/Environment Agency, 2002; CL:AIRE, 2006).

## 6    Comparing contaminant concentrations with risk assessment criteria

If mean contaminant concentrations to which receptors may be exposed exceed SGV or SSAC values and 'pollutant linkages' are intact, the regulator may wish to consider whether a site requires further assessment (which *could* include further exposure assessment, perhaps by questionnaire surveys and/or offering biological sampling of potential receptors if deemed appropriate). If sufficient information is available that suggests a site fulfils the definition of 'contaminated land', it may be 'determined' under Part IIA of the Environmental Protection Act (1990). An options appraisal can then be produced which may include a consideration of remedial works that could be undertaken to reduce the risks (CLR 11, Defra/Environment Agency, 2004). The aim of remedial works is to break the pollution linkages identified in the conceptual model (such as removal of the source, breaking exposure pathways, or removal of receptors). If remedial works are undertaken, verification should be carried out to ensure that remedial objectives have been met (for example, 'clean' topsoil imported onto a site should be tested to ensure that it really is 'clean').

## 7    Conclusion

Assessing the health risks posed by land contamination is a complex process, requiring an understanding of site investigation, exposure modelling and the use of toxicological information. However, environmental/public health practitioners should be familiar with the rudiments of risk assessment, some of which are discussed here. In short, soil sampling and analysis should provide a reliable, representative indication of contaminant concentrations to which receptors may be exposed. These data may then be compared to assessment criteria generated using assumptions appropriate for the land use of a given site, which have been generated using reliable, authoritative toxicological information. Quantitative risk assessment is a powerful tool used in health protection. However, resource limitations, socio-economic factors and gaps in scientific knowledge (along with differences between individuals' perceptions of risk) will result in the need for informed judgements to be made when remedial options (or other interventions) are being appraised.

## 8    References and further reading

CL:AIRE. (2006) Statistical assessment of contaminated land: some implications of the 'mean value test'. Contaminated Land: Applications in Real Environments Technical Bulletin TB 12. Available at: www.claire.co.uk

Department of the Environment. (1994) CLR 4 Sampling strategies for contaminated land. Report by The Centre for Research into the Built Environment, The Nottingham Trent University. Department of the Environment.

Defra/Environment Agency. (2002) Assessment of risks to human health from land contamination: an overview of the development of soil guideline values and related research (CLR7). Available at: www.environment-agency.gov.uk

Defra/Environment Agency. (2002) Contaminants in soil: collation of toxicological data and intake values for humans (CLR 9). Available at: www.environment-agency.gov.uk

Defra/Environment Agency. (2002) The Contaminated Land Exposure Assessment (CLEA) model: technical basis and algorithms (CLR 10).

Defra/Environment Agency. (2002) Contaminants in soil: collation of toxicological data and intake values for humans. Benzo(a)pyrene (Tox report 2). Available at: www.environment-agency.gov.uk

Defra/Environment Agency. (2002) Contaminants in Soil: Collation of toxicological data and intake values for humans. Inorganic Cyanide (Tox Report 5).

Defra/Environment Agency. (2002) Soil Guideline Values for Lead Contamination. Available at: www.environment-agency.gov.uk

Defra/Environment Agency (2004) Model Procedures for the Management of Land Contamination. Available at: www.environment-agency.gov.uk

Defra. (2005) CLAN briefing note 2/05:Soil Guideline Values and the Determination of Land as Contaminated Land under Part IIA. Available at: www.defra.gov.uk

Defra. Circular 01/2006. Environmental Protection Act 1990: Part 2A Contaminated Land. Available at: www.defra.gov.uk

Defra. (2006) CLAN briefing note 6/06 Soil Guideline Values: The Way Forward. Available at: www.defra.gov.uk

Drexler JW, Brattin WJ. (2007) An *in vitro* procedure for estimation of lead relative bioavailability: with validation. *Human and Ecological Risk Assessment* 13: 383-401.

Environment Agency. (2000a) Technical Aspects of Site Investigation in relation to Land Contamination: Vol. 1. R&D Technical Report P5-065/TR.

Environment Agency. (2000b) Technical Aspects of Site Investigation in relation to Land Contamination: Vol. 2. Text Supplements. R&D Technical Report P5-065TR. EA 2000.

Environment Agency. (2005) Environment Agency's Science Update on the use of Bioaccessibility Testing in Risk Assessment of Land Contamination. February 2005. Available at: www.environment-agency.gov.uk

Environment Agency. (2006) CLEA Update 3. Available at: www.environment-agency.gov.uk

Environment Agency and British Geological Survey. (2002a) *In vitro* methods for the measurement of the oral bioaccessibility of selected metals and metalloids in soils: a critical review. R&D Technical Report P5-062/TR/01, Environment Agency, Bristol.

Environment Agency and British Geological Survey. (2002b) Measurement of the bioaccessibility of arsenic in UK soils. R&D technical report p5-062/TR/02, Environment Agency, Bristol.

Ferguson C. (1992) The statistical basis for spatial sampling of contaminated land. *Ground Engineering* June: 34–38.

Gill R, Ramsey MH. (1997) What a geochemical analysis means. In: *Modern Analytical Geochemistry*, ed. Gill R. Longman, Edinburgh.

Goodfellow F, Ouki SK, Murray, V. (2002) Permeation of organic chemicals through plastic water-supply pipes. *Journal of the Chartered Institution of Water and Environmental Management*: 16, 85–89.

Harrison RM. (ed.) (1994) *Understanding our environment: An introduction to environmental chemistry and pollution* (2nd edition). The Royal Society of Chemistry.

Nathanail CP. (2004) The use and misuse of CLR 7 acceptance tests for assessment of risks to human health from contaminated land. *Quarterly Journal of Engineering Geology and Hydrogeology* 27: 361–367.

Nathanail J, Bardos P, Nathanail P. (2002) *Contaminated Land Management Ready Reference*. EPP Publications, Land Quality Press, London.

Oomen AG, Hack A, Minekus M, Zeijde E, Cornelis C, Schoeters G, Verstraete W, van de Wiele T, Wragg J, Rompelberg CJM, Sips AJAM, van Wijnen JH. (2002) Comparison of five in vitro digestion models to study the bioaccessibility of soil contaminants. *Environmental Science and Technology* 36: 3326–3334.

Oomen AG, Rompelberg CJM, Bruit MA, Dobbe CJG, Pereboom DPKH, Sips AJAM. (2003) Development of an in vitro digestion model for estimating the bioaccessibility of soil contaminants. *Archives of Environmental Contamination and Technology* 44: 281–287.

Petts J, Cairney T, Smith M. (1997) *Risk-based contaminated land investigation and assessment.* Wiley, London.

Ramsey MH, Thompson M, Hale M. (1992) Objective evaluation of precision requirements for geochemical analysis using robust analysis of variance. *Journal of Geochemical Exploration* 44: 23–26.

Ramsey MH. (1993) Sampling and analytical quality control (SAX) for improved error estimation in the measurement of Pb in the environment using robust analysis of variance. *Applied Geochemistry.* Supplementary Issue 2: 149–153.

Ramsey MH. (1994) Error estimation in environmental sampling and analysis. In: *Sampling of Environmental Materials for Trace Analysis* B. (ed) Markert VCH, Weinheim.

Ramsey MR, Taylor PD, Lee, J-C. (2002) Optimized contaminated land investigation at minimum overall cost to achieve fitness for purpose. *Journal of Environmental Monitoring* 4: 809–814.

Rayment GE, Sadler R, Craig A, Noller B, Chiswell B. (2003) Chapter 5. Analysis of inorganic parameters. In: *Chemical Analysis of Contaminated Land,* Thompson KC, Nathanail CP. Blackwell Publishing, Oxford.

Ruby MV, Davis A, Schoof R, Eberle S. Sellstone CM. (1996). Estimation of lead and arsenic bioavailability using a physiologically based extraction test. *Environmental Science and Technology* 30: 422–30.

Saikat S. (2006) Bioavailability/bioaccessibility testing in risk assessment of land contamination – a short review. Chemical Hazards and Poisons Report 6: 44–45, Health Protection Agency.

Shifrin NS, Beck BD, Gauther TD, Chapnick SD, Goodman G. (1996) Chemistry, toxicology, and human health risk of cyanide compounds in soils at former manufactured gas plant sites. *Regulatory Toxicology and Pharmacology* 23: 106–116.

Thompson KC, Nathanail CP. (2003) *Chemical Analysis of Contaminated Land.* Blackwell Publishing, Oxford.

## 9  Useful Internet links

Contaminated Land: Applications in Real Environments
www.claire.co.uk

Environment Agency
www.environmentagency.gov.uk

Defra
www.defra.gov.uk

Health Protection Agency
www.hpa.org.uk

Chartered Institution of Environmental Health
www.cieh.org

United Kingdom Accreditation Service (UKAS)
www.ukas.com

# Section 3.4

# Management of incidents affecting drinking water quality

John Gray

## Learning outcomes

At the end of this chapter and any recommended reading the student should be able to:

1. explain the processes and guidelines for the provision of safe water supply in England and Wales;

2. evaluate the roles of the Drinking Water Inspectorate (DWI), local authorities and the water utilities;

3. explain the importance of good analytical support and toxicological advice, plus inter-agency assistance and good communications in the event of the chemical contamination of drinking water supplies;

4. critically discuss examples of chemical water contamination incidents and evaluate the manner in which investigations were carried out, and

5. apply their knowledge in the analysis and management of hazardous situations.

## 1    Introduction

This chapter outlines the arrangements for public water supply in England and Wales and the role of the Drinking Water Inspectorate (DWI) in enforcing regulatory requirements. The management of incidents affecting drinking water quality is described using examples to highlight some of the issues associated with minimising harm to the population. Analytical support, health risks and toxicological advice, interagency assistance and communication are considered.

The need for effective and rapid communications between all relevant bodies in the event of a chemical contamination incident affecting drinking water supplies and the ready availability of an assessment of potential health risks and provision of toxicological advice is highlighted.

## 2    The Drinking Water Inspectorate

### 2.1    Background to the Drinking Water Inspectorate (DWI)

The DWI was formed on 2 January 1990 following the privatisation of the water industry. It provides independent reassurance that public water supplies in England and Wales are safe and acceptable to consumers.

### 2.2    Public water supplies

A public water supply is one which is provided for the purposes of drinking, washing, cooking or food production by a statutorily appointed water company. Inset appointments are when one water company supplies water to part of another water company's area of supply. From December 2005, non-domestic consumers who use at least 50 Ml of water a year were able to purchase water from either their existing company or from a licensed water supplier.

### 2.3    Private water supplies

Water that is not supplied by a statutorily appointed water company is called private water. Local authorities are responsible under the Water Industry Act 1991 for checking the safety and sufficiency of water supplies in their area, including private water supplies. The Inspectorate provides expert technical advice to local authorities but has no regulatory role. Private water supplies make up less than 2% of the total water supply in England and Wales and most such supplies are in rural and remote parts of the country.

### 2.4    Regulatory framework

The Water Industry Act 1991 sets out the regulatory framework and defines the powers and duties under which the Inspectorate operates as well as the responsibilities of water companies. Under the Act, the Secretary of State for Environment, Food and Rural Affairs and the National Assembly for Wales are responsible for regulating the quality of public supplies. These two authorities appoint the Chief Inspector of Drinking Water to act on their behalf to enforce water quality standards and, where appropriate, initiate prosecutions. The Water Act 2003 (section 57) provides for the appointment of the Chief Inspector of Drinking Water and amends the Water Industry Act to allow for the appointment of Inspectors.

### 2.5    Wholesome water

By law (Section 68 of the Water Industry Act 1991) water companies must supply water that is wholesome at the time of supply. Wholesomeness is defined by reference to drinking water standards and other requirements set out in the Water Supply (Water

Quality) Regulations 2000 (2001 in Wales) (the Regulations). Many of these regulations derive from the 1998 European Drinking Water Directive (Council Directive, 1998) which came fully into force on 25 December 2003. Until December 2003, the standards contained within the Water Supply (Water Quality) Regulations 1989 applied.

The standards are directly linked to the World Health Organization guideline values for drinking water quality which are intended to protect public health as well as ensuring that water supplies are aesthetically acceptable to consumers. Under the EC Directive, standards will be subject to revision in the light of new knowledge. The new Regulations contain some new and revised standards; others that are no longer appropriate have been withdrawn. Although the Directive focuses on those parameters of importance to human health, others are included which relate to the control of water treatment processes and the aesthetic quality of drinking water. The Directive allows member states to set additional or tighter national standards to preserve the already good quality of drinking water and to prevent future deterioration.

## 2.6    Testing and reporting

Water companies are required to collect and test samples of the water leaving water treatment works and service reservoirs and from randomly selected consumers' properties. The tests to be carried out and the frequency of testing are detailed in the Regulations. The Inspectorate checks independently that the testing is carried out to the highest standards and that appropriate quality control checks are in place to assure the integrity of the analytical information produced. Water Companies have a duty to make the results of their testing available to consumers and the Inspectorate also publishes summary information on individual companies both in an annual report and on its website.

## 2.7    Water safety

The Regulations also make some provisions for drinking water safety. There are specific requirements concerning *Cryptosporidium*; there is a requirement to adequately treat and disinfect water supplies; and there are controls over chemicals and materials of construction that drinking water supplies might come into contact with.

# 3    Water quality incidents

## 3.1    Incident notification

When events occur that might impact on the quality or sufficiency of the water supplied, water companies are required to notify such events to the Inspectorate under the terms set out in the Water Undertakers (Information) Direction 2004 (DWI, 2004). This duty is enforceable under Section 202 of the Water Industry Act.

The Information Direction requires water companies to inform the Inspectorate of all events that have affected, or are likely to affect drinking water quality or sufficiency of supplies where, as a result, there may be a risk to consumers' health (Box 1). When notified of such events the Inspectorate assesses the water company's provisional information to determine whether the event is an incident. If the event is deemed to be an incident a full report from the company may also be required.

**Box 1** Notification requirements of the Water Undertakers (Information) Direction 2004

Water companies are required to notify the Inspectorate of:

- the occurrence of any event which, by reason of its effect or likely effect on the quality or sufficiency of water supplied by it, gives rise or is likely to give rise to a significant risk to the health of the persons to whom the water is supplied. This will include any event notified by a water undertaker to a local or health authority under regulation 30(5) of the Water Supply (Water Quality) Regulations 1989.

- any other matter relating to the supply of water which:
  - in the opinion of the undertaker is of national significance; or
  - has attracted or, in the opinion of the undertaker, is likely to attract significant local or national publicity; or
  - has caused or, in the opinion of the undertaker, is likely to cause significant concern to persons to whom the water is supplied.

- any reports of disease in the community which it appears might possibly be associated with a water supply.

## 3.2   What should be notified?

The wording of the current Information Direction and its predecessors deliberately leaves it to water companies to decide what to notify. This is because an event that appears significant to a small company could appear to be less so to a larger company. Furthermore the trigger for consumer contacts may be very different between a rural area and a highly populated inner city area. However, the Inspectorate has issued guidance on the type of events that it considers should be notified, the most recent in 1999 (DWI, 1999). The guidance also gave information on the investigation process by which the Inspectorate investigates incidents.

## 3.3   Incident investigation

The Inspectorate assesses the information provided by water companies to determine whether the event meets the criteria of an incident, as defined by the Inspectorate (Box 2).

Most incidents are relatively minor happenings but all are assessed thoroughly (Box 3) and may result in recommendations to the company concerned on the actions needed

**Box 2**  Definition of an incident

An incident can be defined as:

- a non trivial or unexpected breach of Part II of the Water Supply (Water Quality) Regulations 1989, as amended; or
- a breach of Part IV of the 1989 Regulations; or
- an unusual deterioration in water quality; or
- a significant risk to the health of consumers; or
- a significant number of consumers perceiving adverse water quality changes; or
- significant local or national media interest on a water quality issue that could result in consumer concern.

to minimise the risk of future failures. Where the lessons to be learnt might benefit other companies, generic guidance may be issued to the industry. Consideration is given to whether during the incident the company contravened any of the wholesomeness standards set out in the Regulations. The Inspectorate also considers whether the company contravened any other enforceable regulatory duty. If contraventions occurred, the Inspectorate then decides whether the breaches were trivial or likely to recur and whether enforcement action under Section 18 of the Water Industry Act 1991 is required.

These criteria apply only to public water supplies. As mentioned above, the responsibility for monitoring private water supplies rests with local authorities.

The assessment also takes into account the actions taken by the company to protect consumers and whether the company followed the advice given in 'Guidance on Safeguarding the Quality of Public Water Supplies' (Department of the Environment and the Welsh Office, 1989) and whether it followed industry best practice. The Inspectorate will also invite comments from health professionals and any local authority responsible for the area in which the incident occurred as well the Consumer Council for Water and any consumers affected.

**Box 3**  Key components of the Inspectorate's assessment of incidents

During an incident, the Drinking Water Inspectorate assesses:

- what caused the problem and whether or not it was avoidable;
- what the company did in response and how it handled the incident;
- what lessons can be learned to prevent similar incidents in the future;
- if there were any breaches of enforceable regulations; and
- whether the company supplied water that was unfit for human consumption.

## 3.4   Unfit water

The Regulations define water as wholesome if its quality meets the standards contained in the Regulations. Water which breaches those standards is necessarily unwholesome. Depending on the circumstances, DWI may have to consider whether water unfit for human consumption was supplied during the incident. If there is sufficient evidence to show that water unfit for human consumption was supplied (Box 4), that the Company did not exercise all due diligence to prevent the incident from occurring and if it is in the public interest, then prosecution under Section 70 of the Water Industry Act may be considered.

Section 70 of the Act makes it a criminal act for a water company to supply water that is unfit for human consumption. In 1994, the Inspectorate developed a policy that it would consider prosecution of a water company for an alleged offence under section 70 of the Water Industry Act 1991 of supplying water unfit for human consumption.

It will be obvious that a prosecution of a water company for supplying unfit water involves considerable effort in obtaining sufficient and robust evidence that meets the exacting requirements demanded to support a charge in a criminal court.

The definition of "unfit" was clarified in 2000 when, after a legal challenge, it was concluded (Jones, 2000) that either:

> the water if drunk would be likely to, or when drunk did in fact, cause injury to the consumer; or

> the water, by reason of its appearance and/or smell, was of such a quality that it would cause a reasonable consumer of firm character to refuse to drink it or use it in the preparation of food.

Although the Inspectorate may bring a prosecution if it believes that a water company supplied unfit water, it is for the courts to decide whether or not an offence has been committed and, if a company is found guilty of supplying unfit water, what the level of fine should be (up to a maximum of £20,000 per count).

For those incidents that do not justify full Court proceedings the Inspectorate may issue a caution which the Court could take into account in any future offences.

## 3.5   Outcomes of investigations

There are several typical outcomes of an incident assessment by an Inspector:

- a letter sent to the company, copied to other relevant parties;
- a letter sent to the company, copied to other relevant parties, making recommendations for action which the company must take to address deficiencies revealed by the incident;

- enforcement action initiated against the company: a legal process to ensure the company takes all the necessary action to prevent further breaches of either a regulatory duty or a drinking water standard; other relevant parties are informed; and
- initiation of prosecution proceedings against the company or the issue of a formal caution for a criminal offence; other relevant parties are informed.

## 3.6    Number of water related chemical incidents reported to DWI

Between 1990 and 2001 there was a steady year on year increase in the number of notifications received from water companies. This was attributed to the industry becoming more familiar with the process and the type of events that should be notified. In recent years some 60–70% of notifications have been classified as non-incidents. Occasionally the Inspectorate is made aware of a water quality problem by a third party. For example, a health authority may inform the Inspectorate of an increase in the number of reported cases of cryptosporidiosis at the same time as it informs the water company.

Table 1 shows the number of notifications received between 1995 and 2005. It also shows the number that were classified as incidents and the number of cases taken forward for prosecution or for which a caution was issued.

**Box 4** Evidential and other requirements before considering prosecution of a company for supplying unfit water

In order to prosecute a water company for an incident, the Drinking Water Inspectorate must consider:

a) Evidence to demonstrate that:
- (i)    illness or other health effect was experienced by normally at least two consumers which was associated with the quality of the water supplied; or
- (ii)   the quality of the water supplied was such that normally at least two consumers rejected it for drinking or cooking or food production on aesthetic grounds; or
- (iii)  the concentration of a substance in, or value of a property of, the water supplied was at a level at which illness or other health effect may be expected in the long term even though none was manifest in the community at the time; and

b) The Inspectorate considers that the water company does not have the defence that it took all reasonable steps and exercised all due diligence for securing that the water was fit on leaving its pipes or was not used for human consumption; and

c) Whether such a prosecution is regarded as being in the public interest.

**Table 1** Number of notifications made to DWI between 1995 and 2005

| Year | Number of notifications | Number of incidents | Number resulting in prosecutions or cautions |
|------|------|------|------|
| 1995 | 157 | 83 | 3 |
| 1996 | 176 | 76 | 3 |
| 1997 | 197 | 95 | 16 |
| 1998 | 300 | 120 | 17 |
| 1999 | 388 | 166 | 10 |
| 2000 | 429 | 139 | 4 |
| 2001 | 459 | 138 | 0 |
| 2002 | 398 | 130 | 1 |
| 2003 | 353 | 99 | 1 |
| 2004 | 304 | 89 | 2 |
| 2005 | 391 | 92 | 2 |

In earlier years, many of the incidents related to bacteriological failures or problems at water treatment works. In 1997, 33% of incidents related to the supply of discoloured water. This increased to more than 60% in 1998 which was attributed to the condition of the distribution systems and the associated remediation work being carried out. The Inspectorate considered that many of these incidents were avoidable. Since 1998 the number of discoloured water incidents has gradually decreased as companies have responded with improved planning and better operational management.

## 4    Examples of chemical water contamination incidents

### 4.1    Example 1

A consumer reported a petrol-like taste in the water supply which continued for some 30 days. Analytical results confirmed that the value for odour exceeded the standard. A neighbour reported a benzene-like taste in the water supply.

The presence of dissolved hydrocarbons up to a concentration of 31 μg/l was subsequently confirmed. The Local Authority and Health Authority were advised and the latter sought toxicological advice. Bottled water was supplied to consumers in the seven properties affected. Investigations by the company revealed no obvious source of the contamination. The company decided to replace the MDPE (medium density polyethylene) communication pipe and during excavations discovered a layer of bituminous material some 0.5 m thick close to one of the affected properties just under pavement level. This had an odour similar to that found in the consumers' supply and was subsequently shown to contain toluene, kerosene and diesel hydrocarbons.

## 4.2    Example 2

A consumer reported a taste in the water supply. Three affected properties were supplied with bottled water and the consumers were advised not to use the water. The water company sampled on day 2 and confirmed the presence of organic chemicals including 2(methylthio)benzothiazole, dimethyl butanedioic acid and bromohexanol at concentrations up to 0.5 µg/l. Unidentified hydrocarbons at concentrations up to 10 µg/l were also detected.

Toxicological advice related to health risks and toxicology was limited. No specific toxicological information was available for the compounds in question and data were only available for related compounds.

## 4.3    Example 3

The manager at a water treatment works was informed that concentrations of isoproturon, a herbicide, had been detected by on-line organic monitoring equipment at concentrations up to 4.3 µg/l in the raw water source supplying the treatment works. Isoproturon was found in the treated water leaving the works at concentrations of up to 1.3 µg/l. The water company increased the dose of powdered activated carbon to absorb the isoproturon. Subsequent samples taken from the associated service reservoirs and some consumers' properties contained up to 1.5 µg/l isoproturon, in excess of the standard but less than the WHO guideline value.

## 4.4    Example 4

An unknown quantity of chlorpyriphos was discharged into a river, 6 km upstream of the abstraction point supplying a water company's water treatment works. Invertebrate deaths occurred in the river. The company was notified some eight days later and immediately arranged for the analysis of the sample taken the previous day for chlorpyriphos. It also arranged for further samples of the raw water to be taken. Chlorpyriphos was found at a concentration of 0.325 µg/l in the raw water although none was found in the treated water leaving the works. No samples were taken of water in supply.

## 4.5    Example 5

The incident in Wem, Worcestershire, started at about 07.50 during the morning of Friday 15 April 1994 when the Company began to receive customer complaints of an unusual taste and odour in the public water supply to Worcester. It was evident that these were consistent with a problem at Barbourne Water Treatment Works on the River Severn where the Works Operator confirmed that there was an odour and taste in the final water. The Company isolated the treatment works where treatment comprised conventional clarification, filtration and disinfection. Unlike some works, there were no facilities for dosing activated carbon.

Later in the morning the number of complaints had risen to 60 and the decision was made, in collaboration with the Consultant in Communicable Disease Control (CCDC), Worcestershire Health Authority, to advise the customers in the Worcester area not to drink the water. The health risk assessment was made even more difficult by the inconsistency in describing the odour, e.g., sweet, sewage, paint stripper etc. At 1230 hrs a meeting took place of the Worcester Health Emergency Incident Team (HEIT).

A Crisis Management Team was convened at Severn Trent Water and worked in close association with the Worcester Emergency Incident Team. The first press statement issued by the Health Emergency Incident Team advised customers that an organic chemical had entered the water supply system and first indications were that this did not pose any serious threat to health. Until further information became available, the public were advised not to drink the water or to use it in food preparation.

Early on the Saturday, there was a report of a strong solvent smell entering Wem Sewage Works in Shropshire. The identity of one of two chemicals present was confirmed as 2 EMD (2 ethyl 1-4 methyl –1, 3 – Dioxolane). Both chemicals were at sub ppb levels (i.e. very low concentrations) in the potable water supply. The second chemical was identified 13 days later as 2EDD (2 ethyl –5,5-dimethyl-l, 3-dioxane).

Early in the morning the Crisis Management Team met with the Regional Director of Public Health, West Midlands Regional Health Authority. He agreed that the water might taste and smell unpleasant for the next couple of days, but that there was no threat to public health.

It has always been known that certain chemical compounds can cause a highly detectable odour even in trace quantities and the potential impact on potable water systems was thought to be negligible. It was not possible to identify the compound 2EDD by conventional analysis.

Chemical products passing from river sources through water treatment are traditionally removed as part of the process. The organic compounds involved in this incident were not broken down through coagulation, filtration and chlorination. Absorption through carbon treatment can be effective. There was no advanced carbon treatment at the works as Barbourne Treatment Works was due to be shut down.

The public health advice given verbally and early to Severn Trent was that people should be advised not to consume the water. This was confirmed when the Health Emergency Incident Team met later at lunchtime on the Friday. Potentially vulnerable groups such as nursing homes, the Worcester Royal Infirmary, nurseries, play groups, schools and residential homes were all alerted through pre-arranged cascade systems as were all food producers. GP's were contacted through a telephone cascade system.

The two chemicals contaminating the tap water were found at concentrations of less than one part per billion. Medical toxicologists from the National Poisons Centre and the Department of Health advised that these chemicals at the very low concentrations found were not hazardous to health. A press statement was issued at 5.30pm on Friday 15th, assuring the public that the water was safe to drink although taste and smell problems may still occur in some areas.

Severn Trent Water was prosecuted for the above incident for "supplying water not fit for consumption" despite the fact that there was no risk to health and complimentary comments from the Judge on the effectiveness of the emergency response. There were a number of recommendations from the independent report which were aimed at the Water Industry as a whole.

Other examples have been presented and discussed at two conferences, the proceedings of which have been published (Gray and Thompson, 2004; Thompson and Gray, 2006).

## 5    Conclusion and recommendations

Over recent years a number of incidents of chemical contamination of water have been reported in England and Wales. Fortunately, few have resulted in significant adverse health effects. However, experience in responding to these events has shown that to provide effective support to the public and consumers, close links between public health organisations, water companies, the regulators and other related bodies, are essential elements for a successful response. This chapter has addressed some of the common features between the perspectives of medical toxicology, public health, and drinking water quality regulation. From this collaboration it is possible to identify learning needs.

It has been said that the water industry needs to consider planning, preparation and performance when considering the impact of incidents affecting drinking water quality (Jackson, 2004). Planning requires the need to think the unthinkable and plan to deal with it. Preparation must ensure the provision of analytical facilities and appropriate expertise to interpret the results of such analyses. It also requires the ability to assess any impact on public health and to have available safe alternative supplies of drinking water. There is a need to cope with the unexpected and at the same time maintain public confidence. Learning points must be identified after each incident (or emergency) and incorporated into any emergency response plan.

## 6    References

Council Directive 98/83/EC of 3 November 1998 on the quality of water intended for human consumption. *Official Journal of the European Communities*, 5.12.98, L330/32-L330/53. p0032–0054.

Department of the Environment and the Welsh Office. (1989) *Guidance on safeguarding the quality of public water supplies.* London, HMSO.

DWI. (1999) Drinking Water Inspectorate Information Letter 13/99, 28 July 1999.

DWI. (2004) Water Undertakers (Information) Direction 2004. Drinking Water Inspectorate Information Letter 02/2004, 16 January 2004.

Jackson C. (2004) In: Thompson KC, Gray J. (Eds.) *Water contamination emergencies: Can we cope?* Royal Society of Chemistry, Cambridge.

Jones N, QC. (2000) Judgment. Leeds Crown Court, 28 July 2000.

The Water Act 2003. Chapter 37. London, HMSO.

The Water Industry Act 1991. Chapter 56. London, HMSO.

The Water Supply (Water Quality) Regulations 1989. Statutory Instrument No. 1147. London, HMSO.

The Water Supply (Water Quality) Regulations 2000. Statutory Instrument No. 3184. London, HMSO.

Gray J, Thompson KC. (Eds.) (2004) *Water contamination emergencies: Can we cope?* Royal Society of Chemistry, Cambridge.

Thompson KC, Gray J. (Eds.) (2006) *Water contamination emergencies: Enhancing our response.* Royal Society of Chemistry, Cambridge.

## 7    Further reading

Dawson A, West P. (Eds.) (1993) *Drinking Water Supplies: a microbiological perspective.* London, HMSO.

Twort AC, Ratnayaka DD, Brandt MJ, (Eds.) (2000). Water supply. Fifth edition. Arnold, London.

WHO (2004) *Guidelines for Drinking-water quality*, Third edition, World Health Organization, Geneva.

# Section 3.5

# Food additives and contaminants

Diane Benford

## Learning outcomes

At the end of this chapter and any recommended reading the student should be able to:

1. explain the principles of toxicological risk assessment as applied to food additives and contaminants;

2. discuss its use in assessing consumer safety, and in setting regulatory limits for chemicals in food, and

3. apply their knowledge in the analysis and management of hazardous situations.

## 1    Chemicals in food

Food is a complex mixture of chemicals, the vast bulk of which are naturally part of the food. Some are contaminants that are present inadvertently, as a result of environmental pollution, microbial metabolism, cooking or food processing (referred to as process contaminants) (see Box 1). Others are purposefully used or added during food production and processing, including food additives (see Box 2), pesticides and residues of veterinary medicines.

**Box 1** Examples of food contaminants

Environmental pollutants, e.g.
- Dioxins and dioxin-like polychlorinated biphenyls
- Polycyclic aromatic hydrocarbons
- Heavy metals, such as lead and cadmium

Natural toxicants, e.g.
- Aflatoxins
- Shellfish biotoxins

Process contaminants, e.g.
- Acrylamide
- Heterocyclic amines
- Polycyclic aromatic hydrocarbons

**Box 2** Food additives

Food additives have a technological function in food. Important sub-categories are:
- Colours
- Flavour enhancers and flavourings
- Preservatives
- Sweeteners
- Antioxidants
- Emulsifiers, stabilisers, gelling agents and thickeners.

All of these chemicals have the potential to be harmful if ingested in excessive amounts, and the primary aim of the food toxicologist is to determine how much can be consumed without *appreciable* risk to health. This terminology is used in recognition of the fact that it is never possible to guarantee absolute safety but based upon the available evidence any risk is likely to be extremely small. The main difference between these categories of chemicals is that those with an intentional use are subject to regulatory approval processes, and will have a manufacturer or "sponsor" who is responsible for generating the data to support the risk assessment. Therefore the data base of regulatory toxicology studies is normally more complete for additives. In contrast, there may be more mechanistic studies, and sometimes epidemiological studies, available for contaminants than for additives.

## 2    Risk assessment of food chemicals

The general principles of risk assessment were described in Chapter 1.1 of this book. In the first instance, the risk assessment for food chemicals is conducted by scientific advisory committees, which allows separation of the independent assessment of the science from the societal and political influences that need to be taken into account in risk management. The major independent scientific advisory committees that have assessed safety of food additives and contaminants are:

- UK Committee on Toxicity of Chemicals in Food Consumer Products and the Environment (COT) and its sister committees on Mutagenicity (COM) and Carcinogenicity (COC)
- EU Scientific Committee on Food (SCF) (until 2002)
- European Food Safety Authority (EFSA) (since 2002)
- Joint FAO/WHO Expert Committee on Food Additives and Contaminants (JECFA).

The approach taken to risk assessment (or safety assessment) of food chemicals with threshold effects is summarised in Figure 1. In brief, the highest dose that has no observed adverse effect in a study of the most sensitive relevant toxic endpoint is identified (the NOAEL). The NOAEL is divided by uncertainty factors (or safety factors) to allow for inter-species differences if the NOAEL is derived from a study in laboratory animals, and for inter-individual variability in the human population. The aim is to protect the most susceptible subgroups, if that is possible. A combined uncertainty factor of 100 is often used, but a larger factor may be used if key data are missing, and a smaller factor may be used if specific data are available relating to effects in humans. Dividing the NOAEL by the uncertainty factor results in establishment of a health-based guidance value referred to as the Acceptable Daily Intake (ADI) or Tolerable Daily Intake (TDI). The term "acceptable" is used for food additives since they are subject to regulatory approval. The term "tolerable" is used for contaminants and the health based guidance value may be related to weekly or monthly intake for contaminants that have the potential to accumulate in the body. In addition the term "provisional" is conventionally used by JECFA. The ADI and TDI are normally expressed in relation to body weight (e.g. mg/kg bodyweight per day) in order to allow for individuals of different body size, especially children. Regardless of the terminology used, these health-based guidance values are considered to be amounts that can be consumed over an entire lifetime without appreciable risk to health (Box 3).

**Box 3** Health-based guidance values

Additives:
- Acceptable Daily Intake (ADI)

Contaminants
- Tolerable Daily Intake (TDI)
- Provisional Tolerable Weekly Intake (PTWI)

## 3    Regulatory limits for chemicals in food

The approval process for food additives includes consideration of the theoretical intake of the additive assuming that it will be added at the level necessary to achieve its technological purpose in all the foods in which it could be used, taking into account how much of those foods is likely to be eaten. If this exposure assessment indicates that the ADI could be exceeded, then restrictions are placed on the maximum levels or the different food uses, in order to ensure that the intake is below the ADI. These restrictions are specified in international, European Union (EU) and UK regulations.

Whilst contaminants are not subject to an approval process, regulatory limits are applied for some key contaminants to help reduce exposure to below the TDI, where one could be set. The process for establishing regulatory limits for contaminants also takes into account the levels that occur in different types of food, the extent to which it is technologically feasible to reduce the levels, and also what can be reliably measured and therefore enforced. Within Europe the regulations are set by the European Commission, with input from representatives of the national food authorities in member states.

Because of the different ways that regulatory limits are set, a food exceeding the regulatory limit for a particular additive or contaminant will not inevitably result in intakes above the ADI or TDI.

## 4    Implications of exceeding the ADI or TDI

When foods are found to exceed regulatory limits for additives or contaminants, or when assessing levels of unregulated contaminants, it is important to first assess the anticipated intake for average and high level consumers of the foods containing the additive or contaminant. Consideration of children's food consumption is generally important, because young children have a higher caloric requirement, expressed in relation to body weight. If the estimates of total dietary exposure for different subgroups are below the ADI/TDI, then there is not considered to be a health risk. If the ADI/TDI is exceeded by some subgroups, then it is necessary to consider if the available toxicological information allows further conclusions to be drawn. The ADI/TDI is not a threshold of toxicity, and for a substance that does not have acute effects, occasionally exceeding the ADI/TDI is unlikely to be harmful. The greater the degree by which it is exceeded, and the longer the period of potential exceedance, the more likely it becomes that adverse effects will occur. In such situations, action may be taken to withdraw the affected food from sale, and if appropriate, specific advice may be given to subgroups at particular risk.

## 5    Recent issues related to food additives and contaminants

### 5.1    Aspartame

Aspartame is an intense artificial sweetener, which is widely used in beverages and processed foods. Some people have concerns that aspartame could be the cause of a wide range of human illnesses, largely based upon unsubstantiated information available on the internet. In fact, the available evidence on aspartame has been reviewed on many occasions (see EFSA, 2006 for an overview) over the past 2–3 decades. It is metabolised in the gastrointestinal tract into the amino acids, aspartic acid and phenylalanine, and methanol, all of which are present naturally in many foods and in the human body. Ingestion of aspartame at the level of the ADI does not result in elevation of these components within the blood. In the most recent review, EFSA (2006) concluded that intakes of aspartame at the ADI do not lead to toxicologically relevant systemic exposure, and confirmed that there was no reason to revise the previously established ADI. Estimates of intakes, even for high level consumers, are well below the ADI.

### 5.2    Sudan dyes

Sudan dyes have never been approved as food colours in the UK. Although not tested to current standards, the available information indicates that they are genotoxic and carcinogenic. Therefore the expert opinion is that it is not possible to propose a TDI and exposures should be reduced to as low as reasonably practicable. In 2003 it was discovered that they were being used illegally to increase the market value of some spices, such as chilli powder, and legislation was introduced to require testing of chilli and chilli products imported into the EU (EC, 2003). Since then there have been a number of occasions in which Sudan dye adulterated foods have been found on the UK market. At the levels detected the cancer risk is likely to be extremely small, but it is an unnecessary risk that can be avoided if action is taken to prevent these dyes from being added to food.

## 5.3    Acrylamide

Acrylamide has been used as an industrial chemical since the mid-1950s, but its presence in food was only discovered in 2002 (FAO/WHO, 2006). Since then there has been extensive international effort to investigate how acrylamide forms in food, and how formation could be reduced, and also to develop and refine risk assessment for dietary exposure to acrylamide. Acrylamide is known to be neurotoxic in humans as a result of occupational and accidental exposure. Studies in animals have shown that it can cause reproductive effects and is genotoxic and carcinogenic. It is not known whether dietary exposure to acrylamide could cause cancer in humans, but based upon the evidence from the animal studies, it is considered possible. As with the Sudan dyes, the expert opinion is that it is not possible to propose a TDI and intakes should be reduced to as low as reasonably practicable. However because acrylamide is present in a wide variety of cooked foods, it is not possible to have a healthy balanced diet that avoids acrylamide. It is also likely that it has been in our food for generations.

Research is underway to investigate how acrylamide formation can be reduced without incurring other food risks. In the meantime, the Food Standards Agency advises that people should not change their diets because of concern about acrylamide, but should follow the healthy eating guidelines which help to protect against some cancers as well other chronic diseases.

## 5.4    Contaminants in fish

Fish is an important source of nutrients, and most people in the UK eat less than is recommended for health benefits. However, fish also contain contaminants that can be a health concern. There are two main issues: methylmercury accumulates in large predator fish, regardless of whether they are oily or non-oily; persistent organic pollutants, such as dioxins, have the potential to accumulate in oily fish. Fish is the major source of exposure to methylmercury. Dioxins and related compounds are widely present in other foods, although levels have decreased significantly over the past two decades.

The Food Standards Agency asked an expert group of nutritionists and toxicologists to advise on the benefits and risks associated with fish consumption (SACN/COT, 2004) in order to give cohesive advice to consumers. Methylmercury is neurotoxic and the most sensitive effect is impaired neurodevelopmental as a result of pre-natal exposure. Dioxins have a wide range of health effects, the most sensitive of which was considered to be on development of the male reproductive system as a result of pre-natal exposure. The expert group advised that the tolerable intakes set to protect against accumulation of methylmercury and dioxins in a woman's body to levels that could have adverse effects on the foetus, should be applied to susceptible subgroups.

**Figure 1** Derivation of an Acceptable or Tolerable Daily Intake.

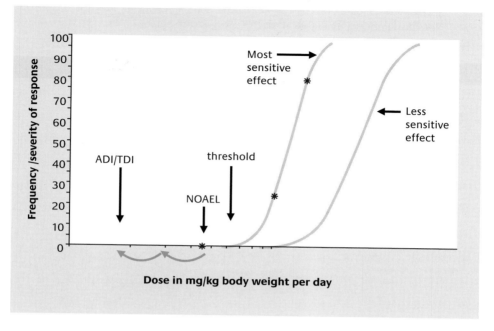

However, as seen in Figure 1, if the most sensitive effect relates to exposure during pregnancy, the TDI could be over-precautionary for people that would not get pregnant. Therefore the COT set additional guidelines, based upon the next most sensitive effect, to be applied for men and for women who would not get pregnant in order to make recommendations on the range of fish consumption at which there would be nutritional benefits without undue risks from the contaminants. Combined with information on the levels of contaminants present in different types of fish and other dietary sources of dioxin-like compounds, this opinion forms the basis of the Food Standards Agency advice to consumers.

## 6    References

EC. (2003) Commission decision 2003/460/EC of 20 June 2003 on emergency measures regarding hot chilli and hot chilli products. *Official Journal of the European Union.* L 154/114.

EFSA. (2006) Opinion of the Scientific Panel on Food Additives, Flavourings, Processing Aids and Materials in Contact with Food (AFC) on a request from the Commission related to a new long-term carcinogenicity study on aspartame. Adopted on 3 May 2006. Available at: www.efsa.europa.eu

FAO/WHO (2006). Safety evaluation of certain food additives. *Food Additive Series* No 56. World Health Organization, Geneva. Available at: www.who.int

SACN/COT. (2004) (accessed February 2008) Scientific Advisory Committee on Nutrition Reports. Available at: www.sacn.gov.uk/reports

## 7    Further reading

Food Standards Agency website: www.food.gov.uk
COT opinions: www.food.gov.uk/science/ouradvisors
SCF opinions: ec.europa.eu/food
EFSA opinions: www.efsa.europa.eu
JECFA procedures and opinions: www.who.int and www.inchem.org

# Section 4

A Review of Some Toxic Agents

# Section 4.1

# Carbon monoxide poisoning

Lakshman Karalliedde, Catherine Keshishian

## Learning outcomes

At the end of this chapter and any recommended reading the student should be able to:

1. explain the manner in which carbon monoxide causes toxicity;
2. describe and discuss common sources of carbon monoxide poisoning and those population groups that are more vulnerable;
3. describe and differentiate between acute and chronic carbon monoxide poisoning;
4. discuss the long-term effects following acute and chronic poisoning;
5. provide basic information for treatment, and
6. apply their knowledge in the analysis and management of hazardous situations.

## 1    Introduction

Carbon monoxide (CO) is a colourless, odourless, tasteless, non-irritant gas which when inhaled in excessive amounts can cause death or serious ill-health. CO poisoning is an important cause of ill-health and death in the UK, causing an estimated 50 fatalities and 200 serious illnesses a year (Department of Health, 1998), although these figures are thought to be underestimated.

In addition, poisoning due to low-level concentrations of CO resulting in chronic symptoms of flu-like illness and cognitive impairment is also a significant health problem. Many cases of chronic illness go undiagnosed and there are no reliable prevalence data to indicate the extent of the problem.

## 2    Sources of carbon monoxide

When there is insufficient oxygen for organic compounds to burn efficiently, there is production of CO. If the oxygen content is sufficient for efficient combustion, carbon dioxide is formed.

The most common source of CO poisoning is from faulty heating or cooking appliances in homes where some defect, such as that in a flue, results in the production of CO when the appliance is in use. Tobacco smoke is also an important source of CO exposure. Other sources include automobile exhaust fumes, camp stoves and lanterns, gasoline power generators and underground mine explosions.

Following the four major hurricanes in the USA during 2004, electric power failures necessitated the use of gasoline powered generators. These appliances caused 167 people to seek treatment for CO poisoning in ten hospitals and there were six deaths attributed to CO toxicity (MMWR, 2005).

A relatively uncommon source of CO poisoning is from the paint stripper methylene chloride which can enter the body by inhalation, ingestion or through the skin. Methylene chloride is metabolised by the human liver to CO. In such instances, due to the continued metabolism and thus production of CO in the body, the time taken for the haemoglobin to free itself from CO may be as long as 12 hours (i.e. twice the time taken following cessation of CO exposure by inhalation from other sources).

## 3    Health effects of acute and chronic carbon monoxide poisoning

There are two well defined forms of CO poisoning. Acute poisonings are usually due to exposure to high concentrations of CO for short durations (minutes or hours). Chronic poisonings are where exposure takes place to lower but nevertheless toxic concentrations of CO over more prolonged periods, such as weeks, months or even years.

### 3.1   Acute carbon monoxide poisoning

#### 3.1.1   Immediate effects

With acute, high-level exposure to CO, headache, nausea and vomiting are early symptoms and there may be rapid progression to dizziness, confusion, shortness of breath, blurred vision, loss of consciousness, fits and death.

Following acute exposures, patients are likely to seek the services of an Emergency Department in a hospital. However, disease progression may be so rapid in certain circumstances that confusion and in-coordination may be severe enough to prevent the patient from seeking the services of an ambulance (dialling 999) or doctor. Death is likely if the person is not immediately evacuated or removed from the source of exposure and treated with high concentrations of oxygen. Oxygen under higher than atmospheric pressure (hyperbaric oxygen therapy) may be used.

Acute poisoning may be severe enough to cause brain damage and damage to the heart muscle. Irregular heart rhythms (arrhythmias) are commonly seen, as are signs and symptoms of heart attacks. In 2005, Satran et al. reported that damage to heart muscle (myocardial injury) is common in patients hospitalised for moderate to severe CO poisoning. The group showed that enzymes which confirmed injury to heart muscle were raised and that there were abnormal changes in the electrocardiogram. They also showed that those who sustained damage to heart muscle died earlier than those who did not.

Many CO poisoned patients have symptoms and signs of abnormal brain function such as impaired memory, tendency to abnormal involuntary movements, gait abnormalities and some disturbances of vision. Twenty-four hours after acute severe exposure to CO, where there has been loss of consciousness, CT scanning may show changes indicative of brain damage. Damage to the basal ganglia is a characteristic of CO induced brain damage.

### 3.1.2  Long-term effects

Following recovery from acute exposure, many patients suffer from a wide range of residual ill-health.

a. The exposure itself may have been so emotionally traumatic that symptoms of post-traumatic stress disorder may occur.

b. The patient may suffer from effects of brain damage due to the lack of adequate oxygen to the brain cells during the period of severe poisoning. These symptoms may range from personality changes to memory loss to deterioration of mental acuity or mental sharpness.

c. The patient may suffer damage to heart muscle which may result in changes in the electrocardiogram and also an elevation of enzymes which are indicative of injury to heart muscle. For example, plasma levels of a structural protein found in the myocardium, troponin, may increase.

d. Damage to muscle cells due to a lack of oxygen to muscle during exposure, may lead to a breakdown of muscle fibres and release of myoglobin, which can damage the kidneys and cause renal failure.

## 3.2  Chronic carbon monoxide poisoning

### 3.2.1  Immediate effects

Chronic carbon monoxide poisoning occurs when there has been long-term exposure (months or even years) to low but toxic doses of carbon monoxide usually in homes, and more rarely at workplaces. It is therefore usual for more than one person to have been exposed to the toxic environment and for other household members, including pets, to present with similar symptoms. Symptoms often improve once the patient is away from their house for a period of time and may worsen over weekends and during the winter months with increasing exposure.

With such exposures death is most unlikely and the patients usually seek assistance from General Practitioners (GPs), often on a very regular basis. It is very difficult to make

## 5.3    Those with pre-existing systemic disease

People with cardiovascular disease including coronary heart disease, angina and anaemia are at significant risk for CO poisoning. Such individuals have compromised blood supply to heart muscle or insufficient haemoglobin to carry oxygen (Karalliedde, 2006). See Chapter 2.3 for more on susceptible populations.

## 6    Treatment

1. Immediate removal from source of exposure.

2. Administer 100% oxygen.

3. Control convulsions if present.

4. Monitor basic physiological parameters – pulse rate, blood pressure, arterial oxygen concentration, electrocardiograph.

5. Measure carboxyhaemoglobin concentration.

6. Consider treatment with hyperbaric oxygen.

For detailed information on treatment for carbon monoxide poisoning, refer to *Toxbase*, the clinical toxicology database of the National Poisons Information Service. www.toxbase.org

## 7    Conclusions

Carbon monoxide is so dangerous because it is undetectable by humans, leaving the individual unaware in most cases that he or she is being poisoned. In high-level exposures, this can lead to death. In low-dose exposures, diagnosis is difficult and can often be missed by doctors, as symptoms are non-specific and mimic other common diseases, and as clinicians may be unaware that such exposures are not infrequent.

Acutely exposed patients require urgent treatment with oxygen (100% or hyperbaric) after immediate removal from exposure to prevent neurological and cardiac sequelae. Acute exposures during pregnancy could harm the foetus and such exposures merit hyperbaric oxygen therapy at lower concentrations of COHb when compared with normal healthy adults who have had exposures.

Long-term low but toxic exposure may lead to protracted ill health primarily because diagnosis is delayed until the source of exposure has been confirmed. These patients require continued care and encouragement for at least three years following cessation of exposure.

Children are more vulnerable to both acute and chronic exposures and tend to suffer ill health at lower concentrations of carbon monoxide when compared to adults. An important aspect is that children who suffer chronic exposures to low concentrations often have difficulty in concentrating in their school work and other activities and thus they tend to show an impairment in their educational progress during an exposure.

Public awareness as well as regular educational activities for health care professionals to raise awareness of this 'silent killer' is a necessity. The public should be urged to install CO monitors and alarms as routinely as they do smoke alarms. It is recommended that all households where gas appliances are used have a CO monitor.

## 8    References

Coburn RF. (1970) The carbon monoxide body stores. *Ann N Y Acad Sci*: 174:11–22.

Copel JA, Bowen F, Bolognese RJ. (1982) Carbon monoxide intoxication in early pregnancy. *Obstet Gynecol* 59:26S–28S.

Department for the Environment, Food and Rural Affairs in partnership with the Scottish Executive, The National Assembly for Wales and the Department of the Environment for Northern Ireland. (2000) *The Air Quality Strategy for England, Scotland, Wales and Northern Ireland.*

Department of the Environment. (1994) Expert Panel on Air Quality Standards. Carbon Monoxide. London: HMSO.

Department of the Environment, Transport and the Regions. (1998). Carbon monoxide. HMSO, London

Department of Health. (2004) Guidance of the effects on health of indoor air pollutants. Committee on the Medical Effects of Air Pollutants.

Department of Health. (1998) Carbon monoxide: The forgotten killer. *Letter from the Chief Medical Officer.* London: Department of Health, PL/CMO/98/5.

HSE. (2005) Workplace exposure limits. Health and Safety Executive EH40/2005.

Karalliedde L. (2006) Carbon monoxide poisoning. *Int J Clin Prac* 60(12):1523–1524.

Longo LD. (1977) The biological effects of carbon monoxide on the pregnant woman, fetus, and newborn infant. *American Journal of Obstetrics and Gynecology* 129: 69–103.

MEDITEXT® Medical Management. Carbon monoxide. In: Klasco RK (Ed): TOMES® System. Thomson Micromedex, Greenwood Village, Colorado (Edition expires (06/2007)) (accessed 02/2007).

MMWR. (2005) Carbon monoxide poisoning from hurricane-associated use of portable generators – Florida, 2004. *Morbidity and Mortality Weekly Report* 54(28): 697–700.

Satran D, Henry CR, Adkinson C, Nicholson CI, Bracha Y, Henry TD. (2005) Cardiovascular manifestations of moderate to severe carbon monoxide poisoning. *J Am Coll Cardiol* 45(9):1513–1516.

Van Hoesen KB, Camporesi EM, Moon RE *et al.* (1989) Should hyperbaric oxygen be used to treat the pregnant patient for acute carbon monoxide poisoning? A case report and literature review. *JAMA* 261:1039–1043.

## 9    Further reading

Flomenbaum NE, Howland MA, Goldfrank LR, Lewin NA, Hoffman RS, Nelson LS. (Eds.) (2006) *Goldfrank's Toxicologic Emergencies.* 8th Edition. McGraw-Hill, New York.

IPCS. (1999) Carbon monoxide. *Environmental Health Criteria* 213. International Programme on Chemical Safety, World Health Organization, Geneva.

Jones A, Karalliedde L. (2006) Chapter 9: Carbon Monoxide Poisoning. In: *Davidson's Principles and Practice of Medicine.* 20th edition. Churchill Livingstone.

WHO. (2000) Carbon monoxide. WHO Air quality guidelines. 2nd edition. World Health Organization, Regional Office for Europe, Copenhagen.

# Section 4.2

# Toxicity of heavy metals and trace elements

Robin Fielder, Lakshman Karalliedde

## Learning outcomes

At the end of this chapter and any recommended reading the student should be able to:

1. discuss the terms 'trace element' and 'heavy metal';
2. explain, with reference to case studies, the source and health effects of some trace elements, e.g. lead, zinc, mercury, arsenic, thallium, aluminium, and chromium, and
3. apply their knowledge in the analysis and management of hazardous situations.

# 1 Introduction

## 1.1 Heavy metals

"Heavy metals" is a somewhat ambiguous term used to describe chemical elements that have metallic or metalloid properties with a specific gravity that is around five times or more than the specific gravity of water. The specific gravity of water is 1 at 4 °C (39 °F). Simply stated, specific gravity is a measure of density of a given amount of a solid substance when it is compared to an equal amount of water. Some well-known toxic metallic elements with a specific gravity that is five or more times that of water are arsenic, 5.7; cadmium, 8.65; iron, 7.9; lead, 11.34; and mercury, 13.546 (Lide, 1992).

There are approximately 23 heavy metals that are important or relevant to health protection and toxicology. Small amounts of some of these heavy metals are necessary for normal body function and good health and are known as "trace elements" (see below), e.g. iron, copper and cobalt, and they are present in the environment and in our diet. Higher amounts do, however, result in toxicity. Others such as lead and mercury have no beneficial effects on health and are toxic at low dose levels. Some heavy metals have the potential to cause disorders of function in the nervous system, kidneys, liver, lung, and in the composition of blood. In addition, allergies may also occur (e.g. to nickel). There are data to indicate that long-term exposures to some heavy metals, e.g. arsenic, cause cancer (CIS, 1999; /AXL 2004).

The heavy metals of particular concern to health are antimony, arsenic, bismuth, cadmium, cerium, chromium, cobalt, copper, gallium, gold, iron, lead, manganese, mercury, nickel, platinum, silver, tellurium, thallium, tin, uranium, vanadium, and zinc (Glanze, 1996).

## 1.2    Trace elements

In the toxicological/biological sciences, "trace elements" are generally considered to be those elements, including some heavy metals, which are essential to health in trace amounts, or where there is some evidence to support claims that they have some benefit to health. These are described as 'essential' or 'probably essential' and are often commercially available in multivitamin products or other food supplements. The Expert Group on Vitamins and Minerals (EVM) listed the following as trace elements: boron, chromium, cobalt, copper, germanium (now withdrawn as a supplement due to toxicity), iodine, manganese, molybdenum, nickel, selenium, tin, vanadium and zinc (EVM, 2003).

## 2    Heavy metal toxicity

In general, heavy metal toxicity is an uncommon clinical entity. However, when it does occur it is not only clinically significant but delays in recognition of toxicity and inappropriate treatment could result in serious ill health (Ferner, 2001).

Symptoms of acute heavy metal toxicity may be more easily recognised if there is a sufficient degree of suspicion and awareness of sources of exposure. In such acute toxic situations, symptoms usually follow rapidly, thus diagnosis and treatment is often prompt (Ferner, 2001). However, symptoms of chronic toxicity can be so vague that the establishment of a cause and effect relationship becomes difficult. The symptoms of chronic toxicity can be so varied – e.g. impairment of brain function (cognitive dysfunction), learning difficulties, nervousness, insomnia, lethargy and general malaise, and they tend to abate from time to time. Therefore, very often there are delays in diagnosis, and in the implementation of appropriate therapy following chronic exposures.

People may be exposed to heavy metals through their everyday applications. In medicine, heavy metals can be used in diagnostic medical applications, such as the direct injection of gallium during radiological procedures, and chromium used in intravenous feeding (parenteral nutrition) (Roberts, 1999). Heavy metals are also commonly used in industrial applications such as in the manufacture of pesticides, batteries, alloys, electroplated metal parts, textile dyes and steel (CIS, 1999). Many products containing these chemicals are also found in our homes and may add to our quality of life when properly used.

Heavy metals may enter the human body through food, water, air, or by absorption through the skin. Ingestion is the most common route of exposure in children (Roberts, 1999). Small children may ingest potentially toxic levels from the hand-to-mouth activity

**Box 1** The concept "As Low As Reasonably Practicable"

### As Low As Reasonably Practicable

In the case of genotoxic compounds for which we assume no threshold, exposures must be kept ALARP, i.e. 'as low as reasonably practicable'. The concept of ALARP involves the consideration of the risks and benefits of the exposure, and so this could mean that some exposures to the chemical may not be permitted at all. For example, such compounds would not be used in household products, cosmetics, food additives and similar products which are frequently used. However, industrial use could be allowed under strictly controlled conditions.

involving contaminated soil by actually eating objects that are not food such as dirt (a phenomenon known as 'pica'), and through sucking and gnawing on old paintwork such as on windowsills. People may be exposed in manufacturing, pharmaceutical, industrial and residential settings; industrial exposure is a common source of exposure for adults. Less common routes of exposure are during radiological procedures, from inappropriate dosing during intravenous (parenteral) nutrition or from a commonly used instrument which is damaged or broken, such as a clinical thermometer (Smith *et al.*, 1997). Heavy metals have been used as agents for both suicide and homicide.

Acute toxicity is more likely to result from inhalation or skin contact of dust, fumes or vapours, or materials in the workplace. However, lower levels of contamination may occur in residential settings, particularly in older homes with lead paint or old lead plumbing.

As with any other potentially toxic agent, a risk assessment is necessary if exposure to heavy metals and trace elements is likely to occur. The main difference with risk assessment of trace elements compared with other toxic agents is the need to consider the minimum amounts that may be necessary for health, in addition to the levels that may be toxic.

Toxic heavy metals with no beneficial effect should be considered as any other toxic substance and, where possible, tolerable daily intakes should be identified, or in the case of genotoxic compounds for which we assume no threshold, exposure should be kept as low as reasonably practicable (see Box 1). This is also true for lead for which the general assumption is that there is no threshold for the adverse effects of lead on the developing nervous system, which may occur in the developing foetus during pregnancy or during infancy or early childhood.

The following sections contain a brief introduction to the toxicity of some of the more common heavy metals.

## 3    Lead

Lead is not required as a trace element in the body. The harmful effects of lead have been recognised for centuries and have even been reported as a contributing factor to the downfall of the Roman Empire. Lead does not have any specific historical medicinal purpose, although it has been used as an ingredient in cosmetic products.

Lead is present in both inorganic and organic forms. Lead has an affinity for bone and acts by replacing calcium. It is deposited in growing bone and will accumulate with repeated exposures. Ingested lead is absorbed at increased levels in children, which makes children more sensitive to the toxic effects of lead than adults: in children, 40% of ingested lead is absorbed, whereas only 5–15% is absorbed by adults (HPA, 2007). Approximately 50–90% of inhaled lead enters the blood. Children under three years are especially vulnerable because they absorb lead more effectively than adults and usually have greater exposures because of their exploratory behaviour and frequent hand-to-mouth activity. As the developing nervous system in children is much more vulnerable to damage than the nervous system in adults, pregnant women are also a high-risk group. Lead follows similar metabolic pathways to calcium in the body, so can pass through the placenta, and infants can also be exposed during lactation.

The toxicology of lead is summarised in the Health Protection Agency (HPA) Compendia of Chemical Hazards Series (HPA, 2007); the summary of the health effects is given below.

## 3.1  Toxicity of lead

Lead is classically a chronic or cumulative toxic substance. Few adverse health effects are observed following an acute exposure at low dose levels. Acute effects including gastrointestinal disturbances (loss of appetite, nausea, vomiting, abdominal pain), neurological effects (encephalopathy, malaise, drowsiness), hepatic and renal damage and hypertension have been reported.

Chronic lead exposure may cause anaemia, basophilic stippling (presence of many blue-staining granules within red blood cells) and decreased haemoglobin synthesis. Neurological effects may also be observed such as fatigue, sleep disturbance, headache, irritability, lethargy, slurred speech, convulsions, muscle weakness, ataxia, tremors and paralysis.

Epidemiological studies in children have shown an inverse relationship between blood lead concentrations above 10 µg/dl and intelligence quotient (IQ). There is some evidence that even lower exposures are also harmful, and it is therefore assumed that there is no completely harmless level of exposure to lead.

Nephropathy (kidney disease) and renal tubule dysfunction (dysfunction in the tubules of the filtering units – nephrons – in the kidney) may arise following chronic lead exposure. Hepatic damage has been reported in a few cases only, following occupational exposure to lead. Gastrointestinal disturbances such as nausea, vomiting, anorexia, constipation and abdominal cramps have also been observed in workers.

Chronic exposure to lead may cause adverse effects on both male and female reproductive functions. Females may experience spontaneous abortion, stillbirths or low birth weight following occupational exposure before or during pregnancy. Males may experience reduced libido, have low semen volumes and sperm counts along with a decrease in sperm motility.

Occupational exposure to lead has been reported to cause an increase in sister chromatid exchange and chromosomal aberrations, although such increases were not observed in environmentally exposed children.

Based on epidemiological and experimental data, the Working Group of the International Agency for Research on Cancer concluded that inorganic lead compounds are probably carcinogenic to humans (Group 2A) (IARC, 2006).

## 3.2   Legislation of lead

The high toxicity of lead has been recognised for many years and has led to a raft of policies to reduce exposures wherever reasonably practical over the past two decades. The elimination of lead in petrol has been of critical importance, though there are concerns about the resultant increased use of benzene, a recognised carcinogen, to sustain high octane ratings, however legislation (in 2000) reduced the maximum amount of benzene in petrol to 1%.

Lead is banned in cosmetics in the EU and any cosmetics marketed in the UK containing lead are illegal, but, nevertheless, they are sometimes brought into the UK from abroad for personal use, so shouldn't be ruled out as a possible source of exposure.

Legislation controlling the marketing and use of lead in paint in the UK came into force in 1992 with the Environmental Protection (Controls on Injurious Substances) Regulations. However, voluntary agreements between the Paintmakers' Association (now called the British Coatings Federation) and the UK Government initially came into being in 1963 (revised in 1974). Under this accord, paints which contained more than 1% of lead in dry film had to be labelled with a warning that they were not to be used on surfaces accessible to children. In practice, however, the UK paint industry had begun to replace its use of white lead (lead carbonate/lead sulphate) in the 1950s with alternatives, such as titanium dioxide, which were technically superior and also considered less hazardous. In the 1960s, lead-drying agents also began to be phased out, along with coloured lead pigments in decorative paints, so that ordinary paints in the UK were virtually lead-free from the 1960s. Some very limited uses of lead did continue, such as in thin primer paints on some prefabricated domestic wooden windows up to the 1980s, and in products intended for professional use. The Lawther Working Party for the then Department of Health and Social Security estimated in its 1980 report that lead-based paints accounted for less than 3% of the current market.

The occupational use of lead is strictly governed by the Control of Lead at Work Regulations 2002 and the Health and Safety at Work (etc.) Act 1974.

The use of lead water supply pipes is no longer permitted in new dwellings, or in repairs to old systems. In areas with a plumbosolvent public water supply (water that is able to dissolve lead), grants have been available from local authorities for the removal of old pipe-work, though these have usually been means-tested and therefore of limited impact.

As a result of these efforts, blood-lead levels in the UK have fallen dramatically in recent decades and surveys indicate that the great majority of UK children are now well below the target level for blood-lead of 10 micrograms per decilitre (µg/dl), set by the international Miami Declaration on Children's Environmental Health, which the UK signed in May 1997.

It is reasonable to expect further reductions in blood-lead levels, as older legislation continues to have an effect and newer actions, such as lowering limits for lead in drinking-water, are introduced. However, it is important to note that the 10 µg/dl level does not denote a concentration at which lead poisoning begins, rather it is a target to minimise the possibility of harm to populations at risk. Indeed recent evidence suggests that some intellectual impairment may occur at levels below 10 µg/dl. The underlying assumption is that no exposure to lead is completely harmless and the aim is therefore to reduce exposure wherever reasonably practicable.

The Housing Act 2004 introduced a new system for rating the 'fitness' of housing. The system is used by local authority environmental health practitioners to secure the remediation of hazards, including domestic lead exposure, such as from old paintwork and lead water pipes. However, the removal of lead paintwork can itself present hazards – from paint dust and vapours from the use of paint-stripping hot air guns. Advice on safe removal is given in a DEFRA advice sheet (DEFRA, 2005).

## 4     Zinc

Zinc is a good example of an essential trace element. It was reviewed by the Expert Group on Vitamins and Minerals in their report *Safe Upper Levels for Vitamins and Minerals* (EVM, 2003).

Meat and cereals are good sources of zinc in the diet. The Committee on Medical Aspects of Food Nutrition and Policy (COMA) has set a Reference Nutrient Intake (RNI) for zinc. An RNI is the amount of nutrient that is enough or more than enough for most (usually at least 97%) of people in a group; if the average intake in this group is at the RNI then the risk of deficiency in the group is very small. The RNI for zinc is 5.5–9.5 mg/day for men and 4.0–7.0 mg /day for women (COMA, 1991).

Zinc is essential as it is a constituent of more than 200 enzymes and is necessary for cell division. Zinc deficiency is associated with a range of adverse effects including poor prenatal development, mental retardation, impaired conduction of impulses in nerves, reproductive failure, dermatitis (inflammatory disorders of the skin), hair loss, diarrhoea, loss of appetite (anorexia), anaemia, susceptibility to infection, delayed wound healing, and macular degeneration (change in the eye which affects vision).

## 4.1    Toxicity of zinc

Symptoms of acute toxicity caused by over-exposure to zinc may include abdominal pain, nausea and vomiting, lethargy, anaemia and dizziness.

Prolonged use of high doses of zinc can result in secondary deficiency of copper, which gives rise to a wide range of effects. These include hypocupraemia (reduced copper content in the blood) and impaired iron mobilisation.

Changes in the blood also occur due to deficiencies in copper, including anaemia, leucopaenia (decreased white cells in the blood), neutropaenia (a decrease in neutrophils – a specific type of white blood cell), increased plasma cholesterol and an increased low density lipoprotein to high density lipoprotein (LDL:HDL) cholesterol ratio . The increase in LDL:HDL ratio is considered harmful as low density lipoproteins are associated with heart attacks, whereas high density lipoproteins are considered protective against heart attacks.

Other toxic effects associated with zinc-related copper deficiency include decreased erythrocyte superoxide dismutase activity, decreased cytochrome C oxidase activity, decreased glucose clearance (decreased removal of glucose in the blood by the kidneys), decreased amount of methionine, decreased leucine enkephalins, abnormal cardiac function and impairment of the pancreatic enzymes: amylase and lipase.

Acute toxicity occurs in humans after oral doses of 200mg of zinc or more. The most sensitive indicator of zinc toxicity is the reduction in copper absorption, measured through effects on the copper-dependent enzyme erythrocyte superoxide dismutase. Repeated daily exposure to 50 mg for several weeks results in effects on this enzyme and a reduction in haematocrit (the blood test which measures the content of cells to volume of plasma) and serum ferritin levels. Doses greater than 100 mg per day have resulted in an altered ratio of LDL:HDL cholesterol. This may be why excess zinc is considered atherogenic, i.e. able to cause the formation of lipid deposits within the lumen of arteries.

The Expert Group on Vitamins and Minerals recommended a safe upper level for daily consumption of 25 mg zinc/day for supplemental zinc (EVM, 2003).

### Metal fume fever

Under occupational exposure conditions, inhalation of zinc compounds (mainly zinc oxide fumes) can result in a condition referred to as 'metal fume fever'. Metal fume fever's unique symptoms have been described in welders/metal workers since the early 19th century. It is an acute, self-limited syndrome characterised by a delayed onset (4–12 hours) after exposure to welding fumes. Symptoms tend to resolve spontaneously in 24–48 hours and treatment is generally supportive and non-interventional. The precise underlying disorders are not known with certainty, and metal fume fever can occur either following the first exposure to metal fumes or after repeated exposures. There is a tendency for attacks to be worse at the beginning of the working week – hence the popular name Monday Morning Fever (Greenberg *et al.*, 2003).

The clinical features of metal fume fever are irritation of the nasal passages, cough, abnormal sounds in the lungs (known as rales) when breathing is heard through a stethoscope, reduced lung volumes, increased rate of breathing (hyperpnoea) and an alteration in the ability of gases to diffuse across the lung to the blood (as detected by carbon monoxide diffusing capacity test), headache, altered taste, fever, weakness, sweating, pains in legs and chest and increases in white blood cells (leukocytosis).

Although metal fume fever occurs in occupationally exposed workers, it is essentially an acute reversible disorder which is unlikely to occur under chronic exposure conditions, when the Workplace Exposure Limit for zinc chloride fumes is 1 mg/m$^3$ over an 8 hour period (HSE, 2005).

Inhalation of zinc chloride may also result in irritation of the nose and throat, shortness of breath (dyspnoea), cough, chest pain, headache, fever, nausea and vomiting. There may be changes in the lung tissues: fibrosis of the lung or inflammation of lungs (pneumonitis).

## 5    Mercury

Mercury has in the past been used as an ingredient in diuretics, antibacterial agents, antiseptic skin ointments, laxatives and hair conditioning agents, and has been used in dentistry for many centuries. Mercurous (calomel) salts were also historically used as a purgative. Mercuric salts (e.g. mercuric chloride) were used as disinfectants and because of their high solubility and acute toxicity, have been used as homicidal agents.

Mercury exists in three forms: organic, inorganic and elemental:

### *Organic mercury*
Organomercury compounds such as methyl mercury are a particular environmental concern because of their formation through the methylation of inorganic mercury by microorganisms in aqueous environments. Methyl mercury is accumulated in the aquatic food chain and the mercury concentrations in predatory fish (e.g. shark, swordfish) are of particular concern to public health (see Chapter 3.5 on food contaminants). Organic mercury is readily absorbed through the gastrointestinal system into the systemic circulation and readily crosses the blood brain barrier; it is concentrated in the brain as well as the kidney, liver, hair and skin. Organic mercury also readily crosses the placenta.

Organic mercury compounds may have significant volatility and may be readily absorbed by inhalation and through the skin as well as orally.

### *Inorganic mercury*
Inorganic mercury, as found in batteries, is absorbed from the gastrointestinal tract, however it is poorly lipid-soluble and only around 10% of an ingested dose would be absorbed. Once absorbed, inorganic mercury is concentrated in the kidney tissues. Inorganic mercury compounds do not in general pose a significant risk by the inhalation route as they are not encountered in a respirable form.

### Elemental mercury

Elemental mercury, as present in mercury thermometers, is not absorbed through the intact gastrointestinal tract to any significant extent, nor through the skin. However, elemental mercury vapour is readily absorbed by inhalation.

Mercury poisoning may often be misdiagnosed as the symptoms are non-specific and insidious in nature. The gastrointestinal system, the nervous system and the kidneys are the most common organ systems affected following mercury poisoning.

The toxicology of inorganic and elemental mercury is summarised in the HPA Compendia of Chemical Hazards Series (HPA, 2007); the summary of the health effects is given below.

## 5.1    Toxicity of mercury

Following an acute exposure to elemental mercury vapour via inhalation, respiratory effects such as cough, dyspnoea (shortness of breath), chest tightness, bronchitis and decreased pulmonary (lung) function may occur. Cognitive, personality, sensory or motor disturbances may also arise, including tremor, irritability, hallucinations, muscle weakness and headaches. Due to the accumulation of mercury in the kidneys, acute renal failure indicated by proteinuria (passage of proteins in the urine), haematuria (passage of blood in the urine) and oliguria (passage of reduced amounts or volumes of urine) is commonly reported. Acute inhalation of elemental mercury may also cause gastro-intestinal effects such as stomatitis (inflammation of the mouth), abdominal pain, vomiting, diarrhoea and ulceration of the oral mucosa, as well as cardiovascular effects such as hypertension (high blood pressure) and tachycardia (increase in heart or pulse rate).

Inorganic mercury compounds are highly irritating to the gastro-intestinal tract and an acute ingestion may cause a metallic taste, abdominal pain, vomiting, diarrhoea and necrosis of the intestinal mucosa, possibly leading to circulatory collapse and death. Ulceration of the mouth, lips, tongue and gastro-intestinal tract may also occur. If patients survive damage to the gastro-intestinal tract, acute renal failure may occur within 24 hours of ingestion. Hypertension and tachycardia have also been reported following ingestion of inorganic mercury compounds.

Acute dermal exposure to elemental mercury vapour can cause erythematous (reddish) and pruritic (itchy) skin rashes, reddening and peeling of skin on palms of hands and soles of feet associated with acrodynia, and contact with soluble inorganic mercury compounds may cause irritation, vesiculation and contact dermatitis.

Chronic exposure to elemental mercury vapour via inhalation may cause neurotoxicity such as decreased psychomotor skills (skills requiring co-ordinated thinking and muscle activity) and neuropsychological symptoms including fatigue, tremor, headaches, depression, irritability, and hallucinations. Nephrotoxicity (toxicity to the kidney) including proteinuria and increased urinary enzyme excretion was observed following occupational exposure to elemental mercury, as well as stomatitis (inflammation of the mouth), sore gums and ulceration of the oral mucosa.

Following chronic ingestion of inorganic mercury compounds, irritability, weakness, insomnia (inability to fall asleep), muscle twitching, swollen gums, excess salivation, anorexia and abdominal pain may occur.

There is little convincing evidence that exposure to mercury causes chromosomal damage or other mutagenic effects. IARC have classified elemental mercury and inorganic mercury compounds as category 3 carcinogens, i.e. not classifiable as carcinogenic to humans (IARC, 1997a).

Conflicting evidence regarding the incidence of spontaneous abortion following inorganic mercury exposure has been presented. Some studies have reported a higher incidence of reproductive failures (spontaneous abortions, still births, congenital malformations) and irregular, painful and haemorrhagic menstrual disorders in occupationally exposed women compared to unexposed women.

### Toxicity of mercury dental amalgams

The toxicity of mercury from dental amalgams is a contentious issue. The views of the Committee on Toxicity of Chemicals in Food, Consumer Products and the Environment (COT) were first sought on this issue in 1986. At that time, the Committee recognised that some mercury may be released from completed dental restorations but was of the opinion that the use of dental amalgam is free from risk of systemic toxicity and that only a very few cases of hypersensitivity may occur (COT, 1986).

The Committee when asked for further advice in 1997, particularly regarding any nephrotoxic or neurotoxic effects arising from dental amalgams, concluded that:

- their former conclusions regarding lack of systemic toxicity and only very few cases of hypersensitivity should remain unchanged.

- nephrotoxicity (toxicity to the kidney) was not associated with exposure of healthy subjects to mercury amalgam from dental restorations. Also, the Committee considered that neurotoxicity (toxicity to the nervous system) caused by exposure to mercury vapour was a matter of greater concern in the occupational setting than in dental patients.

- there was no available evidence to indicate that the placement or removal of dental amalgam fillings during pregnancy was harmful. The Committee was of the opinion, however, that the toxicological and epidemiological data were inadequate to assess fully the likelihood of harm occurring in such circumstances. Until appropriate data were available, they concurred with the view that it may be prudent to avoid, where clinically reasonable, the placement or removal of amalgam fillings during pregnancy.

- further research in a number of areas was recommended (COT, 1997).

## 6    Arsenic

Arsenic is the heavy metal (or metalloid, as it has properties of both metals and non-metals) that has been arguably responsible for the largest number of individuals affected by an environmental chemical. Chronic arsenic poisoning from drinking water has been a threat to approximately 70 million people in Bangladesh and 45 million in West Bengal. Similar health hazards have been reported to exist in Nepal, Thailand, Taiwan, China, Mexico and some other countries in South America. The World Health Organization (WHO) guideline for arsenic content in well water is 10 µg/l.

Historically, arsenic compounds were commonly used as medications for various disorders such as syphilis, acne, malaria and anaemia. In addition, arsenic has been used as a poison since the 15th century and was considered the 'perfect poison' because it is odourless, tasteless, and resembles sugar. Fowler's solution of 1% potassium arsenite was used for over 150 years for the treatment of various ailments including psoriasis, rheumatism, asthma, cholera and syphilis. Arsenicals are still used in the treatment of African trypanosomiasis (sleeping sickness) and in the treatment of rare forms of leukaemia.

Arsenic exists in both organic and inorganic forms. The organo-arsenicals are mainly found in marine organisms or as metabolites in the detoxification pathway in mammals. The Food Standards Agency estimate that the average daily intake of arsenic is 65 µg in the UK, mostly from fish, and that the bulk of this is in the form of organo-arsenicals (DEFRA and EA, 2002). Organo-arsenicals are less toxic than the inorganic compounds and are not considered further in this review.

Soluble inorganic arsenic compounds are well-absorbed following ingestion. Arsenic binds to specific groups of chemicals which are essential for enzyme function, e.g. sulphydryl groups, and thus the activity of many enzymes in the body is inhibited. Hence, very few organs escape the toxic effects of arsenic. Arsenic also replaces inorganic phosphorus in enzymes and thus prevents certain metabolic reactions (e.g. inhibits oxidative phosphorylation).

The toxicology of inorganic arsenic compounds is summarised in the HPA Compendia of Chemical Hazards Series (HPA, 2007); the summary of the health effects is given below.

### 6.1    Toxicity of inorganic arsenic compounds

Single doses of inorganic arsenic may be highly toxic by ingestion and inhalation (70–180 mg orally has been fatal). Trivalent arsenic is, in general, more toxic than pentavalent arsenic.

Inorganic arsenic is a known human carcinogen which acts via a genotoxic mechanism. It is assumed, therefore, that there is no threshold for such effects and that risk management measures should ensure that exposures are prevented whenever possible or, otherwise, kept 'as low as reasonably practicable' (see Box 1 for more on the concept of 'ALARP'). There is sufficient evidence that chronic exposure to inorganic arsenic in drinking water causes non-melanoma skin cancers and an increased risk of bladder and lung cancers in humans.

The effects of inorganic arsenic on the peripheral blood vessels are well documented. Long-term ingestion of contaminated drinking water may lead to Raynaud's phenomenon and acrocyanosis and progression to endarteritis obliterans and gangrene of the lower extremities ("Black foot disease"). An increased incidence of cardiovascular disease has also been noted. Haematologically, anaemia and leucopaenia may occur together with disturbances in haem synthesis.

Chronic exposure to inorganic arsenic compounds may lead to peripheral and central neurotoxicity. Early events may include paraesthesia followed by muscle weakness. In the periphery, both motor and sensory neurones are affected. Characteristic dermal lesions after chronic oral or inhalation exposure may include hyperpigmentation and hyperkeratosis.

Other toxic effects associated with chronic exposure to inorganic arsenic include liver injury, cardiovascular disease and diabetes mellitus.

There is limited data from epidemiology to suggest that inorganic arsenic may be a human developmental toxicant, but it is not possible to draw any definitive conclusions. Administration of high doses of inorganic arsenic by oral, intraperitoneal or intravenous routes may cause embryo-lethality or foetal malformations in laboratory animals.

Inorganic arsenic may cause irritation of the mucous membranes leading to conjunctivitis and pharyngitis and rhinitis after inhalation. Skin irritation and allergic contact dermatitis may occur after exposure to inorganic arsenic compounds.

## 7    Thallium

Thallium is used in small quantities industrially in the production of special glasses used in the electrical and electronics industry. In the past it was used as a rodenticide. Thallium compounds have also been used in suicides and homicides.

Thallium compounds are highly toxic if inhaled, ingested or absorbed through the skin (IPCS, 1996). Following ingestion, the onset of gastrointestinal symptoms may occur after 12–48 hours. These include nausea, vomiting, metallic taste in the mouth, hypersalivation, retrosternal and abdominal pain. Systemic features occur 2–5 days post exposure, the main effects being, in addition to gastroenteritis, a polyneuropathy characterised by numbness around lips, paraesthesia of fingers and toes becoming severe and spreading to arms and legs, and paralysis eventually affecting all muscles. Hair loss (alopecia) occurs at 10–15 days. Death is usually from cardio-respiratory failure and often occurs 10 to 12 days post exposure, although with very high doses death may occur within 24 hours.

An important fact about thallium is that the first systemic symptoms do not occur until 2–5 days post ingestion, though gastro-intestinal symptoms (stomach pains, diarrhoea, vomiting) may occur from 12 hours.

The neurological effects of thallium are believed to be due to impairment of the action of the Na/K pump (the mechanism by which exchange of the ions sodium and potassium occurs in cells), since the affinity of thallium for the enzyme sodium/potassium ATPase is 9–10 times that of potassium.

The characteristic effects of thallium poisoning are often considered the triad gastroenteritis, polyneuropathy and alopecia, but in some cases gastroenteritis and alopecia are not observed (IPCS, 1996).

## 8    Aluminium

Aluminium is the third most prevalent element and the most abundant metal in the earth's crust. Aluminium in the diet is therefore ubiquitous, with very small amounts in food and water, the WHO drinking water standard being 0.2 mg/l The main intakes other than diet are from the use of aluminium-based antacids (grams consumed) and to a lesser extent from aluminium compounds in toothpastes.

Aluminium compounds are poorly absorbed orally and have low acute toxicity by this route. There is some evidence of neurotoxicity following repeated oral exposure in animals particularly when given by injection. Osteomalacia (softening of the bones) has also been produced at high exposure levels. Studies in animals and other experimental systems indicate that aluminium compounds do not have any significant mutagenic or carcinogenic effects or effects on the reproductive system.

It has been suggested that aluminium ingestion may be a risk factor for the development of Alzheimer's disease and impaired cognitive function (thinking) in the elderly, and a large number of studies have investigated this concern (IPCS, 1997). However consideration of all the data from mechanistic studies and from epidemiology suggests that aluminium exposure does not cause Alzheimer's disease or non-specific impaired cognitive function (IPCS, 1997).

Patients with chronic renal failure necessitating prolonged dialysis (a process which takes over the failing kidney's functions regarding waste, salt and fluid removal) for many months are at special risk from the neurotoxic effects of aluminium. This may cause 'dialysis encephalopathy', or a form of osteomalacia or microcytic anaemia (anaemia associated with red blood cells smaller than normal). These effects can be prevented by ensuring that the dialysis water contains less than 30 micrograms of aluminium per litre or by using deionised water.

Possibly the best known environmental toxic episode associated with aluminium in the UK was the Lowermoor incident. In July 1988, 20 tonnes of aluminium sulphate solution was discharged into the wrong tank at the Lowermoor water treatment works in North Cornwall. The total amount of aluminium added in the incident was 850 kg.

Aluminium sulphate is used in the water treatment process as a flocculant to bind suspended solid matter and dissolved organic acids in the raw water before filtration, so some aluminium is usually present in drinking water. The maximum permitted level is 0.2 mg/l. However, following the Lowermoor incident, levels up to 109 mg/l were recorded in the water supply system by the Water Authority and levels up to 720 mg/l were reported in samples taken by private individuals.

The acidity of the contaminated water was sufficient to cause corrosion of metallic plumbing materials, storage tanks and other fittings, leading to the release of increased amounts of copper, zinc, iron and, in some cases, lead into the water supply. Flushing of the mains distribution system to remove the contaminated water resulted in the disturbance of old mains sediments containing iron and manganese oxides and, in some cases, possibly lead and lead salts, which resulted in higher than usual amounts in the water at the tap.

A number of acute effects were reported after the incident by individuals who drank the contaminated water. These included mouth ulceration, skin irritation and gastrointestinal effects such as diarrhoea and abdominal pain. The gastrointestinal effects are almost certainly attributable to the contaminated water, which was reported as tasting very unpleasant. Although the recorded pH values of the water after the incident were not low enough to cause the cases of skin irritation reported, it may be that high concentrations of sulphate and metal salts rendered the water more irritant than would be anticipated from its pH alone.

A number of chronic symptoms have also been reported, including impaired memory, joint pains and/or swelling, tiredness/lethargy, and problems with coordination and concentration. A number of expert groups have been convened by Government over the years to investigate whether chronic effects such as these are likely to have resulted from exposure to the contaminants released during the incident. Full details are given in the draft report of the Committee on Toxicity of Chemicals in Food Consumer Products and the Environment's Subgroup Report on the Lowermoor incident (COT, 2005).

Inquiries to date have concluded that there is no evidence that harmful accumulation of aluminium has occurred, nor that the prevalence of ill-health among those exposed to the contaminated water is greater than usual. The latest enquiry report is due to be published in 2008.

## 9    Chromium

Chromium was reviewed by the Expert Group on Vitamins and Minerals in their report *Safe Upper Levels for Vitamins and Minerals* (EVM, 2003).

Chromium is a trace element that can exist in a number of oxidation states, the trivalent and the hexavalent being the most important biologically. The trivalent form is ubiquitous in nature whilst hexavalent chromium compounds are man-made and do not occur naturally. Chromium in foodstuffs and as food supplements is in the trivalent form with the highest levels in processed meats and whole-grain products.

COMA has not set RNIs for chromium, but has suggested that an adequate level of intake of trivalent chromium lies above 0.025 mg/day for adults and between 0.0001 and 0.001 mg/kg/day for children and adolescents. COMA also noted that no adverse effects were observed at intakes of trivalent chromium of 1000mg–2000 mg per day (COMA, 1991).

Trivalent chromium has been shown to potentiate insulin action and thereby influences carbohydrate, lipid and protein metabolism.

Although referred to as an essential trace element, in humans, deficiency has only been observed in patients on long-term parenteral nutrition (feeding by the intravenous route). The symptoms observed were impaired glucose tolerance and glucose utilisation, weight loss, neuropathy, elevated plasma fatty acids, depressed respiratory quotient and abnormalities in nitrogen metabolism.

In contrast to trivalent chromium, hexavalent chromium has no beneficial effects. It is much more toxic than the trivalent compound and is a mutagen and a carcinogen (see below).

Trivalent chromium compounds are poorly absorbed orally (0.5–2.0%) and absorbed material does not enter blood cells but binds to plasma proteins such as transferrin and is transported to the liver. In contrast, hexavalent chromium does penetrate red blood cells where it is reduced by glutathione to trivalent chromium, which binds to haemoglobin. Excess hexavalent chromium is taken up into the kidneys, spleen, liver, lungs and bone.

There is only limited data on the oral toxicity of trivalent chromium compounds although this appears to be low because of the poor absorption. The Expert Group on Vitamins and Minerals felt unable to derive a Safe Upper Level for trivalent chromium. However, based on one repeated-dose study in the rat where no effects were seen at 15 mg/kgbw/day, they did for guidance purposes suggest a value of 0.15 mg/kgbw/day (EVM, 2003). No recommendations were possible for hexavalent chromium and as this has both mutagenic and carcinogenic properties it is not possible to derive a safe exposure level.

The toxicology of chromium compounds is summarised in the HPA Compendia of Chemical Hazards Series (HPA, 2007); the summary of the health effects is given below.

## 9.1    Toxicity of chromium compounds

The toxicity of chromium depends on the oxidation state, chromium (VI) being more toxic than the trivalent form chromium (III). In addition, chromium (VI) is the more readily absorbed by both inhalation and oral routes.

The respiratory tract is the primary target for inhaled chromium following acute exposure, although effects on the kidney, gastrointestinal tract and liver have also been reported.

Acute ingestion of high doses of chromium (VI) compounds, the exact quantity of which is not usually known, results in acute, potentially fatal, effects in the respiratory, cardiovascular, gastrointestinal, hepatic, renal, and neurological systems.

Due to the corrosive nature of some chromium (VI) compounds, dermal exposure can lead to dermal ulcers. At high doses, systemic toxicity leading to effects on the renal, haematological and cardiovascular system and death has been reported.

Studies of the effects of chronic occupational exposure to chromium compounds have proven difficult due to co-exposures to other toxic substances in the relevant working environments. Occupational exposure to some inhaled chromium (VI) mists may cause nasal septal ulceration and perforation, respiratory irritation and inflammation, dyspnoea, cyanosis, and gastrointestinal, hepatic, renal, haematological effects and lung cancer. Chronic exposure to chromium (VI) compounds can also cause allergic responses (e.g. asthma and allergic dermatitis) in sensitised individuals. Chronic exposure to chromium (III) results in weight loss, anaemia, liver dysfunction and renal failure.

Chromium (VI) compounds are positive in the majority of *in vitro* mutagenicity tests reported and may cause chromosomal aberrations and sister chromatid exchanges in humans. The mechanism of genotoxicity has been proposed to be a result of sequential reduction of chromium (VI) within the cells to chromium (III) and the binding of chromium (III) to macromolecules, including DNA.

Chromium (III) is not considered to be mutagenic in most cellular systems and there is no firm evidence that *in vivo* it is mutagenic to humans or experimental animals. Studies have not shown chromium (III) to be carcinogenic.

Chromium (VI) has been classified as a Group 1 known human carcinogen by the inhalation route of exposure and chromium metal and chromium (III) compounds are not classifiable as to their carcinogenicity to humans (Group 3) due to inadequate evidence in humans (IARC, 1997b).

Potassium dichromate may be toxic to the reproductive system and the developing foetus. There is insufficient evidence to suggest that chromium (III) compounds are reproductive or developmental toxicants.

## 10    Copper

Copper was reviewed by the Expert Group on Vitamins and Minerals in their report *Safe Upper Levels for Vitamins and Minerals* (EVM, 2003).

Copper is an essential trace element, being involved in the function of certain enzymes such as cytochrome C oxidase, amino acid oxidase, superoxide dismutase and monoamine oxidase. Clinical features include anaemia, neutropaenia and bone abnormalities. Less frequent signs and symptoms include hypopigmentation of the hair, hypertonia (increased tone of muscles), impaired growth, increased susceptibility to infection, abnormalities in metabolism of glucose and cholesterol and cardiovascular changes.

COMA has set a RNI for copper of 1.2 mg/day (COMA, 1991).

Food is the major source of copper intake with particularly high concentrations found in nuts (8 mg/kg), shellfish and offal (40 mg/kg).

Copper sulphate is used as a fungicide, an algaecide and in some fertilisers.

The absorption of copper is kept under tight homeostatic control in the body to prevent accumulation of excessive amounts. Where dietary levels are high, absorption is reduced and, in particular, biliary excretion is increased. Copper toxicity only occurs when these defences are overwhelmed.

## 10.1 Acute toxicity

Acute copper toxicity is rare in humans but can occur from contamination of food or drink. The emetic properties (tendency to induce vomiting) and unpleasant taste of copper salts mitigate against frequent accidental or deliberate ingestion. Signs of acute toxicity include salivation, epigastric pain, nausea, vomiting and diarrhoea. Intakes in the range 25–75 mg have been quoted as emetic doses but individual susceptibility varies and lower intakes may produce effects if taken on an empty stomach. Intakes of above about 100 g copper sulphate produce intravascular haemolysis (breakdown of red blood cells), acute hepatic failure, acute tubular renal failure, shock, coma and death.

## 10.2 Chronic toxicity

There are insufficient data in humans to assess the chronic toxicity of copper and only limited data in animals. Studies in human volunteers suggest that daily doses of 7.5–10 mg copper in food or supplements are not associated with adverse effects. In animals, there is marked species variability, with copper salts being relatively well tolerated in pigs and rats, but in sheep, copper toxicosis develops at low dietary intakes.

Copper compounds are believed not to have any significant mutagenic or carcinogenic properties. Reproductive effects have been reported in laboratory animals but these findings were not consistent.

The Expert Group on Vitamins and Minerals used a well conducted subchronic toxicity study in the rat to derive a safe upper limit of exposure. In this study the no observed adverse effect level (NOAEL) was 16 mg/kg bw/day. Higher dose levels resulted in damage to the fore-stomach, kidney and liver. This was divided by an Uncertainty Factor of 100 to give the Safe Upper Exposure level. The recommended safe upper exposure level was set at 0.16 mg/kg bw/day (EVM, 2003).

**11     References**

CIS. (1999) Chapter 7: Metals. *Basics of Chemical Safety.* International Occupational Safety and Health Information Centre (CIS), International Labour Organization, Geneva. Available at: www.ilo.org

COMA. (1991) Committee on Medical Aspects of Food and Nutrition Policy: Dietary Reference Values for Food Energy and Nutrients for the UK. HMSO, London.

COT. (1986) Statement on Dental Amalgam prepared for the Committee on Dental and Surgical Materials. Committee on Toxicity of Chemicals in Food, Consumer Products and the Environment.

COT. (1997) Statement on the toxicity of dental amalgam. Committee on Toxicity of Chemicals in Food, Consumer Products and the Environment. Available at: http://www.food.gov.uk/multimedia/pdfs/committee/cotstatementdentalamalgam1997

COT. (2005) Subgroup Report on the Lowermoor Water Pollution Incident. Lowermoor Subgroup, Committee on Toxicity of Chemicals in Food, Consumer Products and the Environment. Available at: http://cot.food.gov.uk/

DEFRA and EA. (2002) TOX1 Arsenic. *Contaminants in soil: collation of toxicological data and intake values for humans.* Department for Environment, Food and Rural Affairs and the Environment Agency. Available at: http://www.environment-agency.gov.uk/commondata/acrobat/tox1_arsenic_675423.pdf

DEFRA. (2005) Restoration methods and safe working. Advice on lead in old paint – Advice Sheet 3, last updated 16 August 2005. Department for Environment and Rural Affairs. Available at: http://www.defra.gov.uk/environment/chemicals/lead/

EVM. (2003) Safe Upper Levels for Vitamins and Minerals. Expert Group on Vitamins and Minerals (EVM). Available at: www.food.gov.uk

Ferner DJ. (2001) Toxicity, heavy metals. *eMed J* 2(5): 1.

Glanze WD. (1996) *Mosby Medical Encyclopedia.* Rev. edition. Signet, New York.

Greenberg MI, Hamilton RJ, Phillips SD, McCluskey GJ. (2003) *Occupational, industrial and environmental toxicology.* 2nd edition. Mosby, Pennsylvania.

HPA (2007) *Compendium of Chemical Hazards* series. Available at: www.hpa.org.uk

HSE (2005) *EH40/2005 Workplace exposure limits.* Health and Safety Executive, HMSO, London.

IARC (1997a) Beryllium, Cadmium, Mercury, and Exposures in the Glass Manufacturing Industry. *IARC Monographs* Volume 58. International Agency for Research on Cancer, France.

IARC. (1997b) Chromium, Nickel and Welding. *IARC Monographs* Volume 49. International Agency for Research on Cancer, France.

IARC. (2004) Arsenic in drinking water. *IARC monographs* Volume 84. International Agency for Research on Cancer, France.

IARC. (2006) Inorganic and Organic Lead Compounds. *IARC Monographs* Volume 87. International Agency for Research on Cancer, France.

IPCS. (1996) Thallium. *Environmental Health Criteria* No 182. International Programme on Chemical Safety, World Health Organization, Geneva. Available at: www.inchem.org

IPCS. (1997) Aluminium. *Environmental Health Criteria* No 194. International Programme on Chemical Safety, World Health Organization, Geneva. Available at: www.inchem.org

Lide DR. (ed.) (1992) *Handbook of Chemistry and Physics.* 73rd edition. CRC Press, Boca Raton.

Roberts JR. (1999) Metal toxicity in children. In: *Training Manual on Pediatric Environmental Health: Putting It into Practice.* Children's Environmental Health Network, California, US. Available at www.cehn.org

Smith SR, Jaffe DM, Skinner MA. (1997) Case report of metallic mercury injury. *Pediatr Emer Care* 13(2): 114–116.

# Section 4.3

# The toxicology of pesticides

Timothy C Marrs, Lakshman Karalliedde

## Learning outcomes

At the end of this chapter and any recommended reading the student should be able to:

1. define and classify pesticides, and explain the common terminology of the toxicology of pesticides;

2. define and classify insecticides, describe the various types and the main toxic effects of each type, e.g. organochlorines, organophosphorus compounds, pyrethrins and synthetic pyrethroids;

3. discuss insecticides of biological origin other than pyrethrins and nicotine;

4. define and classify fungicides, describe the various types and the main toxic effects of each type;

5. define and classify herbicides, describe the various types and the main toxic effects of each type;

6. define and classify rodenticides and molluscicides and discuss their main toxic effects, and

7. apply their knowledge in the analysis and management of hazardous situations.

## 1    Introduction

The World Health Organization estimates that poor environmental quality contributed to 25% of all preventable ill-health in the world during the past decade. Traditional problems such as contaminated water, poor sanitation, smoky indoor air and exposure to mosquitoes and other animal disease vectors are still the primary environmental factors in ill-health. Across the world, insufficient water supplies, inadequate sanitation and poor hygiene are primarily responsible for global outbreaks of cholera and other diarrhoeal diseases. Diarrhoeal diseases account for 17% of deaths among children under five years worldwide or nearly two million deaths per year (UNICEF, 2007).

Vector-borne diseases affecting more than 700 million in total a year are considered the most sensitive to climate and environmental conditions. Malaria, the best known vector-borne disease, affects more than 500 million people in 90 countries causing 1.1–2.7 million deaths a year, mostly among children under five years of age (UN Millennium Project, 2005).

In the control of vector-borne diseases such as malaria, insecticides have been an invaluable tool that have contributed significantly to the control and, in some instances, the eradication of some vector-borne diseases. Insecticides are a part of the group of substances called pesticides.

However, pesticides, and insecticides in particular (being not completely selective in their toxicity to pests and vectors), have caused 3.5–5 million acute poisonings per year and globally are associated with over 250,000 deaths (WHO, 2006).

Suicide by intentional ingestion of pesticides is a continuing tragedy in developing countries. In rural China, pesticides account for over 60% of suicides. Similarly high proportions of suicides are due to pesticides in rural areas of Sri Lanka (71%), Trinidad (68%) and Malaysia (90%) (Gunnell and Eddleston, 2003; WHO, 2006).

In contrast, occupational acute pesticide poisonings in agricultural workers in less developed countries is 1–4% of the several million cases of occupational injuries and ill-health in agricultural workers worldwide (Litchfield, 2005).

## 2    Definition and a description of pesticides

Pesticides are substances designed to kill unwanted living organisms. Pesticides, and insecticides in particular, have a vital role in killing organisms which affect the production and storage of food, and also in killing insects that transmit diseases (vectors of disease) including malaria. The organisms against which the pesticides are used are referred to as target species. Pesticides are also used on animals to free them of, for example, maggots in sheep, and then such agents may be classified and regulated as veterinary medicines.

Of the pesticides, insecticides in particular achieve their effects by attacking the unprotected nervous system of insects or by altering the metabolism or structures involved in the metabolic processes and/or development of the target species. Unfortunately, many pesticides are not specific in their attack in that they can cause considerable ill-health in humans.

Insecticides are often sprayed on to vegetables and fruits to prevent these food stuffs from being destroyed by insects. They are also used in cotton growing to preserve the quality of the cotton and prevent damage. Human exposure to pesticides may occur whilst pesticides are used in agriculture, including sheep dipping, and are described as occupational exposures.

The main concerns associated with human health are the possible presence of harmful amounts of pesticides in food, safety of individuals using pesticides in agriculture and the use of pesticides with suicidal intent. Protection of exposed individuals can be achieved by removal from the source of exposure and decontamination, and the use of personal protective equipment (PPE) during use. Guidelines for safe storage and disposal are being addressed regularly to improve operator and environmental safety and attempts have been made to find optimal regimens of treatment for poisoned patients and effective antidotes.

## 3     Classification of pesticides

Pesticides may be classified on the basis of their use as follows:

- insecticides
- fungicides
- herbicides
- molluscicides
- rodenticides.

## 4     Insecticides

Insecticides are a large group of pesticides and may be divided on the basis of their chemical structure and mode of action as follows:

- organochlorine compounds, e.g. DDT
- anticholinesterase agents, e.g. organophosphorus compounds, carbamates
- pyrethrins and synthetic pyrethroids
- neonicotinoid compounds
- others.

### 4.1   Organochlorine compounds

Organochlorine compounds such as DDT (dichloro-diphenyl-trichloroethane) and the 'drins' – aldrin, dieldrin and endrin – and related insecticides such as lindane (γ-hexachlorocyclohexane) and endosulfan primarily cause toxicity to the nervous system. This is due to these insecticides interfering with the function of sodium channels (see basic concepts of medicine in appendix for more details) which are needed to function normally for transmission of nerve impulses and for normal activity of the nervous system.

Due to the toxic effects they produce, humans may suffer from tremors, coordination problems (especially with DDT) and convulsions (especially from the 'drins').

Another dangerous aspect associated with this group of insecticides is that they are very persistent, i.e. not easily biodegradable, and therefore they do not break down to non-toxic compounds easily. They tend to persist in human fat and are excreted in the breast milk.

As they are persistent in the environment, they pose a long-term threat to human health.

There have been diverse concerns about ill-health in man attributed to or associated with the use of organochlorine compounds. These concerns, though contentious to date, together with concerns of their persistence in, and effects on, the environment, have resulted in the banning of some compounds, for example organochlorine insecticides such as DDT and the 'drins' in the European Union. There have also been suggestions that exposure to organochlorines may be associated with an increase in the incidence of breast cancer in humans, but detailed consideration of the data indicated that there was no convincing evidence that organochlorine insecticides were associated with the development of breast cancer (COC, 2004).

However, DDT was very effective in destroying mosquitoes, the insects that transmit malaria and the banning of DDT was associated with an increase in the incidence of malaria in several developing countries. Therefore, DDT is still used in some countries to protect public health. Mosquitoes also transmit other infectious diseases such as dengue fever and yellow fever.

## 4.2    Anticholinesterase agents – e.g. organophosphorus and carbamate insecticides

Acetylcholine is a transmitter (chemical messenger) both in the central nervous system and the peripheral nervous system (see basic concepts of medicine in appendix for more details). It is a transmitter in the brain and the only known transmitter at autonomic ganglia, at the post ganglionic nerve endings of the parasympathetic nervous system and some post-ganglionic fibres of the sympathetic nervous system and at the skeletal neuromuscular junctions.

The action of acetylcholine is limited in time and space by the enzyme acetylcholinesterase, which hydrolyses it or inactivates it so that resting nerve activity is restored quickly after the passage of a nerve impulse and is ready to respond to another nerve impulse.

This state is markedly disturbed when acetylcholinesterase is inhibited – it is made inactive by a process called phosphorylation, and can no longer hydrolyse and thereby inactivate acetylcholine. As a result, acetylcholine accumulates at all the sites where it is the neurotransmitter and this accumulation causes several well defined and some undefined clinical syndromes and features.

The main syndromes that follow inactivation of acetylcholinesterase by organophosphorus insecticides and, for that matter, by all organophosphorus compounds that inhibit this enzyme, which includes the chemical warfare agents or nerve agents tabun, sarin and soman are:

1. The acute cholinergic syndrome which follows almost immediately after exposure, where there are increased secretions from all salivary and tear glands (lacrimation), urination, defecation and gastric emesis (SLUDGE) and usually slowing of the heart rate (bradycardia), muscle fasciculations and constriction of the pupils (pin point pupils).

2. The intermediate syndrome which sets in after the acute cholinergic syndrome where there is muscle weakness, particularly of the muscles involved in breathing (muscles of respiration) without fasciculations.

Both these conditions are life threatening and subjects who have been exposed to a large amount of organophosphorus compound(s) often require treatment in an intensive care unit. They also require procedures discussed in Chapter 2.2 on the medical management of chemical incidents such as decontamination, prevention of further exposure, resuscitation and administration of antidotes such as atropine. If the patient survives the initial management, recovery is almost always complete with the acute cholinergic syndrome and the intermediate syndrome.

These organophosphorus insecticides also produce a third syndrome which is not related in any way to inhibition of acetylcholinesterase. This condition, which is not life-threatening, causes weakness of peripheral muscles in the limbs, i.e. the hands and feet. It is a delayed polyneuropathy (organophosphate-induced delayed polyneuropathy, OPIDP), which is attributed to inactivation of the enzyme neuropathy target esterase in the nerve. Unfortunately, recovery from OPIDP is often incomplete and OPIDP causes long-term morbidity. Not all organophosphorus insecticides cause OPIDP. Thus those causing OPIDP are classed as neuropathic organophosphates and they cause a similar weakness or paralysis in hens. It is possible to test for such effects in a toxicity study in the hen and all organophosphates approved for use as pesticides in the UK have been evaluated as negative in this test.

Carbamates produce an identical clinical picture as they too inhibit acetylcholinesterase but the binding of the carbamate to the enzyme is much weaker and thus the duration of inhibition is much shorter. Carbamates do not cause the intermediate syndrome and OPIDP-like muscle weakness.

Some examples of organophosphorus insecticides are chlorpyrifos, dichlorvos, mala-thion (used widely in control of malaria at present), parathion, diazinon and disulfoton. Some OPs, e.g. trichlorfon (under the name metrifonate), are used in tropical medicine.

The related organophosphorus compounds which are grouped as nerve agents used in chemical warfare are discussed in Chapter 4.5 on chemical warfare agents.

## 4.3   Pyrethrins and synthetic pyrethroids

Pyrethrins are natural products of pyrethrum plants (particularly from the flowers of *Tanacetum cinerariaefolium*, a plant of the chrysanthemum family). Synthetic pyrethroids are synthetic analogs that are more stable in sunlight (photostable). These substances are all of low toxicity to humans when taken orally or following dermal exposure. However, they are very toxic to fish.

These agents are broadly grouped into two types on the basis of their parenteral toxicity to rodents. Type 1 are those that produce tremors, for example permethrin and pyrethrins. Type II are those that produce salivation and choreoathetosis (involuntary movements of limbs and fingers), for example deltamethrin, flumethrin and cypermethrin. While of interest to mechanistic toxicologists, these syndromes are of no relevance to the toxic effects in humans, which are largely confined to paraesthesia.

## 4.4   Neonicotinoid compounds

Nicotine and the neonicotinoids (e.g. imidacloprid) also target cholinergic transmission (transmission where acetylcholine is the key chemical messenger or neurotransmitter).

## 4.5   Others

Other insecticides include avermectin, abamectin and Derris which interfere with other chemical messengers (such as gamma aminobutyric acid) or with transport of electrons.

# 5   Fungicides

Fungicides are substances that kill fungi on plants or on wood. The main groups are as follows:

- Metallic fungicides, e.g. copper sulphate used on grape vines (Bordeaux mixture), mercurous chloride and organometals such as methyl mercury sulphate (inorganic and organic mercury compounds were used in the past and have been banned for several years), organotins (fentin), organocopper compounds and organozinc compounds. These are made fat soluble by the process called organification and hence cross over to the brain (cross the blood brain barrier) and most cause toxicity to the nervous system. Some of these compounds can also interfere with the immune system.

- Phenolic fungicides such as pentachlorophenol are acutely toxic and interfere with metabolic processes within the body and may give rise to an increase in body temperature, liver and kidney failure and cause dehydration (lack of fluid in the body). A related compound dichlorophen however has very low oral and repeated dose toxicity. Some have caused cataracts (opacities in the lens of the eye). These have been used in the past as wood preservatives.

- Azole fungicides such as hexaconazole, penconazole and tebuconazole are used in agriculture and horticulture and in human and veterinary medicine. They inhibit some metabolic functions in the fungi (e.g. sterol synthesis). In humans they can affect the liver, thyroid and blood. However, they are well tolerated as drugs for humans.

# 6   Herbicides

Herbicides are substances that kill plants (e.g. weeds) with variable degrees of specificity. The best known are the bipyridilium compounds paraquat and diquat. These are non-selective herbicides, unlike some herbicides which are selective for plants with broad leaves. These compounds are toxic, especially paraquat, which can cause death in humans by toxicity to the small air cells or alveoli in the lungs. Paraquat causes an acute inflammation of lung cells and alveoli which leads to fibrosis of lung tissue and there is no known effective treatment to date. Lethal cases have almost all been the result of ingestion of the agricultural concentrate usually with suicidal intent. Depending on the dose, death occurs up to three weeks after exposure from respiratory failure. If large doses are ingested, death may occur within 24 hours of ingestion.

The local effects of paraquat ingestion are sore throat, pharyngitis, loss of voice (aphonia), eye damage and skin damage. There is no known antidote.

Diquat does not cause lung injury and the organ most affected by diquat is the kidney, with overdoses resulting in kidney failure.

Glyphosate and glufosinate are organophosphoros compounds which are used as herbicides that have no significant anticholinesterase activity.

- Glyphosate kills plants by inhibiting the pathway by which plants produce amino acids. Glyphosate is not very toxic to humans or mammals because the pathway affected by them for the synthesis of amino acids is not present in man. Large doses may cause stomach or gastric irritation, low blood pressure (hypotension) and poor lung function (pulmonary insufficiency). These toxic effects are thought to be due to the other constituents in the formulations and not due to glyphosate itself.

- Glufosinate also affects the synthesis of amino acids in plants. However, the pathway affected by glufosinate is also present in man and overdoses cause toxicity of the nervous system (neurotoxicity) leading to convulsions or fits and tremors.

There are several other herbicides (aniline compounds such as alachlor, propachlor and propanil; triazines such as atrazine and simazine; and triazoles such as amitriole, diuron and linuron). The phenoxy herbicides such as 2,4-dichlorophenoxyacetic acid (2,4-D) are selective for broad leaved plants; their toxic effects include alterations in consciousness, decreased tone of the muscles, metabolic acidosis (increased acidity of the blood), muscle fasciculation and coma. If the urine is made alkaline, there may be increased loss of this herbicide from the body.

## 7    Rodenticides and molluscicides

The rodenticides are substances used to destroy or inhibit the action of rats, mice, or other rodents. Many such substances have been identified. Of particular note are the warfarins and coumarins which act by preventing the clotting of blood. When taken by humans the toxic effects of these are similar and prolonged bleeding disorders usually result. Molluscicides, such as metaldehyde and methiocarb, are used to kill slugs and snails.

## 8    Conclusions

Pesticides are a trade-off between plant health and human health. Human health risk is kept low by an elaborate system of pre-marketing approval. There are rigid guidelines set by health authorities which permit only amounts considered safe for humans to be found as residues on food products. There are also guidelines for users of pesticides in the occupational setting.

## 9    References and bibliography

Ballantyne B, Marrs TC. (1992) *Clinical and experimental toxicology of organophosphates and carbamates*. Butterworth-Heinemann, Oxford.

Bismuth C, Hall AH. (Eds.) (2005) Paraquat poisoning: Mechanisms, Prevention, Treatment. *Drug and Chemical Toxicology* 10. M Dekker Inc, New York.

COC. (2004) Breast cancer risk and exposure to organochlorine insecticides: consideration of the epidemiology data on dieldrin, DDT and certain hexachlorocyclohexane isomers. Committee on Carcinogenicity of Chemicals in Food, Consumer Products and the Environment, Department of Health, UK. Statement COC/04/S3.

Gunnell D, Eddleston M. (2003) Suicide by intentional ingestion of pesticides: a continuing tragedy in developing countries. *J Epidemiol* 23: 902–909.

Hayes WJ, Laws ER. (1991) *Handbook on Pesticide Toxicology*. Volume 1, General Principles. St Louis, Missouri, U.S.A. Academic Press.

Karalliedde L, Feldman S, Henry JA, Marrs TC. (Eds.) (2003) *Organophosphates and Health*. Imperial College Press.

Litchfield MH. (2005) Estimates of acute pesticide poisoning in agricultural workers in less developed countries. *Toxicological Reviews* 24: 271–278.

UN Millennium Project. (2005) Coming to grips with malaria in the new millennium. Task Force on HIV/AIDS, Malaria, TB, and Access to Essential Medicines, Working Group on Malaria, New York.

UNICEF. (2007) Diarrhoeal diseases. *Progress for Children: A World Fit for Children Statistical Review*. Edition 6.

Whitehead R. (Ed.) (2003) *The UK Pesticide Guide*. British Crop Protection Council, Farnham and CABI Publishing, Wallingford.

WHO. (2006) *Pesticides are a leading suicide method*. World Health Organization, Geneva.

# Section 4.4

# Toxicology associated with traditional medicines

Lakshman Karalliedde

---

### Learning outcomes

At the end of this chapter and any recommended reading the student should be able to:

1. discuss the use of traditional medicines, including the growing market in western cultures;

2. explain the concerns and issues associated with traditional medicines;

3. explain the potentially harmful constituents of herbal medicines, including heavy metals, allopathic medicines, toxic plants and plant constituents, animal and human body parts, and pesticides;

4. discuss the herbal traditional medicines to be avoided by vulnerable population groups, e.g. pregnant women, breast feeding mothers, the elderly, the immuno-suppressed;

5. evaluate policies and regulatory systems for traditional medicines, and

6. apply their knowledge in the analysis and management of hazardous situations.

---

## 1    Introduction

The World Health Organization (WHO) defines traditional medicine as 'health practices, approaches, knowledge and beliefs incorporating plant, animal and mineral based medicines, spiritual therapies, manual techniques and exercises applied solely or in combination to treat, diagnose and prevent illnesses or maintain well-being' (WHO, 2003a).

Traditional medicines have and continue to provide an accessible and affordable form of health care in most developing countries of the world.

Of the forms of traditional medicines in use today, Chinese, Ayurveda and Unani (South Asian) medicines are probably the best known as they are used by extremely large populations in China and the Indian subcontinent. Traditional medicines were developed for several thousands of years before the birth of Christ in Egypt, Mesopotamia and Persia (Iran) and were documented by Greek and Roman scientists and physicians. In addition, communities in all parts of the world ranging from South America (the Incas) to Africa and to the Pacific islands have been using forms of medical practice developed by their communities to manage ill-health, poisonings and envenoming (e.g. snake bite, scorpion bite).

Despite the much publicised and scientifically researched benefits of conventional Western (allopathic) medicine, more and more of those living in developed countries such as the United Kingdom (UK) and United States (US) are using traditional medicines today (WHO, 2003b). Estimates suggest that over 50% of the population in developed countries use some form of traditional medical practice at least once during their life times, either in addition to, or instead of conventional medicine. For example, in the US, the Commission for Alternative and Complementary Medicine estimate that approximately 160 million adults are believed to use traditional medicines, spending US$ 17 billion in year 2000 on over 1500 herbal medicines (WHO, 2003a).

The Archives of Internal Medicine reported in 2006 that in the US 21% of adult prescription medication users reported using non vitamin dietary supplements (which includes herbal medicines) and that 69% of those did not discuss this use with a conventional medical practitioner (Gardiner *et al.*, 2006).

A survey among European Union Member States identified about 1400 medicinal plants used in the European Economic Community in 1991. Sales of herbal medicines in the European Union amounted to US$ 6 billion in 1995. The annual national growth rates are 5–22% in Western European countries (Zhang, 1999).

In the UK, a study of Scottish prescription data for 1,891,669 patients in 2003–2004, revealed that 49% of General Medical Practices prescribed homeopathic remedies and 32% of practices prescribed herbal remedies (Ross *et al.*, 2006).

A publication in the British Medical Journal (Waxman, 2006) estimated 'that up to 80% of all patients with cancer take a complementary treatment or follow a dietary programme to help treat their cancer'.

Worldwide, WHO estimates that 70% of the population of Canada and 49% of the population of France have tried complementary or alternative medicine, which often includes herbal remedies (WHO, 2003b). In Japan, 85% of doctors prescribe not only allopathic medicine but also traditional herbal medicine (called Kampo) which is covered by health insurance (Dharmananda, 2003). If patients suffering from a single specific disease state, e.g. HIV/AIDS, are considered, some form of traditional medicine, predominantly of plant origin, is likely to be used by 75% of them, an estimate that is similar for patients in San Francisco, London and South Africa (WHO, 2003b).

As expected, herbal remedies continue to be the first choice of health care in many developing countries. In Africa for example, up to 80% of the population depend on herbal medicines, according to WHO estimates (WHO, 2003a).

One of the key reasons for increased use in developed countries is the generally accepted perception that 'natural' products are safe, have 'stood the test of time' and do not carry the risks inherent in newly developed conventional medicines. There is insufficient awareness that the ingredients that make traditional medicines effective may also be capable of causing serious illness such as allergy, liver or kidney malfunction, blindness, cancer or even death. Herbal medicines should be used with the same degree of caution as conventional medicines but this is difficult given the lack of information available about effectiveness, optimum dose, or adverse effects.

What is important and significant from a health protection perspective and in Public Health is that with the surge in immigration, communities are bringing with them their traditional medical practices. This has the potential to cause difficulties in diagnosis and management by allopathic practitioners in the developed countries to which they have migrated. For example, reports from many Poisons Centres in the US illustrate the difficulties and the numbers of certain migrant populations that have been affected by adverse effects of traditional medicines brought from their countries of origin (Haller *et al.*, 2002). Even in Taiwan, where traditional medicines have been in use for centuries, a Poison Control Centre reported experiencing difficulties in managing patients with poisonings associated with Chinese traditional medicines (Deng *et al.*, 1997).

Thus information, at least on the potential dangers of traditional medicines and herbal medicines in particular, has become a necessity for the provision of appropriate and adequate health care to communities in both developed and developing countries.

## 2    Concerns and issues associated with traditional medicines

Safety and efficacy are major issues associated with any form of medical practice and it is important to be familiar with the issues that influence the safety of traditional medicines, particularly herbal medicines.

The issues are:

1. The presence of intrinsically toxic constituents to which a patient may be exposed whilst using herbal medicines.
2. The potential for adulteration and contamination of herbal products and possible adverse health effects that may result.
3. The disadvantages or dangers of delays in seeking allopathic medical care that may be caused by firstly using herbal medicines that may be of doubtful efficacy for a particular disease state.
4. The vulnerability of some specific population groups to adverse effects of herbal medicines. These include pregnant women, breast feeding mothers, infants and older people and people suffering from some medical conditions that are well-defined in the allopathic medical literature. Such population groups should avoid using herbal preparations or take them only under close supervision.
5. The dangers to patients of not revealing their use of herbal medicines to allopathic practitioners who may prescribe allopathic medicine prior to surgical interventions and investigations or to treat disease. The interaction of allopathic medicine with herbal medicine could render the

allopathic medicine ineffective or could cause life-threatening adverse effects. Herbal medicines have caused complications following surgical operations especially when their use has not been revealed to the surgical and anaesthetic staff.

The rapidly increasing use and growing popularity of traditional medicines in developed countries is intriguing and is to some extent being stimulated by increasing scientific interest in herbal medicine. WHO estimates that of the 35,000–70,000 species of plants that are used for medicinal purposes around the world, only 5,000 have been submitted to biomedical scrutiny (personal communication Shaw). Scientific evidence of efficacy is beginning to emerge from randomised controlled trials in which herbs compare favourably with placebo. Evidence is emerging for herbs such as *St John's Wort* used for mild depression, *ginkgo biloba* used for some forms of dementia, *saw palmetto* used for benign prostatic hyperplasia and *horse chestnut* used for chronic venous insufficiency. Of course, a number of commonly used pharmaceuticals are of botanical origin – aspirin, digoxin and quinine being three well-known examples.

Other concerns relating to traditional herbal medicines are:

1. The therapeutic/toxic constituent/s of the plant may vary in amount due to geographical variations, stage of maturity of the plant or plant component and/or improper storage.
2. Contamination with toxic or harmful elements such as heavy metals may occur during preparation.
3. There may be huge variations in the concentrations of ingredients used in medicines prepared by different manufacturers or at different times and in the potency of those ingredients.
4. Practitioners or manufacturers may deliberately incorporate allopathic medications which may be banned in some countries or are only available on prescription from an allopathic practitioner in developed countries.
5. The labelling of some herbal medicines may be inaccurate, both in indicating the constituents and the amounts of the constituents used, which may be compounded by the fact that the labelling may be in a language not familiar to users or the local medical practitioners.
6. Socio-cultural, religious and other factors may result in different therapeutic regimens or dosages of very similar herbal medicines being used for a particular disease state.
7. There is seldom any biochemical or physiological evidence of the efficacy of a herbal medicine on a disease state.
8. Although many countries have systems for monitoring adverse reactions to herbal medicines, for example, the yellow card system in the UK, adverse effects of many herbs are poorly documented. This is despite encouragement to medical practitioners – both of allopathic medicine and of traditional medicine – and to patients to report adverse effects using the yellow card. Other compounding factors are manufacturers of unlicensed products not complying with normal safety monitoring requirements. In addition, adverse effects may not be attributed to a herbal medicine where the patient had not told their doctor that they

are using such products. Even when an adverse symptom is correctly attributed to use of a herbal product, the identity and the quantity of the constituents may be uncertain.

9. There is less stringent regulation of herbal medicine practitioners when compared to allopathic practitioners. Although schemes for training and assessment of competence and knowledge for the practice of herbal or traditional medicine are being introduced or are already in use in many countries, there are no internationally accepted standards.

The preparation, distribution and marketing of traditional medicines are largely unregulated (though this is changing in some countries). Although many of the issues listed above make it difficult to regulate herbal medicines and practitioners, it is disappointing that there has been so little progress in implementing regulation in those countries such as the UK which have had well-developed systems for regulating allopathic medicines and practitioners in place for decades. Health authorities need to develop guidelines and analytical facilities to ensure safety of imported herbal medicines and to develop mechanisms to monitor and assess the practice of traditional medicines. The publication in the BMJ (Waxman, 2006) suggests 'that the alternative medicines industry should be subject to the level of scrutiny that defines pharmaceuticals'. The author Dr Waxman, goes on to suggest reclassifying these agents as drugs – for this is after all how they are marketed – and that in this context, the current EU initiative to bring forward legislation on this matter is welcomed. The current regulatory situation in the UK is discussed in the following section.

## 3    Regulation of traditional medicines in the UK

Whereas effective and extensive legislation exists for the import and use of allopathic medicines (by the Medicines and Healthcare products Regulatory Agency) and food (Food Standards Agency), there is currently only weak regulation of traditional medicines in the UK. Traditional herbal medicines sold or made available in the UK are not tested unless there has been report of ill-health or some other reason for concern.

The Medicines and Healthcare products Regulatory Agency (MHRA) are developing and implementing several measures to ensure the safety of traditional medicines. These are numerous and varied in nature. The MHRA have identified three possible routes by which a herbal remedy can reach a consumer in the UK:

1. Unlicensed herbal remedies: Products which do not have to meet specific standards of safety and quality and may not be accompanied by the necessary information for safe use, such as contraindications and safety warnings. However, by April 2011 all manufactured herbal medicines will be required to have either a traditional herbal registration or a product licence.

2. Registered traditional herbal medicines: A simplified registration scheme. The Traditional Medicines Registration Scheme began on 30th October 2005. This ensures that products meet specific standards of safety and quality and have information on usage based on traditional usage and

systematic patient information. Thus this regulatory measure informs users of the indications for use.

3. Licensed herbal medicines: These herbal products have a product licence or the authority to market like any other medicine which indicates that considerations such as safety, quality and efficacy have been scrutinised and the guidelines for safe use by consumers are available. Such products can be identified by a distinctive nine digit (distinctive nine digit Product Licence (PL) number) Product Licence (PL) number on the product container or packaging which is prefixed by the letters PL.

It is necessary to emphasise that products made available with no or unconfirmed details of all constituents and the quantities present of each constituent, often in languages which cannot be read by consumers or medical practitioners, are most likely to cause ill-health, which would be difficult for health professionals to diagnose and treat effectively.

More information on the regulation of traditional medicines can be found on the MHRA website.

## 4    Potentially harmful constituents of herbal medicines

Diverse potentially toxic or harmful constituents have been identified in samples of herbal medicines (Ernst, 2002; Ko, 1998; Steenkamp *et al.*, 2000). These include:

- heavy metals (e.g. lead, mercury, cadmium, arsenic, silver)
- allopathic medications – prescription only and over the counter medications
- toxic plant constituents (e.g. alkaloids and whole or parts of toxic plants)
- animal and human body parts
- pesticides.

### 4.1    Heavy metals

One of the earliest published cases of heavy metal poisoning due to the use of a traditional medicine was in 1975 (Tay and Seah, 1975). Since then there have been a large number of such poisonings published.

A survey of 5,536 exposures to traditional medicines and food supplements reported to the National Poisons Unit in London from January 1983 to March 1989 and in 1991 included 657 (12%) reports of symptomatic cases and five confirmed cases of heavy metal poisoning resulting from use of contaminated traditional remedies (Perharic *et al.*, 1994). The same Unit reported 12 cases of poisoning with lead, arsenic or mercury between 1991 and 1995, nine of which were associated with herbal remedies from India, and three with use of Indian cosmetics (Shaw *et al.*, 1995).

In 1988, traditional medicines were found to account for nearly 16% of all acute poisoning in Pretoria, South Africa and the associated mortality was 15% (Venter and Joubert, 1988).

In 2005, a review from the UK found 31 published cases of poisoning by lead, arsenic, mercury and magnesium resulting from the use of Indian traditional medicines (Lynch and Braithwaite, 2005). The reports came from the UK, USA, Canada, Australia, India, Israel, Germany, Netherlands, and Qatar. 71% of these patients were of an Indian ethnic origin and 10% were of white ethnic origin. The patients' ages ranged from 9 months to 70 years.

## 4.2    Allopathic adulterants

### 4.2.1   Prevalence of allopathic adulterants

Prevalence of allopathic medicines in herbal preparations has been of particular concern in Asian countries with large Chinese populations.

The Taiwanese Food and Drugs Administration reported that 30% of the antirheumatic and analgesic herbal products that they sampled contained allopathic drugs including paracetamol, aminopyrine, caffeine, chlormezanone, chloroxazone, diazepam, diclofenac, ethoxybenzamide, hydrochlorothiazide, ibuprofen, indometacin, ketoprofen, mefenamic acid, papaverine, phenylbutazone, piroxicam, prednisolone and salicylamide (NLFD, 1991). Aminopyrine and phenylbutazone are no longer prescribed in the UK.

Another study in Taiwan analysed 2,609 samples and found that 26% contained at least one adulterant (Huang *et al.*, 1997). The most common adulterants included caffeine, acetaminophen, indometacin, hydrochlorothiazide, prednisolone, chlorzoxazone and ethoxybenzamide. Several of these medications could cause serious adverse side effects resulting in fatal or debilitating medical disorders.

In Hong Kong, the Government Laboratory carried out 65,748 tests on Chinese medicines in 2004 (GovHK, 2004). Many of the proprietary Chinese medicines on sale for treatment of obesity and impotence caused the most concern. They were found to contain sidenafil, tadalafil, sibutramine and N-nitrosofenfluramine. The problem appears to be increasing: the number of Chinese proprietary samples for the treatment of obesity and impotence submitted to the laboratory for analysis increased six fold between 2003 and 2004.

In Malaysia in 1991, 83% (25 out of 30) of anti-arthritis preparations seized from Chinese medicine shops contained phenylbutazone (an aspirin-like anti-inflammatory drug) in amounts ranging from 0.6–198 mg per pill or capsule. "Black pills" for arthritis known as "Zhui Feng Tou Gu Wan" or "Black Pearls" have also been reported to contain phenylbutazone (Ries and Sahud, 1975).

Adulteration is a widespread practice and has been reported from Australia, Belgium, Canada, The Netherlands, New Zealand, UK and USA. In 1999, 8 out of 11 Chinese herbal creams available in London for treatment of eczema, were found to contain dexamethasone at concentrations inappropriate for use on the face or in children (Keane *et al.*, 1999). The 1998 Californian survey of imported Asian patent medicines revealed that of the 257 products that were analysed for pharmaceuticals, 17 products contained pharmaceuticals that were not declared on the label (most commonly ephedrine, chlorpheniramine, methyltestosterone and phenacetin) (Chan, 2003).

In India, 38% of 120 samples of alternative medicines that had been dispensed to patients suffering mainly from asthma and arthritis were found to be adulterated with steroids (Gupta *et al.*, 2000).

### 4.2.2    Dangers of allopathic adulterants

The rather complex combinations of allopathic and traditional herbal medicines could lead to one or more of the following scenarios:

1. The herbal drug being taken in excess of the prescribed dose or for an extended duration leading to the safe dose of the allopathic constituents being unknowingly exceeded.
2. The herbal medicine containing an amount of allopathic medication capable of producing toxic or adverse effects.
3. Exposure to the allopathic constituent within the herbal medicine exacerbating the disease state for which the herbal medicine is taken.
4. Harmful interaction(s) occurring between the allopathic constituent in the herbal medicine and allopathic medicine(s) prescribed by a general practitioner or other allopathic medical practitioners.
5. An undeclared allopathic constituent of a herbal medication producing a complication or adverse effect, the diagnosis of which being delayed or completely missed, resulting in severe ill health. This is particularly so in long-term consumers of herbal medicines.

In 1975 a subject who was taking Chinese herbal medicines for the relief of arthritis and back pain developed agranulocytosis (dangerously low levels of neutrophils, cells that protect against infections) and life-threatening infections with bacterial sepsis resulting in death (Tay and Seah, 1975). The herbal medicines were shown to contain substantial amounts of undeclared aminopyrine and phenylbutazone, drugs that are well known causes of agranulocytosis.

Slimming agents in particular have caused severe liver disease including liver failure due to the allopathic constituent (Corns, 2002).

Inclusion of animal and human products in traditional herbal medicines can have two possible consequences. Firstly, they may transmit infections to the user. For example, the ingredients of Nu Bao include human placenta (*Placenta hominis*), deer antler (*Corna cervi pantotrichum*) and donkey skin (*Colla cori astin*), which are potential sources of bacteria and viruses that could cause infection.

Secondly, some constituents that are used medicinally are potentially toxic, where the toxin is part of the medicine. For example, venom extracted from skin glands of certain species of toads (*Bufo marinus, Bufo alvarius*) is used in some aphrodisiacs and some other Chinese medications (e.g. chan su). The venom contains bufotoxins, which have similar molecular structure and pharmacological effects as digoxin. These preparations can cause symptoms and clinical findings very similar to digitalis overdose and toxicity (e.g. persistent nausea and vomiting, light headedness, slowing of the heart rate, palpitations, insomnia, seeing yellow halos around lights) and have led to dangerous alterations in heart rhythm and even death.

## 4.3    Toxic plants and toxic constituents of plants

Some plants have always been known to be toxic to man and even to cause death. These naturally occurring toxins present in plants are commonly referred to as phytotoxins. Whilst most of the information on the toxicity of plants remains anecdotal, studies on toxic components of plants have also resulted as a result of serious 'unexplained' adverse effects in agricultural livestock or when similar disease processes do occur in groups of humans who have received a particular form of herbal treatment. For example, the occurrence of kidney disease or liver disease in groups of patients who had received a particular form of herbal treatment, has at least within the past three decades provoked or 'kick-started' study of toxic constituents of herbs.

Obviously, concentrations of the toxic constituents in herbal preparations are an important consideration. The presence of a toxic component does not always imply that an adverse effect would follow intake. Thus concentrations of the toxic component, the dosages of the herb taken and the duration of intake are all important factors in the discussion of toxicity of plants.

For example, with herbal teas and honey, the amount or frequency of consumption is important. The fact that large quantities may be consumed over a long period is an important factor in the toxicity.

Toxicological studies on herbal teas have been limited. It is possible that some herbal teas, during the course of their preparation or formulation may lead to concentration of some toxic constituents. This would of course be true of water soluble toxic constituents.

Of the known toxic constituents of plants, arguably the best known are the pyrrolizidine alkaloids. Other toxic constituents belong to the chemical classes such as glycosides, glycoalkaloids, saponins and psoralens. An important consideration is that some biologically inactive toxic constituents or phytotoxins may become toxic following metabolism in the human body. Further, some constituents may have the potential to cause changes in genes (mutagenicity) or cancers (carcinogenicity).

In addition, some plants such as soya and peanut contain allergens. Also, there is a possibility that some plants may have chemicals that alter the secretion and function of hormones in the body which are then referred to as endocrine disruptors.

According to Chan and Critchley (1996), preparations containing aconite, podophyllin or anticholinergics are the cause of nearly all serious poisonings associated with plant constituents of herbal medicines in Hong Kong.

As an example of target organ toxicity, some effects on the kidney are listed below:

- **Herbs with direct renal toxicity:** Many traditional medicines and foods especially in the tropical regions of Africa and Asia contain plants that can cause renal toxicity. One of the better known plants is the djenkol bean. A traditional remedy in South Africa called "Impila", made from the roots of *Callilepis laureola*, has marked liver and kidney toxicity.

- **Herbs that cause kidney toxicity due to oxalic acid content:** Some herbs high in oxalic acid content such as rhubarb and star fruit may increase the formation of kidney stones.

- **Herbs that cause changes in electrolyte (e.g. sodium and potassium) exchange in the kidney:** Licorice root in high doses for prolonged periods causes retention of sodium, which has the potential to increase blood pressure, and a loss of potassium, which leads to hypokalaemia and possibly symptoms such as muscle weakness. It also increases the toxicity of allopathic drugs such as digoxin.

- **Herbs with high potassium content:** The juice from the noni fruit (*Morinda citrifolia*) can cause an increase in blood and body potassium due to its high potassium content. Dandelion, stinging nettle, horsetail and alfalfa are also high in potassium.

- **Herbs that cause an increase in volume of urine (diuresis):** Juniper berry, parsley, dandelion, horse tail, asparagus root, lovage root, golden rod, uva ursi, stinging nettle leaf and alfalfa have been used traditionally as diuretics. These drugs should be used cautiously by patients who have compromised kidney function, particularly by those patients who require frequent renal dialysis.

- **Herbs in patients with renal transplants:** The success of renal transplants could be compromised by drugs such as St John's Wort, which decrease the effectiveness of immuno-suppressants such as ciclosporin. Echinacea is an immune system modulator and caution is required in patients using immuno-suppressants.

**Sources:** Karalliedde and Gawarammana, 2007.

## 4.4    Pesticides and other toxic contaminants – animal and human body parts

Samples of green tea recently analysed have proven to be contaminated with DDT and DDT-like pesticide Dursban, raising concerns about tea's possible role in the development of breast cancer (Barbee, 2006). Even though the association between breast cancer and DDT is contentious at best (see chapter on pesticides), this illustrates the presence of pesticides in herbal preparations.

In a recent publication (Tagami *et al.*, 2008), 56 pesticides were detected in natural medicines with a simple rapid sample preparation method.

The 2004 Annual Report of the Government Laboratories in Hong Kong reported that about 1% of the Chinese herbal medicine samples were found to contain levels of pesticides that were of concern (GovHK, 2004). Contamination with pesticides such as quintozene and hexachlorobenzene may have resulted from improper use of pesticides during cultivation or from environmental pollution. In early 2004, some ginseng powder products imported from Taiwan were found to be contaminated with organochlorine pesticides. Since then, all ginseng powder products imported from Taiwan have been screened for the presence of pesticide residues. Contamination of ginseng was also reported in 2002 on the ConsumerLab.com website. Of the 21 ginseng products tested, two had levels of pesticides 20 times more than allowed levels (Aschwanden, 2001).

Cumin is commonly used in Egypt for childhood coughs, aches or itching. A sample of seeds purchased from a local Egyptian market was found to contain the organophosphorus insecticide profenfos at a concentration of 0.37 g/kg which was nearly twice the residue the WHO and Codex Alimentarius Commission permit in vegetables (Karalliedde and Gawarammana, 2007). This finding was of concern as children's low body weights may make them vulnerable to the toxicity from the pesticide.

In the UK, DEFRA's *SID 5* project developed the following techniques for assay of pesticides in food products/nutrients (DEFRA, 2005). Analytical methods based on rapid extraction/dispersive SPE cleanup were successfully developed and validated for the quantitative confirmation of 50 pesticides in curry powder and 40 pesticides in chilli powder at 0.5 mg/kg. For most of the remaining pesticides, the recovery data indicated that the methods were suitable for screening purposes. The validation data obtained for the pesticides requested by the Pesticide Safety Directorate (carbendazim, methomyl, methamidophos, monocrotophos and procymidone) showed that all were validated in curry powder, and either validated or considered suitable for screening in chilli powder. A combination of GC-MS/MS and LC-MS/MS is required for comprehensive analysis and monitoring of all of the pesticides in spices.

The methods described represent a significant advance in the multi-residue deter-mination of spices and should be suitable for the analysis of pesticides in spices for future PRC monitoring purposes. The results obtained demonstrate that the methodology is suitable for the purpose of enforcing the proposed EU MRL for ethofumesate in spices. The results obtained suggest that the methodology is also suitable for the detection of most of these pesticides at 0.1 mg/kg, but further work is required to achieve validation of all analytes at or below that level.

The methodology has been shown to give good recovery of most pesticides added to samples of dried spices. Further work is required to test extraction efficiency for samples with incurred residues. The scope of the methods could also be extended to include other pesticides. An abstract of a poster covering the GC-MS/MS part of the validation work was accepted for presentation at the European Pesticides Residues Workshop (EPRW) 2006.

There are several traditional remedies that contain animal and human body parts (e.g. toad skin, human placenta) and these are potent sources of infection. Some animal constituents in particular contain very toxic constituents.

More details on the toxic effects of pesticides can be found in Chapter 4.3.

## 5    Drugs to be avoided by vulnerable population groups

Examples of three vulnerable populations are discussed below. More details on susceptible groups are given in Chapter 2.3.

### 5.1   During pregnancy

The following groups or classes of herbal medicines should be avoided during pregnancy:
1. Those with a tendency to promote or regulate menstruation (emmenagogues) and also cause abortions (abortifacients).
2. Those that either directly or indirectly produce contractions of the smooth muscle of the uterus – e.g. laxatives, essential oils and bitters. These may also cause adverse effects on the developing systems in the foetus such as the nervous system.
3. Those that produce hormonal effects which would either cause feminising of a male foetus or masculinisation of a female foetus – oestrogenic and androgenic herbs.
4. Those that could cause malformation in the foetus – teratogens or teratogenic drugs.
5. Those that could cause changes in the genetic make-up of the foetus- mutagens.

### 5.2   During breast-feeding

As a general rule, breast-feeding mothers should avoid:
1. Remedies containing high doses of herbs containing alkaloids, particularly those that may affect the nervous system, e.g. Chinese herbs – coptis, phellodendron (berberine alkaloids), sophora root (oxymantrine), ma-huang (ephedrine) and evodia (rutecarpine).
2. Remedies containing high doses of herbs known to have hormonal effects e.g. fennel, anise, liquorice.
3. Herbs containing plant alkaloids known to cause liver and/or kidney damage. For example some herbs that contain toxic pyrrolizidine alkaloids are known to cause liver failure.
4. Strong purgatives, e.g. aloe or rhubarb root, that can cause diarrhoea or colic in the infant.
5. Herbs with a powerful immunosuppressive effect – e.g. tripterygium.

## 5.3   The elderly

Any form of drug therapy in the elderly, whether with allopathic or herbal medicines, is associated with the following risks or dangers, many of which increase the risk of side effects having more serious consequences.

1. The risk of drug interactions is greater as older people tend to suffer from several disease states and are required to take multiple medications.
2. Most functions of the vital organs are decreased and if kidney function is decreased, drugs are likely to be got rid from the body more slowly, there is risk of accumulation of drugs and thus of adverse effects and toxicity.
3. The metabolism of some drugs may be reduced in the elderly.
4. Mouth lesions are likely both due to lack of oral hygiene and due to retention of medications in the mouth when there is some difficulty in swallowing.
5. Altered mental activity often occurs in old age due to nerve cells having been lost or damaged or due to some defect in the production and effects of the chemical messengers (neurotransmitters). The loss of nerve cells results in many elderly patients becoming more sensitive to drugs that act on the nervous system, particularly nervous system depressants such as sedatives and pain killers.
6. Drugs which affect the heart and blood vessels increase the risk of adverse effects such as low blood pressure and dangerous changes in heart rhythm as a result of their use in the older age group. This is due to loss of elasticity of the blood vessels, degenerative changes in blood vessel walls and in heart muscle cells that occur with ageing.
7. Adverse reactions to drugs may present in the elderly in an unusual manner – vague symptoms should not be ignored. Confusion is often the presenting symptom.
8. Since falls are likely to have serious consequences for the elderly, all precautions should be taken to minimise side effects that might result in falls, such as decrease in blood pressure or confusion.

## 6   Conclusions

There is little controversy that several traditional herbal remedies in particular have stood the test of time. There is also no controversy that documentation of efficacy and adverse effects, particularly of carcinogenicity and mutagenicity, is sparse when compared to allopathic medications. The variations in preparations, doses and routes of intake are all influenced by cultural, social and religious factors. Though herbal medicines will continue to provide affordable and accessible health care to the vast majority of the world population, there is a public health issue. In addition from a health protection and public health perspective, it is necessary to be aware that 'epidemics' of most unusual disease states may occur due to the undeclared use of traditional herbal medicines.

Much of the information for this chapter was obtained from the book *Traditional Herbal Medicines – Guide for Safer Use* (Karalliedde and Gawarammana, 2007).

## 7    References

Aschwanden C. (2001) Contamination problems. *Bulletin of the World Health Organization* 79 (7):692.

Barbee M. (2008) Excerpt from "Politically incorrect nutrition" – Vital Health Publishing quoted in Worldwide Health.com 28.3.2008. Available at: www.worldwidehealth.com

Chan K. (2003) Some aspects of toxic contaminants in herbal medicines. *Chemosphere* 52:1361–1371.

Chan TY, Critchley JA. (1996) Usage and adverse effects of Chinese herbal medicines. *Hum Exp Toxicol* 15(1):5–12.

Corns C, Metcalfe K. (2002) Risks associated with herbal slimming remedies. *J R Soc Promotion Health* 122(4):213–219.

DEFRA. (2005) Project SID 5. Department for Environment and Rural Affairs. Available at: www.defra.gov.uk

Deng JF, Lin TJ, Kao WF, Chen SS. (1997) The difficulty in handling poisonings associated with Chinese traditional medicines: a poison control centre experience for 1991–1993. *Vet Hum Toxicol* 39(2):106–114.

Dharmananda S. (2003) Kampo Medicine – The Practice of Chinese Herbal Medicine in Japan. Institute for Traditional Medicine, Oregon, US. Available at: http://www.itmonline.org/arts/kampo.htm

Ernst E. (2002) Toxic heavy metals and undeclared drugs in Asian herbal medicines. *Trends in Pharmacological Science* 23:136–139.

Gardiner P, Graham RE, Legedza TR, Eisenberg DM, Phillips RS. (2006) Factors associated with dietary supplement use among prescription medication users. Arch *Intern Med.* 166(18):1968–1974.

GovHK. (2004) Government Laboratory Annual Report 2004, Government of Hong Kong.

Gupta SK, Kaleekal T, Joshi S. (2000) Misuse of corticosteroids in some of the drugs dispensed as preparations from alternative systems of medicine in India. *Pharmacoepidemiol Drug Saf* 9(7):599–602.

Haller CA, Dyer JE, Ko R, Olson KR. (2002) Making a diagnosis of herbal-related hepatitis. *West J Med* 176(1):39–44.

Huang WF, Wen KC, Hsiao ML. (1997) Adulteration by synthetic therapeutic substances of traditional Chinese medicines in Taiwan. *J Clin Pharmacol* 37:344–50.

Karalliedde L, Gawarammana I. (Eds.) (2007) *Traditional herbal medicines – a guide to their safer use*. Hammersmith Press, London.

Keane FM, Munn SE, du Vivier AW, Taylor NF, Higgins EM. (1999) Analysis of Chinese herbal creams prescribed for dermatological conditions. *BMJ* 318:563–564.

Ko RJ. (1998) Adulterants in Asian patent medicines. *N Engl J Med* 339(12):847.

Lynch E, Braithwaite R. (2005) A review of the clinical and toxicological aspects of traditional (herbal) medicines adulterated with heavy metals. *Expert Opinion Drug Safety* 4:769–778.

NLFD. (1991) Annual report of National Laboratories of Food and Drugs, Taiwan 1990–1991.

MHRA. Medicines and Healthcare products Regulatory Agency. Available at: www.mhra.gov.uk

Perharic L, Shaw D, Coldbridge M, House I, Leon C, Murray V. (1994) Toxicological problems resulting from exposure to traditional remedies and food supplements. *Drug Safety* 11:284–294.

Ries CA, Sahud MA. (1975) Agranulocytosis caused by Chinese herbal medicines. Dangers of medications containing aminopyrine and phenylbutazone. *JAMA* 231(4):352–355.

Ross S, Simpson CR, McLay JS. (2006) Homeopathic and herbal prescribing in general practice in Scotland. *Br J Clin Pharmacol* 62(6):647–652; discussion 645–6. Epub 2006 Jun 23.

Shaw D. (2007) Medical Toxicology Unit, Guy's and St Thomas's NHS Foundation Trust. Personal communication.

Shaw D, House I, Kolev S, Murray V. (1995) Should herbal medicines be licensed? *BMJ* 311(7002):451–452.

Steenkamp V, Stewart MJ, Zuckerman M. (2000) Clinical and analytical aspects of pyrrolizidine poisoning caused by South African traditional medicines. *Therapeutic Drug Monitoring* 22:302–306.

Tagami T, Kajimura K, Satsuki Y *et al.* (2008) Rapid analysis of 56 pesticide residues in natural medicines by GC/MS with negative chemical ionization. *J Natural Med* 62(1): 126–129.

Tay CH, Seah CS. (1975) Arsenic poisoning from antiasthmatic herbal preparations. *Med J Aust* 2(11): 424–428.

Venter CP, Joubert PH. (1988) Aspects of poisoning with traditional medicines in Southern Africa. *Biomed Environ Sci* 1:388–391.

Waxman J. (2006) Shark cartilage in the water. Personal view. *BMJ* 333:1129.

WHO. (2003a) Traditional medicine. *Factsheet* 134. World Health Organization, Geneva.

WHO. (2003b) Traditional medicine – Report by the Secretariat. *56th World Health Assembly* A56/18. World Health Organization, Geneva.

Zhang, X. (1999) Traditional medicine worldwide: the role of the WHO. *Drug Info J* 33:321–328.

# Section 4.5

# Chemical weapons: deliberate release of chemical agents

David Baker

---

## Learning outcomes

At the end of this chapter the student should be able to:

1. discuss the history, nature and classification of chemical warfare agents;
2. explain the essential properties of chemical agents and how these determine the management of an incident and the management of the patient;
3. describe and discuss the pathophysiological effects, signs and symptoms of exposure to chemical agents;
4. explain the military and civil approaches to incident management;
5. evaluate and discuss policies for the management of the incident and the management of the patient, and
6. apply their knowledge in the analysis and management of hazardous situations.

---

## 1    Introduction

Most health professionals in developed nations today have little or no experience of managing victims of chemical warfare. In the early 20th century in Europe the situation was quite different. Chemical warfare was widely used along the static battlefield conditions of the First World War and caused many hundreds of thousands of casualties on all sides. During this time, military doctors, nurses and ambulance teams, most of whom had come from civil life, would have been very familiar with the effects of chemical agents. This experience persisted into the period between the two wars. Although chemical weapons were not used in the Second World War in Europe there was considerable concern that they would be, particularly against civilians by aerial bombardment. During the brief years of peace the experience gained in the First World War (WW1) was put to use and there was detailed planning for managing gas attacks by the mass provision of respirators to civilians.

Following the Second World War (WW2) public awareness of chemical weapons gradually diminished. Although they remained a major threat during the Cold War this was only seen to be a military problem. Elsewhere, civil defence was abandoned and a generation of health practitioners worked without any training to manage chemical warfare victims other than that which they might have gained during military service, which was itself becoming a rarity, particularly in the United Kingdom.

Against this, chemical weapons were used in a number of campaigns around the world, often with considerable effect, particularly against unprotected civilians. Because of a growing fear of an unknown quantity and the atmosphere of widespread civilian involvement and fear that characterised the Cold War, chemical agents were increasingly seen as 'weapons of mass destruction' in the same light as nuclear and biological agents. It was believed that there was little that could be done for the mass casualties that would be the result of an attack using chemical agents on crowded cities. This view has persisted and has been fuelled by the use of a chemical warfare agent by terrorists, highlighting again the vulnerability of civil populations.

This situation is however at odds with reality. Release of chemicals in the urban environment is almost an everyday occurrence managed routinely by the emergency services. However, when dangerous chemicals are released deliberately as a result of terrorist action, the incident takes on an aura that is disproportionate to the real hazards present. There is an element of fear and turbulence that surrounds any report of a possible urban chemical attack which is fuelled by unfamiliarity and mass reporting. Targeted civil populations are vulnerable as a result of lack of organisation, protection and understanding of the real risks, and thus chemical releases lead to a multiplication of panic which amplifies the effects of the incident. For the terrorist this is a desirable outcome and so the attractions of the release of chemical agents which are relatively easy to produce are magnified.

The objective of this chapter is to present the realities of chemical warfare agents in a simple way from the point of view of the immediate and longer term hazards to health that they present in a civilian setting. The classical and newer agents will be discussed in terms of their characteristics and their effects on the body. Management of any chemical release involves both management of the incident and the management of the patient and a clear understanding of both is essential if health professionals are not to become casualties themselves and the lives of victims are not to be lost as a result of inadequate or inappropriate medical care. Thus the importance of protection and decontamination and the management of casualty flow will be considered, together with the essentials of life support and specific therapy.

## 2    Chemical warfare agents and weapons

### 2.1    Definitions

A chemical warfare agent may be defined as a chemical substance that is released deliberately to kill, seriously injure or otherwise incapacitate man through pathophysiological effects. For a chemical to cause harm either accidental or deliberate release is necessary; chemical warfare agents and industrial chemicals are not harmful when confined. There are many highly dangerous substances used in industry every day which cause no harm due to correct handling. This follows the source-pathway-receptor model (see Chapter 2.3). In the military context, release of a chemical to cause harm is achieved by the use of a weapon to distribute it. Shells, bombs and aerial spraying are classic methods employed to disperse chemicals. Recent experience has shown that chemical agents can be released directly in a civil setting by terrorists.

## 2.2 Classifications

Chemical warfare agents have conventionally been considered along with biological and nuclear weapons as 'weapons of mass destruction'. A biological agent may be defined as a self-replicating organism (e.g. bacteria or viruses) deliberately released to cause harm to man by infection. This results in a deliberate, calculated epidemic. Nuclear weapons cause harm by a massively powerful explosion which is accompanied by the release of large quantities of radiation and radioisotope contamination.

After WW2, chemical weapons were classified along with biological and nuclear devices as Nuclear, Biological and Chemical (NBC) agents. This classification has now been expanded to Chemical, Biological, Radiological and Nuclear Weapons (CBRN) to include radioisotopes that may be released deliberately using a small conventional explosive charge.

It is important to realise that all CBRN weapons do not cause casualties in the same way. Chemical and biological agents are quite different in their properties, particularly in the time they take to act. Radiological agents are really chemicals that cause harm as a result of the effects of the radiation they release. Nuclear weapons cause harm in another substantially different way. They produce serious physical damage to man and his environment from the effects of the powerful explosion in a similar way to high explosives but with secondary effects from the released radiation.

## 3. Poisoning in peace and war

Most health professionals are familiar with individual poisoning, either deliberate or suicidal. The use of chemical substances for this end has been known through the ages and is still a feature of modern life. Poisoning is often different from chemical agent release in that medical responders are not usually at risk from the poison. This is a different situation from chemical agent release where medical teams may be in danger of themselves becoming casualties by being exposed to the released agent that persists on the casualty or his location. Chapter 2.2 discusses management of chemical incidents in healthcare settings in detail.

The use of chemicals in warfare had been considered for many centuries but it was not until WW1 that mass release of chemicals was used as part of military activity. Over 113,000 tons of chemicals were used in that war. Mass casualties were often caused when there was an element of surprise. The first major chemical attack was on 22nd April 1915, when chlorine released as a cloud caused 15,000 Allied wounded with 5000 fatalities. However with the introduction of protective masks such mass fatalities were not usually repeated. The Russians however, who had little or no protection, suffered over 500,000 casualties from chemical warfare, a fact that had great bearing on the subsequent organisation of their army in later times. Box 1 outlines the development of chemical agents.

Early chemical attacks in WW1 probably fuelled the idea of chemical agents being weapons of mass destruction. In fact the ratio of dead to wounded was less than 8% and was lower than any other weapon systems used during that war. Explosive shells on the other hand, had a dead to wounded ratio of over 15% and were the cause of 59% of all fatalities on both sides. In later wars where chemical weapons were used, the dead to wounded ratio fell further. In the Iran-Iraq War in the 1980s the ratio among 27,000 casualties was less than 1%. By the time of the terrorist chemical attack on the Tokyo subway in 1995 the dead to wounded ratio was 0.25% among 5000 casualties. These figures highlight the fact that if modern respiratory and antidote care is available, casualties from chemical warfare agents can be successfully treated.

**Box 1** Development and use of chemical weapons

| | |
|---|---|
| 1915 | Chlorine, phosgene used |
| 1916 | Hydrogen cyanide used |
| 1917 | Mustard gas used |
| | (many other compounds were tested during the period of WW1) |
| 1919 | Lewisite weaponised, but not used |
| 1925 | International treaty banning the use of chemical weapons |
| 1936 | Mustard gas used in Abyssinia |
| 1936–1945 | Nerve agents such as sarin developed and weaponised |
| 1945–1991 | Soviet development of nerve agents and new toxic agents |
| 1980s | Mustard gas and nerve agent use in Iran – Iraq War |
| 1988 | Use of chemical agents against a civilian population in Hallubjah, Iraq |
| 1995 | First use of a chemical warfare agent by terrorists (Tokyo) |
| 2000–? | Further development of urban chemical agents and toxins by terrorists |

## 3.1    Medical and civil chemical releases

Most use of chemical agents has been in battle. Where used against unprotected civilians in countries with little or no medical resources such as Abyssinia in 1936 and Kurdistan in 1988, there has been considerable loss of life. This highlights the major differences between chemical agent use in military and civil situations. These differences are outlined in Table 1.

## 3.2    Hazards and threats

Hazard and threat are often used interchangeably in the media but have distinct meanings in relation to the dangers from chemical weapons. As noted previously, hazardous chemicals are not dangerous while confined. For a chemical agent to cause

**Table 1** Comparison of military and civilian exposures to chemical agents

| Characteristics | Military | Civil |
|---|---|---|
| Chemical agent | Limited range of identified chemical warfare agents. | Large range of toxic industrial chemicals – urban release of chemical warfare agents also possible. |
| Nature of release | Expected and detected – deliberate attack. | Unexpected and variable detection – accidental release or deliberate urban attack. |
| Detection and identification | Tuned battlefield alarm system and identification systems. Evidence of attack from weapon characteristics. | No fixed detection systems – mobile identification possible. Detection of release usually based on presenting toxidromes. |
| Response | Trained and protected physically fit population. Organised and protected medical response. | Untrained, unprotected population. Fear of attack a strong panic multiplier fuelled by media. Limited protected medical responses in some areas. |

harm it must be (1) available to the user, (2) be deliverable through a weapon system, and (3) the assailant must have the intention and the ability to use it. Thus threat is a function of a number of factors which may be expressed as follows:

Threat = f (available hazard + delivery means + intention).

## 3.3    Chemical and biological hazards

Chemical and biological weapons (CBW) are usually considered to be separate. However they can be regarded as a spectrum of hazards, ranging from low to high molecular weight substances through to self-replicating organisms (Box 2). The advantage of this concept medically is that agents with different physical properties can be grouped according to pathophysiological effects and medical responses that are available for treatment.

Examples of pathophysiological effects of CBW agents are:

- cellular disruption – DNA cross linking;
- toxic pulmonary oedema;
- receptor binding (NMJ, nerve ion channels, GABA), and
- bacterial toxin release.

**Box 2** The chemical and biological weapon (CBW) spectrum

**Chemical agents** ——— **Toxins** ——— **Biological agents**

| small molecular weight, simple e.g. sarin | higher molecular weight, complex e.g. botulinum toxin | self-replicating organism e.g. smallpox |

**i.  Uses of the CBW spectrum**

Chemical and biological warfare agents are usually viewed as being separate weapons but in terms of their effects in man they may be viewed as a continuous spectrum of hazards. The spectrum ranges from low molecular weight chemical agents through to self-replicating organisms such as viruses and bacteria. Toxins, which are chemicals with molecular weights ranging between 1000 to about 1,000,000, are chemical substances usually of biological origin (e.g. from bacteria, animals or plants). The value of the CBW spectrum is that agents from different parts of the spectrum have common mechanisms or act at the same site. A good example of this is the nerve agents such as the chemical sarin which block the neuromuscular junction, and botulinum toxin (produced by the organism *Clostridium botulinum*), which does the same but at a different receptor site. In terms of medical management, both lead to a failure of transmission of nerve impulses to muscle fibres and paralysis and require common emergency life support measures.

**ii.  Properties of agents of the CBW spectrum**

Agents in the CBW spectrum each possess four distinct properties: toxicity, latency of action, persistency and transmissibility.

- **Toxicity and latency of action:** determined by toxicodynamics and toxicokinetics
- **Persistency and transmissibility:** determined by physico-chemical properties

Expressions of toxicity for CW agents are discussed in the main text. Latency may be expressed as $L_{50}$, the time taken for signs to develop in 50% of an exposed population. This covers a time span ranging from seconds to hours for chemical agents and days in the case of biological agents (a period most familiar as 'incubation time'). Persistency and transmissibility are related to the physical properties of the agents and characterise the ability of agents to remain where they have been released and the risk of contamination or infection being passed to others. Toxicity and latency determine the management of the patient whereas persistency and transmissibility determine the management of the chemical agent released.

## 4    Toxicology of chemical warfare agents

Chemical warfare agents have been extensively tested over the years in laboratory animals but there are very little direct toxicological data available for humans. Thus expressions of toxicity in terms of $LD_{50}$ are derived from experimental data (see chapter 1.3 for details of determining toxicity experimentally). An expression commonly used for toxicity of inhaled agents is $LCt_{50}$. This is the chemical concentration in $mg/m^3$ multiplied by the time of exposure in minutes to cause death in 50% of an exposed population. The problem with the expression is that the amount of agent inhaled depends on the rate and depth of breathing: persons breathing quickly and deeply will inspire a greater quantity of agent than those breathing normally. However, $LCt_{50}$ is a useful comparison of the effective toxicity to man of different chemical warfare agents. Toxicity values of a range of chemical agents are shown in Box 3.

### 4.1    Pathophysiological effects of chemical warfare agents

Chemical warfare (CW) agents have effects on all the functional systems of the body including the central and peripheral nervous systems, the skin and mucus membranes, the gastrointestinal and urinary systems, the blood and bone marrow, and the cardiac and respiratory systems. The effects on the respiratory system are the most important since these lead to respiratory failure and subsequent cardiac arrest. Effects on the

**Box 3** Chemical warfare agents: expressions of toxicity

**Expressions commonly used to measure toxicity:**

- $LD_{50}$ – Lethal dose required to kill 50% of test animals, extrapolated to humans. Expressed as weight of chemical per kilogram bodyweight (mg/kg).
- $LCt_{50}$ – Lethal dose required to kill 50% of test animals over time. Usual expression for inhalational pathway. Expressed as concentration x time for 50% lethality ($mg.min/m^3$) The product of concentration x time is known as the 'lethal index'.

**Toxicity of CBW agents in $LCt_{50}$ values ($mg.min/m^3$)**
- GA (Tabun): 150
- GB (Sarin): 70–100
- GD (Soman): 40–60
- Phosgene: 3200
- Sulphur mustard: 1500
- Lewisite: 1200
- Hydrogen cyanide: 3000

Botulinum toxin
- Based on experimental toxicology BoTx is 15,000 times more toxic than VX and 100,000 times more toxic than GB

respiratory system may be on the airway, alveolar gas exchange or on the control and muscular activity of diaphragm and chest wall movement. Such effects are mediated via the autonomic and voluntary nervous system. Respiratory failure is the final pathway leading to death from CW agents.

## 5    Classes of chemical warfare agent

It is convenient to consider CW agents in terms of the conventional military classification but it should be remembered that this classification serves just as well as models for many industrial chemicals that cause similar pathophysiology. Box 4 lists the conventional military classification.

**Box 4** Classification of chemical warfare agents

- **Nerve agents**
  Tabun, Sarin, Soman, VX

- **Lung damaging agents (choking agents)**
  Chlorine, phosgene

- **Agents affecting tissue respiration ('blood' agents)**
  Hydrogen cyanide, cyanogens

- **Vesicants**
  Mustard gas, Lewisite

- **Disabling and knockdown agents**
  Tear gases, ?opioids

### 5.1    Nerve Agents

These are highly toxic organophosphate (OP) compounds developed as CW agents from pesticide research by Schrader in 1936. Following secret development during WW2 nerve agents became a major threat during the Cold War. A nerve agent was almost certainly used in the attack against Kurds in Hallabjah, Iraq, in 1988. The nerve agent sarin was used in the terrorist attack in Tokyo in 1995.

*Actions*
Acetyl cholinesterase (AChE) is a key enzyme at all sites in the nervous system where acetyl choline is the chemical transmitter. Chemical nerve agents can cause non-reversible inhibition of AChE throughout the cholinergic system. This causes a build up of acetyl choline (ACh) and a continuous overstimulation of the synapses. This results in increased concentrations of ACh at muscarinic and nicotinic sites and signs and symptoms related to the basic pharmacology of the cholinergic nervous system (see Basic Concepts appendix for further information). As a result there are acute, intermediate and long term effects of OP poisoning. Acutely excessive stimulation of the autonomic nerve system produces excess secretions with airway blockage,

bronchospasm, bradycardia, gastric and urinary effects. Excessive stimulation of the neuromuscular junction produces initial fasciculation (twitching of groups of muscle fibres) and flaccid (depolarising) muscle paralysis requiring ventilation, which may resolve following oxime therapy.

Following an initial recovery there may be renewed paralysis after 24 hours in 20% of cases. This may last several days and is of a different type to the initial paralysis (non-depolarisation paralysis).

### Toxins

Neurotoxins can block the transmission of impulses along the nerves. Many natural neurotoxins are produced by insects, reptiles and marine organisms but few are feasible as CBW agents. An example is saxitoxin which is produced by a small marine organism and which blocks the sodium channels in the nerve upon which normal transmission of impulses depends.

Botulinum toxin, from the bacterium *Clostridium botulinum*, acts by inhibition of release of ACh at the nerve terminal causing failure of cholinergic nerve transmission. The classic pattern of botulism is a gradual paralysis setting in several hours after eating contaminated food. Botulinum toxin is the most toxic substance known to man but toxicity is greatly reduced by life support and antitoxin intervention.

## 5.2    Lung damaging agents (pulmonary oedemagens)

Lung damaging agents were used as chemical weapons during the First World War. Chlorine was first used in 1915 and was followed by phosgene, the properties of which are described in Box 5. They caused both upper and lower damage to the airways and lungs and were fatal due to the onset of pulmonary oedema, where the lung alveoli fill with fluid and normal oxygenation of the blood fails. The lung damaging agents were eclipsed during the Cold War by more toxic agents such as nerve agents but a new threat arose from per-fluoro isobutylene (PFIB), which is known in the civil context as a by-product of heating Teflon.

There are many toxic industrial chemicals which cause pulmonary oedema. Both phosgene and chlorine are widely used in the chemical industry. In addition, isocyanates are also used in many synthetic processes. A release of methyl-isocyanate in Bhopal, India (1984) caused over 5000 deaths from pulmonary oedema.

## 5.3    Vesicant agents

Chemical warfare agents which attacked the skin and mucous membranes were also developed and used during the First World War. The most well-known, mustard gas (which is actually an oily liquid at normal temperatures), caused many hundreds of thousands of casualties, mostly with disabling rather than fatal injuries. Mustard gas was used again in the Iran – Iraq War during the 1980s.

**Box 5** Properties of phosgene

**Uses of phosgene:**
- Chemical warfare gas and major industrial use
- Liquid/vapour can be formed accidentally by decomposition of chlorinated hydrocarbons

**Symptoms of phosgene exposure:**
- Acute and chronic exposure causes toxic pulmonary oedema (PE)
- Exposure causes initial upper respiratory symptoms of pronounced cough, dyspnoea, and 'choking'
- The latent period between exposure and symptoms is dose dependent:
  - high dose: 1–4 hours
  - low dose: 8–24 hours

**Toxic effects and dose:**
- 1 ppm chronically: chronic lung disease (N.B. below odour threshold)
- >25 ppm.min: acute lung effects
- 50–150 ppm.min: initial inflammatory response, which may be followed by PE
- >150 ppm.min: clinically significant and life – threatening PE
- 800 ppm for 2 minutes: lethal

The signs and symptoms of mustard gas poisoning are shown in Box 6. Characteristic effects include severe conjunctivitis, vesication and ulceration of the skin, an example of which can be seen in Figure 1.

**Box 6** Signs and symptoms of mustard gas poisoning

- Early smell of garlic, then latent sign-free period.
- After 2–6 hours: nausea, fatigue, headache, eye inflammation and pain, lachrymation, blepharospasm, photophobia and rhinorrhoea.
- Hoarse voice and development of erythema to skin.
- Exacerbation of above symptoms with blister formation to inner thighs, perineum and other sweat areas.
- Development of chemical bronchiolitis in high temperature exposure.

## 5.4 Agents affecting tissue respiration (cyanides)

Cyanide agents include the gas hydrogen cyanide (HCN) and the cyanogens. Following inhalation they act very quickly (short latency) and in high concentrations cause death by interfering with the normal function of oxygen at the mitochondria in the body cells. Early antidote therapy is essential for management. This involves either producing a variant of haemoglobin in the red cells of the blood (methaemoglobin) which binds to cyanide and renders it ineffective or accelerating the breakdown of HCN by the enzyme rhodonase which can be achieved by providing sodium thiosulphate. Another approach is to use dicobalt edentate. HCN combines with heavy metals and the cobalt ions in this compound act to remove HCN in this way. The properties of cyanide are described in Box 7.

**Figure 1** Mustard gas vesication with ulceration. Courtesy of Ministry of Defence, London, 1987.

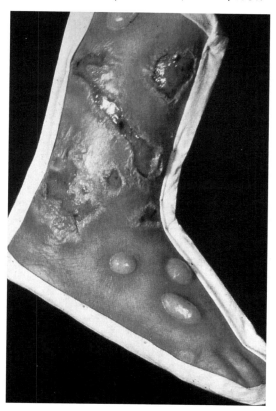

## 6    Practical realities for emergency medical management of chemical casualties

Exposure to chemical warfare agents is a rare event which is unfamiliar to most emergency responders in the UK. However there are many lessons which apply to the management of accidental chemical release in the civil arena which are direct parallels of the measures required for the safe management of chemical warfare agent casualties. The key issues are (1) to ensure the safety of the responders and to prevent secondary casualties, and (2) to provide essential life support and antidotes to casualties to prevent loss of life from respiratory failure.

Chemical agent release management can therefore be divided into (1) management of the incident, and (2) management of the patient.

**Box 7** Actions of hydrogen cyanide

- Short latency.
- Binds to $Fe^{3+}$ atom on cytochrome oxidase in mitochondria, uncoupling electron receptor action of oxygen, and disrupts production of ATP.
- Cellular tissue oxygen concentrations are initially normal.
- Advanced life support measures may not be effective. Early antidote therapy essential.

The key steps in management are:

- planning;
- incident management;
- protection;
- triage;
- resuscitation and immediate therapy;
- decontamination, and
- continuing care.

## 6.1    Chemical incidents: the civil Hazmat response

To respond safely to contaminated casualties following chemical agent release, protection of the medical responders is essential. Medical and paramedical staff are now trained and equipped in many countries to be able to wear level C protection (Figure 2). This consists of a filtration respirator, which filters the contaminated atmosphere through activated charcoal, and a protective suit and gloves. The length of time such a suit can be worn in a contaminated zone depends on the level of contamination. The level C suit is the civilian equivalent of the military NBC suit which is worn to protect troops against the most toxic CW agents.

In the civil context, chemical releases are managed by describing zones around the release. These are (1) the hot zone around the site of release, where direct contamination risk is highest, (2) the warm zone outside the hot zone where contamination is usually secondary and transmitted by contaminated persons leaving the hot zone, and (3) the cold zone outside the warm zone where contamination is minimal. Between the warm and cold zones is the decontamination unit where patients are decontaminated before being evacuated further. Figure 3 shows the standard arrangement of these zones following chemical agent release in the civil setting.

The hot zone contains the highest level of contamination. Victims are rescued by protected fire personnel and taken to the warm zone to await decontamination. Here protected medical responders may have to provide essential life support before patients are decontaminated: this is the basis of the UK Hazardous Area Response Teams (HART), who provide early treatment dynamically integrated with decontamination. The HART teams, which were set up in 2006, provide specially trained and equipped paramedic teams who can operate safely in a contaminated zone (Figure 4). They are trained to administer specific antidotes for chemical agents and to provide airway and ventilatory support. Equipment includes a full range of protective equipment, antidotes, airway management devices and an automatic ventilator designed to operate in a contaminated zone (Figure 5).

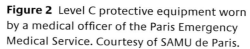

**Figure 2** Level C protective equipment worn by a medical officer of the Paris Emergency Medical Service. Courtesy of SAMU de Paris.

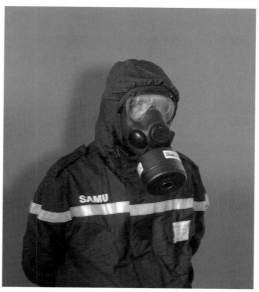

**Figure 3** Arrangement of contamination and zones following a chemical release.

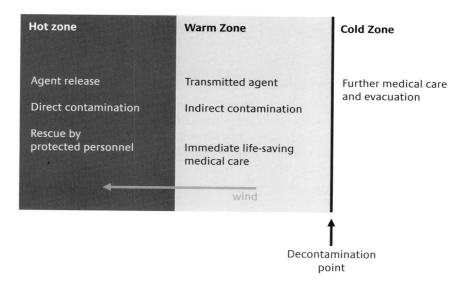

| Hot zone | Warm Zone | Cold Zone |
|---|---|---|
| Agent release | Transmitted agent | Further medical care and evacuation |
| Direct contamination | Indirect contamination | |
| Rescue by protected personnel | Immediate life-saving medical care | |

wind

Decontamination point

**Figure 4** HART team response vehicles 2006. Courtesy of London Ambulance Service.

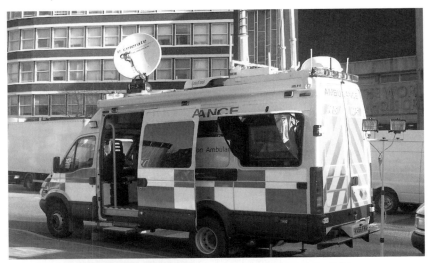

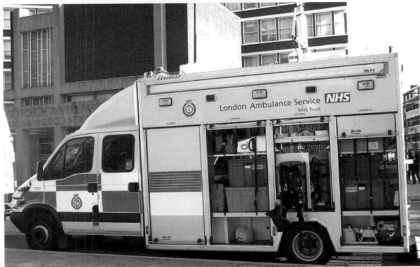

**Figure 5** Life support in a contaminated area 2007: the Pneupac VR1 ventilator with patient circuit filtration. Courtesy of Smiths Medical International Ltd, Hythe, UK.

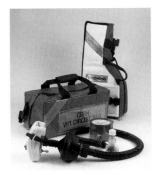

## 6.2    Practical aspects of treatment for chemical casualties

Early advanced life support and antidote therapy must be provided by specially trained medical and paramedical personnel working in the contaminated zone wearing level C protection. This care includes essential provision of airway and ventilatory support for victims with impending respiratory arrest which is the main cause of death following chemical agent exposure. Triage of patients is also required in the contaminated zone to give priority for decontamination and evacuation to those who are most seriously injured.

Care given prior to decontamination is termed TOXALS (the provision of advanced life support in a contaminated area). This is an extension of the familiar ABC (airway, breathing and circulatory support) of basic and advanced life support. The elements of TOXALS are shown in Box 8.

Once a patient has been decontaminated and stabilised, continuing airway, ventilatory and antidote treatment through to the hospital, emergency room and, for severely affected cases, the intensive care unit is essential.

**Box 8**  Life support for CW agent casualties (TOXALS)

> **A**ssessment (patient and site)
> **A**irway
> **B**reathing (requirement for artifical ventilation)
> **C**irculation
> – control of haemorrhage and cardiac abnormalities
> **D**isability (level of unconsciousness)
> **D**rugs and antidotes
> **D**econtamination
> **E**vacuation

## 7    Chemical agent release in a civil setting: some lessons from recent history

In recent years, chemical agents have been used by urban terrorists. Chemical agent exposure should therefore now be regarded as a civil as well as a military hazard. Examples are:

- Tokyo, 1995, where the nerve gas sarin was released into the underground railway system (Box 9).

- USA, 2001, where anthrax spores were sent through the post. Anthrax is a biological warfare agent which kills by producing anthrax toxin. This can also be considered a chemical agent in its own right.

**Box 9**  The Tokyo sarin release, 1995

---

**Case study: the Tokyo sarin incident, 1995**

**Primary casualties:**

- 688 victims were transported to hospitals by ambulance.
- >4,000 casualties reached hospitals either on foot or by private transport.
- 5,510 sought medical attention in 278 hospitals and clinics.
- 12 patients died from respiratory failure.

**Occupational health consequences:**

- Of 1,364 fire emergency personnel who were at the incident, 135 (9.9%) showed acute symptoms and received medical treatment.

- 23% of staff at St Luke's Hospital had secondary exposure and developed signs and symptoms:
  - 39.3% of nurse assistants
  - 26.5% of nurses
  - 21.8% of doctors
  - 18.2% of clerks.

**Medical lessons learnt from the Tokyo sarin incident:**

1.  Many contaminated patients left the release site and came to hospital where they contaminated the medical and nursing staff.

2.  Careful cordon control of contaminated persons is required and decontamination should be carried out before sending patients on to hospital.

3.  Strain on medical and ventilation resources may occur. The most severely injured patients require life support with artificial ventilation to survive.

4.  Patients with severe and moderate poisoning require follow-up with evaluation to determine long term adverse health effects including neurotoxic and behavioural effects.

5.  Disaster planning should include mass casualties from chemical exposure: both acute and chronic effects.

---

- Moscow, 2002, where, in order to end a siege by terrorists in a theatre, security forces used a chemical compound producing rapid onset of unconsciousness (a knock down agent) which was claimed to be an opioid of the fentanyl class, a compound used widely during general anaesthesia. The agent was non-persistent but responders wore protective equipment and respirators. Due to poor management of casualties, there were deaths among both terrorists and hostages from acute respiratory failure.

These incidents, and the continuing concern that terrorists will strike again using chemical agents, underline the importance of understanding the risks and management of chemical agent releases by all health care workers.

## 8    Conclusions

Chemical agents are part of a chemical – biological toxic agent spectrum. Release of CBW agents by terrorists in civilian settings has been shown to be possible and medical services should be prepared to respond using medical HAZMAT protocols. The essential characteristics of toxic agents determine both the incident and casualty management, and careful site management is essential to avoid secondary casualties. CBW casualties can be managed using standard medical skills but protection and training of emergency and healthcare personnel is essential. Good incident management and early life support affects the prognosis and can break the link between mass injury and mass loss of life.

## 9    Further reading

Harris R, Paxman J. (1982) *A higher form of killing*. Chatto and Windus, London.

Marrs TC, Maynard RL, Sidell FR. (Eds.) (2007) *Chemical warfare agents: toxicology and treatment*. 2nd edition, John Wiley and Sons, Chichester, UK. Chapter 13, pp.277–286.

Ministry of Defence (1987) *Medical Manual of Defence Against Chemical Agents* D/Med (F and S)(2)/10/1/1 p1–1. HMSO, London.

Zaitchuk R, Bellamy RF. (Eds.) (1997) *Medical Aspects of Chemical and Biological Warfare*. Department of the Army, Office of the Surgeon General, Borden Institute.

# Appendix

# Appendix

## Basic medical concepts

Lakshman Karalliedde, David Baker and Virginia Murray

### Learning outcomes

At the end of this chapter and any recommended reading the student should be able to:

1. understand the structure and function of the systems of the human body;
2. understand how body systems are vulnerable to toxic substances;
3. use the knowledge gained to better understand the content of other chapters of this book, and
4. apply their knowledge in the analysis and management of hazardous situations.

## 1 Introduction

This appendix is designed to provide basic knowledge about the structure and function of the human body for those who have received no formal education in medicine, biological sciences or human biology. Readers will find this section useful for understanding the terminology used in the main body of the book, and by the lecturers/teachers on the *Essentials in Toxicology for Health Protection* course. The section is also designed to stimulate interested health professionals to learn more of the disease states and disorders of organs and systems in the body that follow exposure to toxic chemicals.

The human body can be divided into a number of systems on the basis of both structure (anatomy) and function (physiology). Each of these systems can be affected by exposure to toxic agents and some play an essential role in combating toxic effects.

The information presented in the following sections will describe the essentials of normal function of the body and so provide reference points for the toxic effects described in other chapters. The areas to be considered are:

1. The cell.
2. The nervous system – central nervous system and peripheral nervous system (including the autonomic nervous system [sympathetic and

parasympathetic nervous systems], neurotransmitters, neuromuscular junction).

3. The respiratory system – lungs and breathing (including transport of oxygen and carbon dioxide).
4. The heart and circulation – the cardiovascular system, including a section on blood and blood components, blood pressure and blood vessels.
5. The gastro-intestinal system – stomach, intestines.
6. The liver – normal functions and the metabolism of foreign substances (xenobiotics).
7. The kidney.
8. The endocrine system – the production and role of hormones in the body.
9. The immune system and body defence mechanisms.

## 2    Cells: the fundamental building blocks of body systems

Man has evolved from life forms that were originally just single cells. The function of the whole body depends on providing each of its 30 trillion cells with a suitable chemical environment, water and oxygen. The cells of the body require a constant environment which is independent of changes in the outside world. For the amount of a substance in the body to remain constant, the amount gained each day must not exceed the amount required by the cells to function and excreted or lost from the body each day.

If intake exceeds the daily amounts required by cells to function normally and that of loss, there will be an imbalance. The amount of this imbalance will determine whether the cells will function abnormally (dysfunction or malfunction), or whether the cells would decrease in size (atrophy) or increase in size (hypertrophy). It will also determine whether cells would multiply abnormally (producing growths – tumours or malignancies) or die. This is the basis of toxicology, where the amount taken by the body is in excess of its needs and/or exceeds the amount that can be lost from the body by normal mechanisms, resulting in malfunction, disease or death. Rarely, chemical agents can produce direct local effects on the tissues with which they come into contact. A good example is the corrosive effect of acids and alkalis on the skin.

The amounts of foreign substances that enter the body depend on diet, the amounts inhaled (taken in during breathing), and the amounts absorbed through the skin. Toxic substances can also enter by other means, such as when venomous animals bite or sting.

One of the most important 'defence' mechanisms of the body rests with the organs by which either excessive amounts are eliminated (e.g. kidney, liver, intestine) or where excessive amounts are altered to a non-toxic state or metabolised (e.g. liver, intestine). The lungs also have an important role in elimination of toxic substances, and toxic substances may also be eliminated through the skin.

## 3    The nervous system

The main functions of the nervous system are to monitor, integrate (process) and respond to information from inside and outside the body. The nervous system controls or regulates many body functions essential to life such as breathing (respiratory centre), circulation (vasomotor centre), hormonal secretions, temperature, and indirectly the activity of the lungs, blood vessels, heart, kidneys and several other organs. Fundamentally, the role of the nervous system is to maintain normal body function by making the necessary adjustments or responses to changes which may eventually cause harm or ill-health.

The nervous system controls body functions and receives information from the outside world by means of transmission of electrical impulses passing along nerve cells (neurons) and their processes. In various parts of the system these signals are passed from cell to cell by special relay stations called synapses, where the signal is passed by a chemical messenger. These chemical messengers are called neurotransmitters. Special synapses are found at the end of nerves which pass a signal directly onto an organ, also through a neurotransmitter.

Overall, the nervous system consists of the central nervous system (CNS), comprising the brain and spinal cord, and the peripheral nervous system (PNS), which is composed of nerves extending to and from the CNS. The major constituent systems of the central and peripheral nervous systems, shown in Box 1, are described in the following sections.

**Box 1** The major parts of the nervous system

**Central nervous system**

Peripheral nervous system $\longrightarrow$ autonomic $\longrightarrow$ sympathetic

$\longrightarrow$ parasympathetic

$\longrightarrow$ somatic

### 3.1    The central nervous system

The brain and spinal cord are made up of dense accumulations of nerve cells and their associated fibres. The cell bodies give rise to grey matter, and the fibres, with a special coating called myelin, make up the white matter. The whole central nervous system is carefully protected. Three connective tissue membranes called meninges enclose the brain to varying lengths and the spinal cord. These meninges also cover the nerves entering and leaving the brain and the spinal cord. The meninges also enclose blood vessels and venous sinuses (chambers to which blood drains from veins from the nerve cells). Meninges retain cerebrospinal fluid (CSF), which is a watery liquid similar, but not identical, in composition to blood plasma, which supports, cushions and nourishes the brain. The meninges form partitions within the skull and brain. Inflammation of these lining membranes gives rise to the serious condition called meningitis whilst inflammation of the brain tissue itself (nerve cells) is referred to as encephalitis.

The major regions of the brain are the cerebrum, the midbrain, pons, the medulla oblongata and the cerebellum, which are shown in Figure 1.

**Figure 1**  Diagram of the brain. Not to scale.

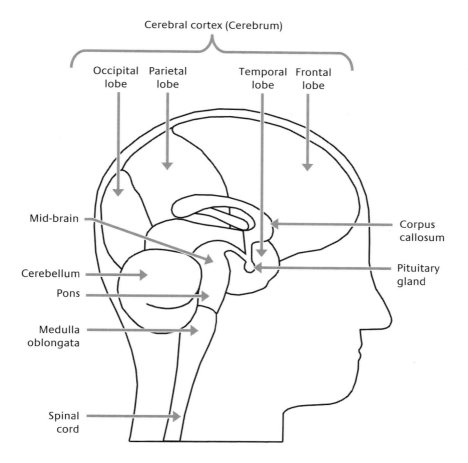

### 3.1.1   The cerebral hemispheres (cerebrum)

The cerebral hemispheres are the uppermost (superior) part of the brain, and are separated by the longitudinal fissure formed by the meninges to the right and left hemispheres. They make up approximately 83% of total brain mass and are collectively referred to as the cerebrum.

The cerebral cortex (cerebrum) constitutes a 2–4 mm thick grey matter surface layer. Because of its many convolutions, the grey matter accounts for about 40% of total brain mass. It is responsible for conscious behaviour and contains three different functional areas: the motor areas, sensory areas and association areas. Also located internally in the cerebral cortex are the white matter, responsible for communication between cerebral areas and between the cerebral cortex and lower regions of the CNS, as well as the basal nuclei (or basal ganglia), involved in controlling muscular movement and several bodily functions. CSF is contained in the lateral ventricles located in the cerebral hemispheres.

The corpus callosum connects right and left hemispheres to allow for communication between the hemispheres. The frontal lobe is associated with cognition and memory. The parietal lobe processes sensory input mainly whilst the occipital lobe has the visual perception area. The temporal lobe is associated with hearing.

The diencephalon is located centrally within the forebrain (the anterior or front part of the brain). It consists of the thalamus, hypothalamus and epithalamus, which together enclose the third ventricle (a sac containing cerebrospinal fluid found within the brain which is connected to the lateral ventricles in the cerebral hemispheres and to the 4th ventricle in the brain stem). The thalamus acts as a grouping and relay station for sensory inputs (inputs such as pain, touch and temperature from the periphery), ascending to the sensory cortex and associated areas. It also mediates motor activities, cortical arousal or wakefulness and memories. The hypothalamus, by controlling the autonomic (involuntary) nervous system, is responsible for maintaining the body's homeostatic balance that is commonly referred to as maintaining the internal environment ('the milieu interior'). This is the environment in which the cells function by maintaining the appropriate balance of electrolytes, ions, temperature, hormones and all other factors that are associated with normal function. Moreover, the hypothalamus forms a part of the limbic system, the 'emotional' brain. The epithalamus consists of the pineal gland and its connections.

### 3.1.2   Midbrain, pons and medulla

The midbrain, pons and the medulla oblongata lie below the diencephalon and are part of the continuing pathways from the cerebral hemispheres to the spinal cord and its nerves. This part of the brain contains collections of neurons which are referred to as 'nuclei' or 'centres', which control several vital functions such as cardiac (heart) activity and respiration (breathing).

The midbrain, which surrounds the cerebral aqueduct (the duct that conveys the cerebrospinal fluid to the sub-arachnoid space via the fourth ventricle), provides fibre pathways between higher and lower brain centres, contains visual and auditory reflex and subcortical motor centres. The pons is mainly a conduction region, but its nuclei also contribute to the regulation of respiration and nuclei of some cranial nerves. Cranial nerves comprise twelve pairs of nerves which arise directly from the brain and not from the spinal cord and leave the brain through apertures or foramina in the skull.

The medulla oblongata has an important role as an autonomic reflex centre involved in maintaining vital body functions. In particular, nuclei in the medulla regulate respiratory rhythm (the respiratory centre), heart rate (cardiac centre), blood pressure (vasomotor centre) and contain the nuclei of several cranial nerves. Moreover, the medulla oblongata provides important conduction pathways between the spinal cord and higher brain centres.

### 3.1.3  Cerebellum

The cerebellum, which is located behind the pons and medulla, accounts for about 11% of total brain mass. Like the cerebrum, it has a thin outer cortex of grey matter, internal white matter, and small, deeply situated paired masses (nuclei) of grey matter. The cerebellum processes impulses received from the cerebral motor cortex, various brain stem nuclei and sensory receptors in order to 'fine-tune' skeletal muscle contraction (the muscles that control movement-walking, running etc.), thus giving smooth, coordinated movements.

### 3.1.4  Spinal cord

The spinal cord is the direct continuation of the brain from the brainstem into the vertebral column. It contains the nerve pathways through which messages are sent from the brain (efferent pathways) and to the brain (afferent pathways). Like the brain itself, the spinal cord is composed of central grey matter containing nerve cells and white matter which comprises nerve fibres. Not all messages controlling the body have to go up to the brain and return. The nerves of the grey matter in the cord can act on

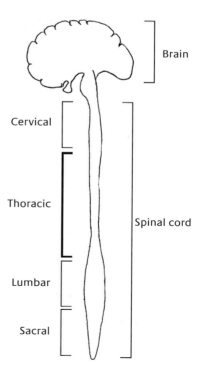

**Figure 2** Diagram of the spinal cord. Not to scale. The spinal cord is an extension of the brain itself and is divided into cervical, thoracic, lumbar and sacral sections according to the vertebrae which surround and protect it.

their own in response to a sensory stimulus. This action is known as a 'spinal reflex' and the knee jerk is perhaps the best known example.

The structure of the spinal cord and its connections are shown in Figures 2, 3 and 4.

**Figure 3** Diagram of the somatic nervous system and visceral nervous system. Not to scale. Impulses are received via afferent nerves – the cells of the afferent nerves are in the dorsal horn. Transmission of impulses from the dorsal horn to cells in the ventral horn takes place via connecting neurones. The cell in the dorsal horn which sends impulses to the nerve fibre or axon is called the internuncial cell. The ventral horn cell and its nerve fibre (axon) sends impulses (efferent) to skeletal muscle cells to help us move.

Impulses from viscera (e.g. intestines) are sent to the spinal cord via afferent nerves with the cell in the dorsal root (dorsal root ganglion) – the central process enters the spinal cord (grey matter). Connecter cells are in the grey matter. The connector fibres or pre-ganglionic fibres pass to a peripheral ganglion. From these peripheral ganglia (which may receive more than one pre-ganglionic fibre), nerves arise to supply the viscera. These are therefore post-ganglionic fibres.

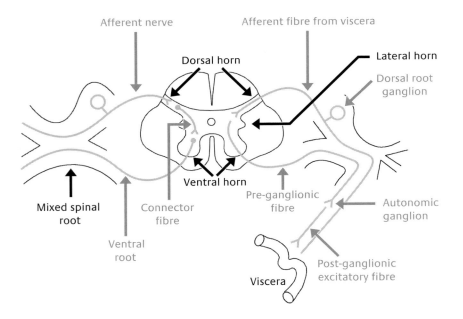

**Figure 4** Diagram of efferent pathways from the spinal cord. Not to scale. These are either autonomic (sympathetic and parasympathetic ) or somatic (the nerves controlling muscles). The autonomic system goes through a series of relay stations called ganglia, some of which lie alongside the spinal cord itself, e.g. the sympathetic chain.

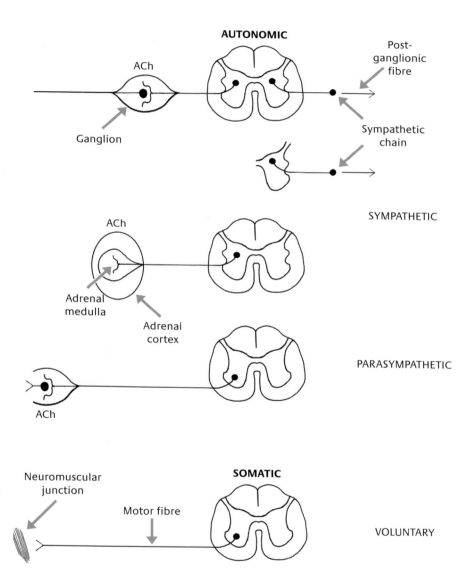

This contains motor nerves that control voluntary movement together with sensory nerves that carry information concerning touch, pain, temperature and position to the brain.

Nerves arise from nerve cells and the basic structure of a nerve cell is shown in Figure 5.

**Figure 5** Diagram of the nerve cell. Not to scale.

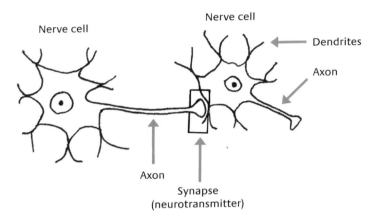

Nerve cells have a cell body, dendrites and an axon. The nerve cell and its processes are called neurons. The nerve cell and its processes behave like a small electrical battery: the resting voltage inside the nerve cell is -70 mV, one millivolt being one thousandth of a volt. The fluid inside the nerve cell, like that of other cells in the body, contains a high concentration of potassium ions (K+). In contrast, the nerve cell is surrounded by tissue fluid which contains mainly sodium chloride, which gives rise to sodium ions (Na+). In the resting state, the sodium ions are removed from the interior of the cell by the sodium pump. The pump effectively exchanges sodium ions for potassium ions. Both sodium ions and potassium ions diffuse across the cell membrane. Potassium diffuses much more rapidly than sodium thus generating the resting membrane potential of about -70 mV (interior negative to exterior).

A nerve impulse is a transient event which for a very short period of time alters the permeability of the cell membrane and allows sodium ions to enter the cell. These positively charged sodium ions change the potential inside the cell from -70 mV to +40 mV – a process called depolarisation. The sudden change from negative to positive voltage inside the cell is termed an action potential, and is propagated along the cell membrane. Each action potential corresponds to a nerve impulse or message which is conveyed to its destination by the membrane, changing its 'behaviour' along the whole nerve causing a propagation of the nerve impulse.

A nerve impulse lasts about one millisecond and each nerve impulse in both motor and sensory nerves (i.e. nerves that carry messages or impulses to the spinal cord and brain from the peripheral tissues as regards pain, temperature, touch) is associated with sodium entering and potassium leaving the cell momentarily. Following the action potential, i.e. during the resting phase, there is gradual expulsion of the sodium that had entered the nerve cell. The maximum rate of discharge from an anterior horn cell is considered to be approximately 200 impulses a second.

The rate of propagation of the nerve impulse or nerve conduction varies with the size of the nerve fibre, the large nerve fibres having a diameter of 20 μm have a velocity of conduction of 120 metres per second. These large fibres have a sheath made up mainly of fatty material called myelin (i.e. the nerves are myelinated), and the gaps in this sheath called Nodes of Ranvier enable a nerve impulse to 'leap-frog' down the nerve as the exchange of sodium and potassium ions only occurs at these interruptions in the myelin sheath.

The smaller fibres such as those that convey pain impulses to the brain are about 1 μm in diameter and are not individually myelinated. Therefore they are able to conduct impulses only at about 5 metres per second.

## 3.2.1   Autonomic nervous system

The part of the peripheral nervous system that supplies smooth muscles (in contrast to the striated or skeletal muscles found in our limbs etc.) is termed the autonomic nervous system. The autonomic nervous system also controls the heart, the digestive and urinary systems and the secreting glands such as sweat and salivary glands. In general, the autonomic nervous system is concerned with *involuntary* nerve impulses. The part of the peripheral nervous system that controls *voluntary* actions, such as movement, is known as the somatic nervous system.

The autonomic nervous system is subdivided into:
1. the sympathetic nervous system,
2. the parasympathetic nervous system.

These systems differ in the chemical transmitter involved in the transmission of impulses at synapses. In the sympathetic nervous system the chemical transmitter is predominantly noradrenaline, whereas in the parasympathetic nervous system, the chemical messenger is acetyl choline. The actions of these two sections of the autonomic nervous system are shown in Table 1 and Figure 6.

**Table 1** Actions of the autonomic nervous system

| Organ supplied | Sympathetic activity | Parasympathetic activity |
|---|---|---|
| Pupil of the eye | Dilates | Constricts |
| Air passages, bronchi and bronchioles | Dilates | Constricts |
| Salivary glands | | Increased salivary secretion and dilatation of blood vessels |
| Heart | Speeds up, increases force of ventricular contraction | Slows heart rate |
| Digestive tract | Reduces motility | Increases motility |
| Sphincters of the digestive tract | Constricts | Relaxes |
| Rectum | Allows filling | Empties and relaxes anal sphincters |
| Bladder | Allows filling | Empties and relaxes internal sphincter |
| Blood vessels | Vasoconstriction | Nil (except salivary gland and external genitalia-vasodilatation) |
| Sweat glands | Sweating | Nil |

### 3.2.1.1 The sympathetic nervous system

The sympathetic nervous system is active in states of emotional excitement and stress. The system gives rise to what has been called the 'flight or fight' reaction. Increased sympathetic nerve activity causes the heart to beat faster and also increases the force of contraction of the ventricles of the heart (the force with which the heart muscle contracts) and these effects cause an increase in the output from the heart (cardiac output) and therefore the blood pressure increases. In addition, the pupils of the eye dilate, the air passages increase in diameter allowing an individual to breath in more air, and also contracts the muscles associated with sweat glands and skin causing the hair to 'stand on end' and form goose pimples. The rate at which breathing occurs also increases and this is due to excitement of the respiratory centres in the brain. In addition, sympathetic stimulation slows down the contractions of the digestive tract.

***Structure of the sympathetic nervous system***

The nerve cell (the neuron) in the spinal cord (lateral horn) sends a fibre (axon), referred to as the pre-ganglionic fibre, to the ganglion (a collection of nerve cells and their fibres), which is called the sympathetic ganglion. A second fibre starts from the synapse within the ganglion and terminates in the organ (e.g. smooth muscle) it supplies. The preganglionic fibre is covered by a white fatty sheath made of myelin. For

**Figure 6** Diagram of the autonomic nervous system and the organs it controls. Not to scale.

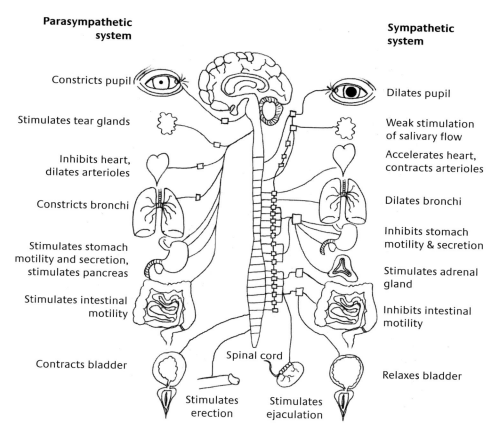

| Parasympathetic system | Sympathetic system |
|---|---|
| Constricts pupil | Dilates pupil |
| Stimulates tear glands | Weak stimulation of salivary flow |
| Inhibits heart, dilates arterioles | Accelerates heart, contracts arterioles |
| Constricts bronchi | Dilates bronchi |
| | Inhibits stomach motility & secretion |
| Stimulates stomach motility and secretion, stimulates pancreas | Stimulates adrenal gland |
| Stimulates intestinal motility | Inhibits intestinal motility |
| Contracts bladder | Relaxes bladder |
| Spinal cord | |
| Stimulates erection | Stimulates ejaculation |

this reason, the bundle of pre-ganglionic fibres is called the white ramus. The fibre after the ganglion is termed the post-ganglionic fibre and does not have a myelin sheath, therefore is grey in colour and referred to as the grey ramus.

In the spinal cord, the pre-ganglionic outflow takes place between the first thoracic segment and the second lumbar segment. The cells of origin are in the lateral horn of the spinal grey matter in these segments and the fibres leave the spinal cord with the nerves to the voluntary or skeletal or striated muscles. All the fibres from these cells in the lateral horns run to a chain of neurons called the sympathetic chain which lies very close to the spinal cord. The sympathetic trunk extends upwards towards the neck to the angle of the jaw (superior cervical ganglion of the sympathetic chain) and extends downwards across the back of the thoracic and abdominal cavities to the pelvis.

The chemical transmitters found in the sympathetic nervous system are adrenaline (epinephrine) and noradrenaline (norepinephrine). Chemically, noradrenaline and adrenaline are amines of the benzene derivative catechol and are referred to collectively as catecholamines. Noradrenaline is rapidly removed after release, mainly by re-uptake into the nerve so that the target organ is capable of responding to further nerve impulses. However, the neurotransmitter at the site between the pre-ganglionic and post-ganglionic fibres (the ganglion) is acetylcholine.

### Effects of sympathetic nervous activity

Over-activity of the sympathetic nervous system leads to narrowing of blood vessels (vasoconstriction) and consequently a reduction of the blood supply to the organ or tissue. If it is widespread, the narrowing of the blood vessels will lead to an increase in blood pressure (hypertension), profuse sweating and dilatation of the pupils.

Sympathetic nerve fibres can cause either contraction or relaxation of the smooth muscle of the innervated structure. When noradrenaline causes contraction, the receptor responding to the neurotransmitter is referred to as an alpha receptor. If the action of the sympathetic nerve system is to cause relaxation, the receptor concerned is called a beta receptor. The alpha and beta receptors found in the sympathetic system are called Ahlquist receptors. These can be blocked selectively by either alpha or beta blockers which are classes of drugs used in medical treatment. Blockade of beta receptors in the heart is used to reduce blood pressure. Stimulation of beta receptors in the airways is used in the treatment of asthma to dilate or increase the lumen through which air can move in the small airways or bronchioles of the lung.

In addition there are ganglion-blocking drugs that block transmission at the sympathetic ganglia, thereby preventing the transmission of the nerve impulse from the pre-ganglionic fibre to the post-ganglionic fibre. These ganglion blockers are used to treat very high blood pressure in cases of emergency.

### 3.2.1.2 Parasympathetic nervous system

The parasympathetic fibres originate in the cranial nerves and from the lower end of the spinal cord (the sacral region). The twelve cranial nerves have the cells of origin in the brainstem. The third, seventh, ninth and tenth cranial nerves all contain parasympathetic fibres. The tenth cranial nerve or the vagus nerve is the principal parasympathetic nerve and its stimulation causes a slowing of the heart amongst many other effects, such as those on the stomach and stomach secretions, oesophagus and the small airways of the lungs.

As in the sympathetic system, the parasympathetic nervous system has two neurons which give rise to the pre-ganglionic and post-ganglionic nerves. However, the post-ganglionic nerve is usually very short. In the heart, the ganglion and the post-ganglionic nerves lie within the organ of innervation, the cardiac muscle.

The neurotransmitter at ganglions (synapses), which are junctions between the pre-ganglionic fibres and the post-ganglionic fibres, in both the parasympathetic nervous system and the sympathetic nervous system is acetylcholine (see Figure 4 of the peripheral nervous system). Acetylcholine is also the neurotransmitter at the post-ganglionic nerve endings of the parasympathetic nervous system, and acts as the neurotransmitter at some post-ganglionic nerve endings of the sympathetic nervous system.

Acetylcholine (ACh) has two distinct actions within the autonomic nervous system and at the neuromuscular junction, which are described as nicotinic or muscarinic. These terms were used since early experimenters applied the two chemicals nicotine or muscarine (found in toadstools) directly to autonomic nerves. ACh activity in the ganglia of the parasympathetic systems and the neuromuscular junction is called nicotinic, while the activity at the junction between the end of the nerve and the organ supplied, other than skeletal muscle, is termed muscarinic.

Like noradrenaline, the effects of acetylcholine are terminated very quickly after its release. However, with acetylcholine it is due to the activity of the enzyme acetylcholine esterase (AChE). Inhibition of this enzyme is the basis of poisoning by organophosphate pesticides and nerve gases.

In most parts of the body, the action of the parasympathetic nervous system is the opposite of that of the sympathetic nervous system (Table 1). Thus it slows the heart rate, lowers blood pressure, constricts the pupils and constricts or narrows the airways. In addition, the parasympathetic nervous system speeds up digestion and plays an important role in defaecation and emptying of the bladder and increases secretions from several glands such as the salivary glands and tear glands.

## 3.3   Neurotransmitters

In 1921, the Austrian scientist Otto Loewi discovered the first neurotransmitter. In his experiment (which came to him in a dream), he used two frog hearts. One heart (heart 1) was still connected to the vagus nerve. Heart 1 was placed in a chamber that was filled with saline. This chamber was connected to a second chamber that contained heart 2. Fluid from chamber 1 was allowed to flow into chamber 2. Electrical stimulation of the vagus nerve caused heart 1 to slow down. Loewi also observed that after a delay, heart 2 also slowed down. From this experiment, Loewi hypothesised that electrical stimulation of the vagus nerve released a chemical into the fluid of chamber 1 that flowed into chamber 2. He called this chemical "Vagusstoff". We now know this chemical as the neurotransmitter – acetylcholine.

Neuroscientists (scientists who study the nervous system) consider the following criteria necessary for a chemical to be termed a neurotransmitter:

- the chemical must be produced within a nerve cell;
- the chemical must be found within a nerve cell;
- when a nerve cell is stimulated, the nerve cell must release the chemical;
- when the chemical is released it must act on a specialised area, usually in the adjacent or neighbouring nerve cell (the post-synaptic nerve cell) and cause a biological effect where usually there is a change which alters the movement of ions across a cell membrane;
- after the chemical is released it must be inactivated. This may occur due to re-uptake of the chemical by the nerve cell that released it or by an enzyme which alters its chemical structure and therefore prevents further action at the receptor or specialised nerve ending; and

- if this chemical is applied on the post-synaptic membrane (i.e. the membrane of the adjacent nerve cell), it should produce the same effect as when the chemical is released by a nerve cell.

There are many types of chemicals that act as neurotransmitters. The more common neurotransmitters and those of particular interest in toxicology are:

- acetylcholine;
- norepinephrine or noradrenaline;
- epinephrine or adrenaline;
- dopamine;
- serotonin;
- histamine;
- gamma amino butyric acid (GABA);
- glycines, and
- glutamate aspartate.

Acetylcholine is found in both the central and peripheral nervous systems. Choline is taken up by the neuron. When the enzyme choline acetyltransferase is present, choline combines with acetyl coenzyme A (CoA) to produce acetylcholine.

Dopamine, norepinephrine and epinephrine are a group of neurotransmitters called 'catecholamines'. Norepinephrine used to be known as 'noradrenaline' and epinephrine as 'adrenaline'. Each of these neurotransmitters is produced in a step-by-step fashion by different enzymes.

Neurotransmitters are made in the cell body of the neuron and then transported down the axon to the axon terminal. Molecules of neurotransmitters are stored in small packages called vesicles. Neurotransmitters are released from the axon terminal when their vesicles 'fuse' with the membrane of the axon terminal, spilling the neurotransmitter into the synaptic cleft.

Neurotransmitters will bind only to specific areas (receptors) on the post-synaptic membrane that recognise them.

### 3.3.1 Some neurotransmitters and their effects

***Norepinephrine (Noradrenaline)***
Norepinephrine functions in:
- Arousal, energy, drive
- Stimulation
- Fight or flight

Norepinephrine deficiencies result in:
- Lack of energy
- Lack of motivation
- Depression

### *Dopamine*

Dopamine functions in:

- Feelings of pleasure
- Feelings of attachment/love
- Sense of altruism
- Integration of thoughts and feelings

Dopamine deficiencies result in:

- Anhedonia: the loss of the capacity to experience pleasure. Anhedonia is a core clinical feature of depression, schizophrenia, and some other mental illnesses
- Lack of ability to feel love, sense attachment to another
- Lack of remorse about actions
- Distractibility

### *Serotonin*

Serotonin functions in:

- Emotional stability
- Reducing aggression
- Sensory input
- Sleep cycle
- Appetite control

Serotonin deficiencies result in:

- Irritability
- Irrational emotions
- Sudden unexplained tears
- Obsessive-compulsive disorder
- Sleep disturbances

### *Gamma-aminobutyric acid (GABA)*

GABA functions in:

- Control of anxiety
- Control of arousal
- Control of convulsions
- Keeps brain activity 'balanced'

GABA deficiencies result in:

- 'Free-floating' anxiety
- Racing thoughts
- Rapid heart
- Inability to fall asleep
- Constant 'fight or flight' state
- Panic

## 3.4   The neuromuscular junction

The junction between the motor nerve and the skeletal muscle fibre which it supplies is the neuromuscular junction. This is very important both in health and disease for several reasons. Firstly, there is a gap between the nerve fibre endings and the muscle fibres and the messages across this gap are carried by the neurotransmitter acetylcholine. The acetylcholine is synthesised in the nerve fibre and is discharged when an impulse reaches the end of the nerve fibre. This chemical messenger reaches specialised parts of the muscle fibre called end plates, which contain specific receptors through which sodium ions pass into muscle fibre and produce a change in membrane potential which is called the end plate potential. This movement of ions – depolarisation – spreads to the whole muscle fibre (propagated action potential) causing calcium ion release, and muscle contraction follows.

Acetylcholine stays only for a very brief period at the neuromuscular junction as it is quickly hydrolysed or inactivated by the enzyme acetylcholinesterase. This enables the next impulse to release acetylcholine again and cause another muscle contraction.

The neuromuscular junction functional activity is vulnerable to many toxic substances. Firstly toxic substances can interfere with the production and release of the chemical messenger acetylcholine. The specialised parts of the muscle fibres may be damaged or altered in disease states such as myasthenia gravis. The enzyme cholinesterase, which restricts acetylcholine in time and space, can be inactivated by several toxic substances, of which the best known are the pesticides belonging to the class of compounds called organophosphates. Some chemical warfare agents (nerve agents) such as sarin, tabun and soman are also organophosphates and produce the same effect.

Importantly in medical practice particularly in the speciality of anaesthesia, drugs are used to prevent transmission at the neuromuscular junction and thus produce muscle relaxation (the drugs used being called muscle relaxants) to facilitate surgery. Historically the Indians of South America used a substance as an arrow poison to paralyse their prey during hunting and this arrow poison was refined to become one of the best known muscle relaxants: curare or tubocurarine.

Every muscle in the body consists of muscle fibres which are the units that cause muscles to contract and enable us to move, run, talk or do whatever we wish to do. Every muscle fibre needs a nerve supply in order to contract. The origin of these nerves to muscle are from cells in the spinal cord (anterior horn cells) and as there are more muscle fibres than nerve cells, each nerve cell or anterior horn cell innervates more than one muscle fibre. For example in the leg, as many as 200 muscle fibres may share a single anterior horn cell. Where eye muscles are concerned, only about five muscle fibres would share one anterior horn cell.

These nerves leaving the anterior horn cell are called axons or motor nerves and branch to supply a group of muscle fibres on reaching the muscle. The anterior horn cell and the muscle fibres supplied by this neuron are called the motor unit. The motor unit forms the basis for voluntary movement (movements which are intentional). If the motor nerve or axon is cut or damaged, paralysis of muscles occurs.

Nerves from the anterior horn cells carry nerve impulses or messages which enable the muscle fibres to contract. If an anterior horn cell discharges slowly or at a very low frequency, the muscles tend to be relaxed or flaccid. When the rate of discharge from the neurons increases, one may see co-ordinated contractions. However, these motor neurons are capable of discharging at very fast rates, usually in disease states leading to either tremulous contractions-clonus or sustained contractions-tetanus. Tetanus is also the name given to an infection (lock-jaw) caused by the tetanus bacillus (*Clostridium tetani*), which occurs when wounds become contaminated with soil/faeces which contains the bacteria, and has been a serious sequel of accidents and war injuries before immunisation against the disease became available.

## 4    The heart and circulatory system – the cardiovascular system

The heart and the cardiovascular system are involved in the transport of blood. Blood is transported through the body via a continuous system of blood vessels. Blood vessels that carry blood away from the heart are called arteries and vessels that bring blood to the heart are called veins. Arteries usually carry oxygenated blood away from the heart into capillaries supplying tissue cells. The exception is the pulmonary artery which carries venous blood from the right side of the heart to the lungs. Veins collect the blood from the capillary bed and carry it back to the heart and usually carry 'dirty' blood, except of course for the pulmonary vein which brings oxygenated blood from the lungs to the left side of the heart (Figure 7).

The circulatory system is divided into:
- the pulmonary circulation, which takes unoxygenated blood from the right side of the heart to the lungs and returns to the left side of the heart with oxygenated blood;
- the systemic circulation, which takes oxygenated blood from the left side of the heart to all cells in the body and returns unoxygenated blood (i.e. blood from which the cells have extracted the necessary oxygen and carrying the carbon dioxide returned by the cells ) to the right side of the heart.

The circulation or the cardiovascular system also:
- carries food from the digestive tract to the cells to provide nutrition for growth and energy;
- carries waste products from cells in the body to the kidneys to enable the body to get rid of (excrete) these unwanted products in the urine;
- carries hormones from the glands that produce them (endocrine glands) to other organs of the body, and
- carries heat from parts of the body where heat is produced to the skin so that surplus heat can be given off.

### 4.1    The heart

The heart is an organ consisting essentially of two pumps, right and left, which circulate blood round the body. Each pump has two chambers, the atrium which collects the blood either from the lungs (the left atrium) or from the tissues (right atrium) and then passes through valves to the major pumping chambers  – the ventricles. The left ventricle pumps the blood with oxygen which has entered the chamber from the

**Figure 7** Diagrammatic representation of the circulatory system. Not to scale.

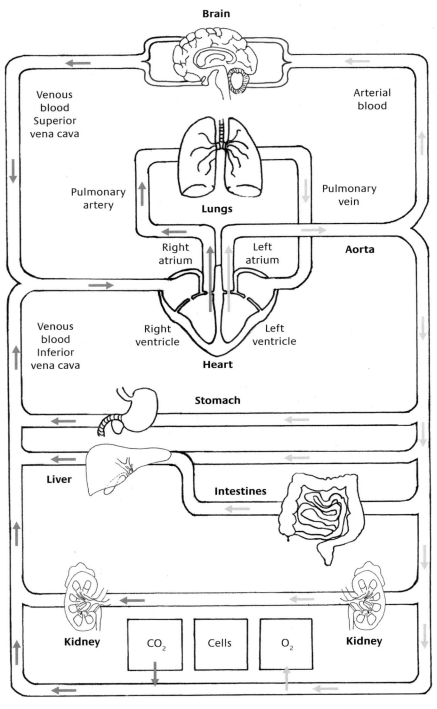

left atrium (diffused through the small air sacs or alveoli in the lungs and bound to haemoglobin and also oxygen dissolved in the blood [in solution] to the tissues), whilst the right ventricle pumps the blood that has returned from the cells or tissues (after extraction of oxygen and nutrients and containing greater amounts of carbon dioxide than in the blood which reached the cells from the left ventricle)) to the lungs to get rid of the waste products such as carbon dioxide.

Each time the heart beats, each ventricle pumps out about 70 ml of blood, and this volume is termed the stroke volume. The heart beats about 70 times a minute, which is termed the heart rate; this is usually measured in patients by counting the pulse rate at the wrist.

## 4.2   Blood vessels and blood pressure

From the left side of the heart, oxygenated blood is pumped by the left ventricle to the aorta which carries blood to the whole body. From the aorta arise the large arteries or branches which carry the oxygenated blood to the various parts of the body. For example, the carotid arteries arising from the aorta supply the brain, and the renal arteries arising from the aorta supply the kidneys. From the aorta, blood goes to the arteries, the next group of blood vessels that carry oxygenated blood, and then to arterioles as it nears organs or cells to which the blood supply is intended. From arterioles the blood goes into the very thin-walled capillaries which travel between cells and give out oxygen and allow carbon dioxide to come into the blood vessel. Now the blood, which has provided oxygen and nutrition to the cells, passes from the end of the capillaries to the venules, veins and then to the larger veins – the superior and inferior vena cava.

The capacity of the venous side of the circulation is much greater than that of the arterial side and often accommodates 75% of the blood volume. This is because the walls of the vessels on the venous side are not as thick and contain less muscle than the vessels on the arterial side. The left ventricle contracts each time the blood is pushed into the aorta and this flow of blood causes a wave of flow commonly referred to as a pulse. This pulse can be felt only in arteries which are often not visible, but on the contrary veins are often visible and a pulse cannot be felt in veins as the flow in them is not pulsatile. It is the fluctuation of the blood pressure in the artery between the systolic pressure (e.g. 130 mm Hg) and the diastolic pressure (e.g. 80 mm Hg) that gives rise to the pulse.

**Blood pressure** is the force applied to the wall of the arteries as the heart pumps blood to the cells in the body through the arterioles and capillaries. The measurement of blood pressure is dependent on the amount of blood pumped, which in turn is dependent on the volume of blood in the body (blood volume), the force with which the heart pumps the blood and the diameter and elasticity of the arteries. This pressure from behind (driven by the left ventricle) is termed in Latin *vis a tergo*.

In order to have a blood pressure there has to be a flow from the heart – **cardiac output** – and a resistance to flow on the arterial or systemic side of the circulation. This resistance (the peripheral resistance) determines the blood pressure according to the equation:

## Blood pressure = cardiac output × peripheral resistance

The resistance to blood flow is mainly in the small arterioles as it is the smaller diameter vessels that offer the greatest resistance to flow through them.

There are two components to a measurement of blood pressure. The first is the maximum pressure exerted when the heart is pumping the blood – the systolic pressure. The second represents the pressure in the arteries when the heart is at rest – diastolic pressure. In 'normal' people these measurements are recorded as 130/80 mm of Hg.

The arterioles have smooth muscle in their walls, which is arranged circularly. When the muscle contracts it makes the blood vessels smaller. The sympathetic nervous system provides a nerve supply to these vessels and stimulation of this system causes contraction of the smooth muscle in the walls and thus vasoconstriction and an increase in peripheral resistance and hence of blood pressure. When the arterioles are relaxed or when the sympathetic nerve stimulation is not present, the vessels are vasodilated or there is vasodilation. The diameter of these vessels is directly under the control of the sympathetic nerve outflow regulated by the vasomotor centre in the medulla oblongata of the brain.

There are many nerve cell groupings that influence the activity of the vasomotor centre. The best known are the baroreceptors which are found in a special area, the carotid sinus, of each carotid artery (arteries supplying blood to the brain). The higher centres in the brain (regions of the brain where conscious thoughts occur) also influence the activity of the vasomotor centre. Emotional stress and excitement cause stimulation of the vasomotor centre and an increase in blood pressure. Carbon dioxide content in the blood also influences vasomotor centre activity. When the carbon dioxide content and tension is low, as in patients who are breathing rapidly, the activity of the vasomotor centre is reduced. A shortage of oxygen, in contrast, would increase the activity of the vasomotor centre.

There are several factors affecting blood pressure. These include disease of arteries such as thickening or loss of muscle fibres (arteriosclerosis, which usually occurs with ageing), psychological factors such as stress, anger and fear, kidney disease, and pain. Certain hormonal disorders are also associated with a high blood pressure. An increase in blood pressure may occur during pregnancy in some individuals.

## 4.3 The blood (haematopoietic system)

An adult has approximately 5 litres of blood in the body. A new born baby has only 300 ml (80 ml per kg body weight). Blood is composed of cells (45%) and plasma (55%). Blood cells are formed in the bone marrow, which is found in cavities of bones. Blood cells can be broadly divided into red and white blood cells and platelets.

### Red blood cells

There are approximately 5 million red blood cells per cubic mm of blood that contain the pigment haemoglobin, which is bright red in colour when combined with oxygen and is purple-blue in colour when no oxygen is present. Every 100 ml of blood has about 15 g of haemoglobin and this haemoglobin plays an important role in the carriage of not only oxygen but also of carbon dioxide. The life span of the red cell is about 100 days. For the formation of red blood cells (and also of proteins), iron is required, and deficiency of iron would lead to iron deficiency anaemia. Other requirements for the formation of red blood cells are vitamin B12 and folic acid. Lack of vitamin B12 and folic acid leads to the formation of abnormally large red blood cells and a state called megaloblastic anaemia.

The hormone erythropoetin which is formed in the kidney also plays a role in the production of red blood cells as this hormone is produced in increased amounts when the body is lacking in oxygen, often for long periods of time. This hormone stimulates the bone marrow to produce more red blood cells.

### White blood cells

There are three types of white blood cells – lymphocytes, granulocytes and monocytes.

The lymphocytes produce antibodies which are able to react with foreign substances called antigens and destroy the antigens. Thus they are an important protective mechanism of the blood and of the body.

The granulocytes are larger than the lymphocytes in size and are so called as they contain granules. Some of these granules take up the red stain eosin more readily and are called eosinophils whilst others take up the basic stain haemotoxylin and are called basophils. Those that do not take up either the acidic or the basic stain are called neutrophils. The nuclei of the granulocytes are divided into many connected parts and are therefore called polymorphonuclear cells. The most important aspect of granulocyte activity is their ability to ingest foreign particles that enter the blood – a process called phagocytosis. The granules contain enzymes which are able to digest these engulfed particles, which may include bacteria and other organisms capable of causing infections.

Monocytes are the largest in size of the white blood cells and are able to engulf foreign particles – i.e. are capable of phagocytosis, like the granulocytes.

The granulocytes make up about 70% of the white blood cells (neutrophils 65%, eosinophils 4% and basophils 1%). The lymphocytes make up about 25% of the total white cells and monocytes the remaining 5%.

### Platelets and blood clotting

Platelets have two main functions in the human body. They are able to clump together and block small holes in the blood vessels by forming platelet plugs. This is a very important step in preventing loss of blood or bleeding from blood vessels, particularly after injuries.

Blood clotting is a process by which the body prevents loss of blood from blood vessels following injury. It is initiated by a platelet plug and also by the breakdown of platelets which causes the release of a factor called thromboplastin which converts a component of the blood called prothrombin to thrombin in the presence of calcium ions. Thrombin when formed, acts on another component in the blood called fibrinogen, and changes the fibrinogen to fibrin which is actually the blood clot.

There are a few inherited diseases where the clotting of blood is affected due to lack of specific substances in the person's blood. These diseases include haemophilia and Christmas disease.

### Plasma

Plasma is the straw-coloured fluid in which the blood cells are suspended. It consists of a watery solution of plasma proteins and plasma electrolytes and all the substances transported in the blood. It also contains the factors or ingredients necessary for blood clotting. If the factors necessary for blood clotting are removed from plasma, the remaining fluid is called serum.

### 4.4    Common medical terms used to describe symptoms and signs of heart and blood vessel disorders

**Hypotension:** is an abnormally low blood pressure which can occur following blood or excessive fluid loss, failure of the heart to pump efficiently (heart failure) or as a result of toxic effects on the arterioles causing a decrease in peripheral resistance. Abnormally low blood pressure is seen in the clinical state referred to as shock. Hypotension may also follow loss of plasma, as in burns.

**Hypertension:** is defined as a sustained normally high blood pressure. Transient high blood pressures are part of a normal circulation. Hypertension causes a strain on the left ventricle which has to pump the blood against a higher pressure. Initially the heart muscle increases in size (left ventricular hypertrophy). This can then lead to failure of the heart to maintain normal function, i.e. heart failure. High blood pressure may also cause blood vessels to burst and this may occur in the blood vessels to the brain, i.e. stroke. If this occurs, it may result in paralysis on the side opposite to the site where the blood vessel burst, due to the anatomy of the nervous system and brain circulation.

**Ischaemic heart disease:** is a disease of the blood vessels to the heart which results in an insufficient supply of oxygen to the heart muscles, which is severe enough to cause temporary strain, or even permanent damage to the muscle – i.e. death of muscle fibres.

**Myocardial infarction:** is a term used to describe irreversible injury to heart muscle, which results in loss of function or inability of the muscle to pump blood. Common symptoms include crushing central chest pain that may radiate to the jaw or arms. Chest pain may be associated with nausea, sweating and shortness of breath.

**Angina:** is a chest pain that occurs secondary to the inadequate delivery of oxygen to the heart muscle. It is often described as a heavy or squeezing pain in the midsternal area of the chest. When the blood supply to the heart muscle is reduced, due usually to a partial or complete obstruction of the blood flow in the arteries supplying the heart muscle (coronary arteries), the pain that arises is called angina pectoris. It is a tight constricting pain round the chest but may also be felt on the inside of the arms or in the neck.

**Dyspnoea:** is difficult or laboured breathing; shortness of breath. Dyspnoea is a sign of serious disease of the airways, lungs, or heart.

**Oedema:** is the presence of abnormally large amounts of fluid in the intercellular tissue spaces of the body, usually applied to demonstrable accumulation of excessive fluid in the subcutaneous tissues. Oedema may be localised, due to venous or lymphatic obstruction or to increased vascular permeability (which may follow stings from insects), or it may be more widespread due to heart failure or renal disease. Collections of oedema fluid are designated according to the site, for example ascites (peritoneal cavity), hydrothorax (pleural cavity) and hydropericardium (pericardial sac). Oedema due to heart failure is usually first detected as a swelling around the ankles (ankle oedema). Oedema may also occur at the back in front of the end of the spinal cord (sacral area), where it is referred to as sacral oedema.

## 5    The respiratory system

Respiration or breathing has three main functions:

1. to deliver oxygen to the cells;
2. to eliminate carbon dioxide and
3. to regulate the pH of the blood.

The oxidation of carbon and hydrogen from food in order to produce energy and heat requires oxygen from the air, obtained through breathing. In the cells, oxygen is delivered to the mitochondria – intra-cellular structures which are the 'powerhouses' of the cells. Mitochondria have cytochromes which combine the oxygen, hydrogen and carbon atoms to generate energy in the form of adenosine triphosphate (ATP), and produce water and carbon dioxide as a waste product.

At rest, 250 ml of oxygen are absorbed per minute during breathing to satisfy the metabolic requirements of the body. The energy requirements depend on the level of activity of the individual. For example during heavy exercise, the oxygen requirement may be as high as 5000 ml of oxygen per minute.

The lungs fill the thoracic cavity. During breathing, the thoracic cavity expands and the lungs also expand. This creates a negative pressure inside the chest which sucks air in through the structures shown in Figure 8. This is referred to as inspiration. When the thoracic cavity returns to its normal (resting) size, the lungs also decrease in size and the air is forced out through the respiratory tract. This is called expiration.

Physiologically, four phases of respiration are recognised:

1. Ventilation: the movement of air to and from the lungs.
2. Distribution: air entering the lungs is distributed to all parts including the small air sacs (alveoli) where gas transfer to and from the blood takes place.
3. Diffusion: the oxygen from the air diffuses through the walls of the alveoli to the adjacent blood vessels and carbon dioxide from the blood vessels diffuses back into the alveoli.
4. Perfusion: blood rich in carbon dioxide and low in oxygen is pumped to the lungs via the pulmonary arteries, by the right ventricle of the heart. Blood low in carbon dioxide but loaded with oxygen is returned to the heart via the pulmonary veins. Matching of ventilation and perfusion (i.e. blood supply to the alveoli – air sacs) within the lung ensures normal gas exchange.

The alternating increase and decrease in the size of the chest during normal breathing is under the control of collections of nerve cells in the medulla oblongata (the respiratory centre). Nerves from the anterior horn cells in the cervical and thoracic regions of the spinal cord supply the muscles of respiration. The main muscles involved are the diaphragm and the intercostal muscles (the muscles between the ribs). These muscles are all striated (skeletal) muscles, which are muscles that are usually under voluntary control (by the somatic nervous system). For this reason, the normal reflex action of breathing can be overridden by voluntary activity, such as taking a deep breath.

The respiratory system can be affected by a wide range of agents including drugs such as morphine (commonly grouped as opiates which are agents derived from or containing

**Figure 8** Diagram of the respiratory system. Not to scale.

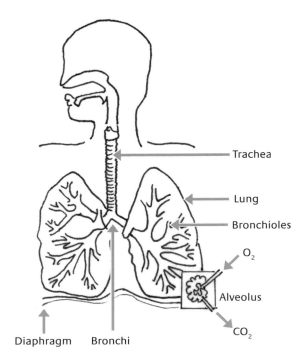

Hypoxia may be due to decreased amount of oxygen in the air breathed in (inspired oxygen) as at high altitude, or may be due to lung disease when the oxygen cannot enter the red blood cells in the blood that flows through the lungs.

In contrast to asphyxia, where an individual will struggle to breathe with all the available resources in the body, in hypoxia, the individual will soon lose control and become unconscious.

If the supply of oxygen to the brain cells is interrupted for more than three minutes (as seen when the heart ceases to pump blood effectively [commonly referred to as cardiac arrest]), the nerve cells in the brain may be irreversibly damaged and may lead to 'brain death'. If there is a deficiency of haemoglobin to transport the oxygen, as is seen in anaemic patients due to either poor nutrition or prolonged blood loss, as with heavy menstruation or bleeding piles, the term used is anaemic hypoxia. The hypoxia associated with carbon monoxide poisoning is an anaemic hypoxia as there is insufficient haemoglobin to transport the oxygen due to its preferential binding with carbon monoxide, which has an affinity about 250 times greater for haemoglobin than oxygen.

If blood flow is very slow, there would be insufficient oxygen for the cells to function. This is referred to as stagnant hypoxia.

Finally the cells may be unable to utilise the oxygen brought to them by the blood due to the enzymes within the cells being inactive or destroyed. This occurs in cyanide poisoning, where vital enzymes such as the cytochromes are destroyed by the cyanide and the cells cannot extract the oxygen in the blood.

### 5.3.3  Pulmonary oedema

In the lungs, the pulmonary arterial pressure is usually 25 mm Hg compared to about 130 mm Hg in arteries arising from the aorta from the left ventricle. When the pressure in the left atrium or pulmonary veins is elevated (for example when the atrium cannot empty its contents to the left ventricle either because the atrium muscle is not contracting in the normal manner or when there is an obstruction to the flow of blood from the atrium to the ventricle such as narrowing/stenosis of the valve between the two chambers, commonly referred to as mitral stenosis), the pressure in the pulmonary capillaries could be exceeded to such an extent that fluid would pass from the capillaries into the alveoli. This fluid would interfere with diffusion of gases. The presence of fluid in the alveoli or in the lung is referred to as pulmonary oedema. Pulmonary oedema leads to difficulty in breathing (as there is insufficient oxygen and accumulation of carbon dioxide, which are both stimuli for the respiratory centre) and the patient would become dyspnoeic – that is being conscious of breathing and difficulty in breathing – and would be breathless. Pulmonary oedema may also occur due to the action of poisonous gases such as chlorine or phosgene, where the structure of the alveolar walls and capillaries are damaged leading to a leakage of fluid into the alveoli. If the left side of the heart fails, the heart muscle on the left side of the heart does not function or contract adequately and there is a build up of pressure in the pulmonary veins bringing blood from the lungs; this would also cause pulmonary oedema.

### 5.3.4  Cyanosis

Cyanosis is a bluish discolouration, especially of the skin and mucous membranes, caused by an excessive concentration of deoxygenated haemoglobin (haemoglobin not bound to oxygen) in the blood. A point of interest to those particularly in countries where anaemia is very common, is that the haemoglobin levels may be so low that the amount of haemoglobin without oxygen (deoxygenated haemoglobin) would be insufficient to cause cyanosis.

## 6    The gastro-intestinal system

Food or water entering the body through the mouth passes down the oesophagus and then to the stomach. From the stomach, partially digested food passes on to the duodenum, jejunum and ileum (small intestine). That which has not been absorbed proceeds to the caecum, ascending, transverse, descending and sigmoid colon (large intestine), the rectum and finally to the anal canal (Figure 10).

**Figure 10** Diagram of the gastro-intestinal system. Not to scale.

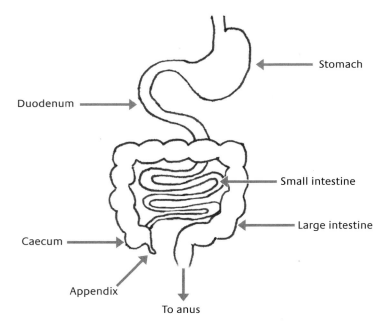

In the mouth, saliva is produced by three paired salivary glands: parotid, submandibular and sublingual. Saliva is secreted by these glands, usually in response to the thought, site, taste or smell of food. Secretion of saliva is under control of the parasympathetic nervous system. Thus when there is over-activity of the parasympathetic nervous system and there is more secretion of the neurotransmitter of that system (acetylcholine), there will be excessive secretions, for examples as in organophosphorus insecticide poisoning. If the action of acetylcholine on the receptors is blocked by drugs such as atropine, dryness of the mouth results.

The food formed into a bolus in the mouth passes down the oesophagus due to propulsive contractions of the muscle of the oesophagus, which are controlled by another parasympathetic cranial nerve, the vagus. Then the food enters the stomach which not only acts as a storage organ but also promotes digestion by secretions (pepsin for digestion of proteins, and hydrochloric acid) from the cells lining the stomach wall. The secretions of the stomach are also under the control of the vagus nerve and also a hormone called gastrin.

At regular intervals of minutes, small quantities of food pass through an opening at the distal end of the stomach, called the pyloric sphincter, to the duodenum. The contents of a stomach usually empty in about four hours. However, with a very fatty meal, the emptying of the stomach becomes much slower due to the release of a hormone called enterogastrone.

Stomach ulcers or duodenal ulcers, commonly referred to as peptic ulcers, occur because pepsin, which aids in digesting proteins, acts on the cells of the stomach wall. Digestion of stomach wall cells is aided by the presence of hydrochloric acid, also secreted by the cells lining the stomach.

The stomach also has a role in vitamin B12 metabolism. Loss of the stomach or a large part of it can lead to a condition known as pernicious anaemia, which is due to lack of vitamin B12.

## 6.1    The pancreas

The pancreas is a gland which sends its secretions to the blood stream and also into the duodenum. The secretion of insulin and glucagons, which are necessary for the control of blood sugar in the human body, is from the pancreas. The juices from the pancreas which enter the duodenum, known as the pancreatic juices, contain the enzymes trypsinogen and chymotrypsinogen, which are precursors of the protein splitting enzymes trypsin and chymotrypsin.

Pancreatic secretion is also under control of the vagus nerve. Insulin secretion is from the Islets of Langerhans. Failure to produce sufficient insulin results in diabetes mellitus.

Secretions from the liver also enter the duodenum via the bile duct. The bile is stored and concentrated in the gall bladder, which also contracts due to the action of the vagus nerve, and can also contract due to the action of some hormones. The bile constituents may concentrate and give rise to gall stones, and inflammation of the gall bladder is referred to as cholecystitis.

## 6.2    The small intestine

The small intestine is concerned primarily with the absorption of sugars or carbohydrates and produces the related enzymes maltase, sucrase and lactase. Though the nerve supply to the small intestine is both from the parasympathetic and sympathetic nervous systems, these nerves regulate motility or contractions of the small intestine (peristalsis) and have no role in the production of the digestive enzymes. The absorption of food takes place mainly in the small intestine. Amino acids and fats are also absorbed here.

## 6.3    The large intestine

The large intestine absorbs mostly water so that the water content that reaches the large intestine is ultimately reduced by about two thirds. The large intestine is not essential to life. However, the bacteria present in the large intestine are important in the provision and production of vitamins, particularly those of the vitamin B group.

## 6.4    Common medical signs and symptoms and terms used for gastro-intestinal disorders

**Dyspepsia:** is the impairment of the function of digestion, usually applied to epigastric discomfort following meals.

**Peptic ulcer:** is an ulcer in the wall of the stomach or duodenum resulting from the digestive action of the gastric juice on the mucous membrane, when the latter is rendered susceptible to its action.

**Cholecystitis:** is acute or chronic inflammation of the gallbladder.

**Gall stones:** are stones within the gall bladder, usually of cholesterol (non-opaque) or of calcium bilirubinate (bilirubin), opaque and commonly associated with haemolytic anaemia (Sickle cell disease, spherocytosis, thalassaemia). Gall stones are considered to have an increased incidence in individuals commonly referred to as having the 4 Fs: fat, female, fertile, flatulent.

**Pancreatitis:** is an acute or chronic inflammation of the pancreas, which may be asymptomatic or symptomatic and which is due to autodigestion of pancreatic tissue by its own enzymes. It is caused most often by alcoholism or biliary tract disease, less commonly it may be associated with hyperlipidaemia (increased fat content in blood), hyperparathyroidism (increased activity of the parathyroid glands), abdominal trauma (accidental or operative injury), vasculitis or uraemia (increased content of urea in blood usually due to kidney disease).

**Ileus:** is distension of the intestines, usually due to an obstruction such as a tumour. When a lesion causes a cessation of peristaltic movements in the intestines, the term paralytic ileus is used.

**Pyloric stenosis**: is most often a congenital disorder affecting neonates, where the pylorus is thickened causing obstruction of the gastric outlet to the duodenum. This is more common in males. Symptoms of projectile vomiting begin several weeks after birth. Incidence is approximately 1 in 4,000 live births. Pyloric stenosis may occur in adults due to a tumour at the pyloric end of the stomach.

## 7    The liver

The liver is the chemical factory of the body, both producing essential molecules and modifying and detoxifying ingested toxic substances (Figure 11).

**Figure 11** Diagram of the liver and biliary system. Not to scale.

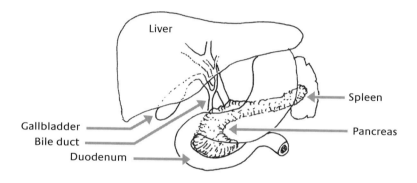

The main functions of the liver are given below.

- Production of essential proteins such as albumin.
- Synthesis of factors that are involved in the clotting of blood.
- Maintaining the level of sugar in the blood. The excess carbohydrate absorbed by the blood from food is converted to glycogen which is also formed from excess fat and protein. The liver glycogen maintains the normal blood glucose level in the blood when glucose is used up by the cells.
- Formation of urea from the ammonia which collects after amino acids have been used up (deaminated). The urea is eliminated through the kidney.
- The bile salt produced by the liver along with products from an anatomically closely related organ, the pancreas, plays a vital role in digestion and absorption of fat. It also stores fat soluble vitamins (A and D).
- The destruction of used red blood cells and removal of the breakdown product of haemoglobin (bilirubin) in the bile via the bile duct to the intestine (duodenum). The liver stores vitamin B12 which is necessary for the maturation of blood cells.
- In relation to toxicology, the liver plays a vital role by modifying the toxicity of foreign substances (toxins, drugs) that gain entry into the body by any route. Some drugs used in medical treatment are administered as pro-drugs which depend on the liver to produce the active drug through

the action of liver enzymes. The liver also has the ability to bind toxic substances to other compounds to make them more water soluble and thus enables the kidney to excrete them from the body.

## 7.1   Jaundice

One of the important roles of the liver, as noted above, is the formation of bilirubin from the red cells that die. Approximately 200 mg of bilirubin are made each day, which is insoluble in water. It is bound to albumin and brought to the liver, where the albumin is replaced by glucuronic acid (an acid made from glucose) which makes the bilirubin water soluble. The water soluble complex passes down the bile duct, which is the channel through which the liver eliminates its waste products, into the intestine (duodenum). Water-soluble bilirubin is responsible for the characteristic colouration of the faeces.

The failure to excrete bilirubin gives rise to yellowish discolouration of the whites of the eyes, the skin and nails and mucosal membranes, which is called jaundice. Jaundice is essentially a sign of liver failure. Several toxic compounds such as some pesticides, solvents such as carbon tetrachloride and dry cleaning fluids, damage the liver cells and prevent them from functioning normally to bind the bilirubin to the glucuronide. There are many drugs used in the treatment of disease which also damage the liver cells and are termed hepatotoxic. For example, very high doses of the common drug paracetamol can cause liver damage, liver failure and jaundice. Another common and important cause of damage to liver cells which often results in liver failure is excessive alcohol (ethanol) consumption.

Therefore in liver failure, jaundice occurs, the blood urea falls (as urea is no longer formed from ammonia), there is insufficient production of proteins, of which albumin is the most important, which may lead to swelling of ankles or oedema (as proteins are essential to maintain plasma osmotic pressure which keeps fluid within capillaries) and blood clotting will be impaired. The most important effect is that the blood will not have sufficient glucose for the cells to function normally.

In addition, when the liver cells fail to function properly, their ability to make foreign substances less toxic by metabolic enzymes fails and the toxicity of some drugs used in medicine such as morphine is increased.

## 7.2   Role of the liver in metabolism of xenobiotics

Man is constantly and unavoidably exposed to foreign chemicals or xenobiotics, which include both man-made and natural chemicals such as medical drugs, industrial chemicals, pesticides, pollutants, plant alkaloids and plant metabolites and toxins produced by moulds, plants and animals.

The physical property that enables many xenobiotics to be absorbed through the skin, lungs or gastrointestinal tract is their fat solubility or lipophilicity. Lipophilicity is also an obstacle to their elimination as they can be readily reabsorbed. Another important consideration is that lipophilicity facilitates the entry of toxic substances into cells. Therefore, the elimination of xenobiotics often depends on their conversion to water soluble compounds by a process called bio-transformation, which is catalysed by enzymes in the liver and other tissues. An important result of biotransformation is the conversion of a lipophilic substance to one that is more water soluble (hydrophilic) (see Phase 1 and Phase 2 reactions below).

This transformation is probably one of the most important defence mechanisms of the body. Xenobiotics such as drugs exert beneficial effects and others may cause deleterious effects as in the case of poisons. The effect a xenobiotic produces in the human body is dependent on its physicochemical properties and thus the results of xenobiotic exposure would be altered by this process of biotransformation.

Some drugs must undergo biotransformation to be effective because the metabolite of the drug and not the drug itself produces a therapeutic or beneficial effect. Similarly, some xenobiotics undergo biotransformation to produce their harmful or toxic effects. However, in the vast majority of situations, biotransformation terminates the effectiveness of the xenobiotic in the human body, be they beneficial or harmful. In the context of toxicology, this means that many potentially toxic substances are made relatively innocuous by biotransformation by liver enzymes. These are predominantly the cytochrome P450 group of isoenzymes which are responsible for the majority of oxidation reactions which xenobiotics undergo.

The enzymes catalysing biotransformation reactions often determine the intensity and duration of the action of drugs and play a key role in chemical toxicity. The xenobiotic biotransforming enzymes catalyse two types of reactions. These are:

**Phase I reactions:** addition of a functional group (e.g. -OH, -NH2, -SH or -COOH) to produce a slight increase in water solubility or hydrophilicity.

**Phase II reactions:** include glucuronidation, sulfation, acetylation, methylation, conjugation with glutathione and conjugation with amino acids (e.g. glycine, taurine, glutamic acid). These reactions cause a large increase in water solubility and thus increase the excretion of the xenobiotic. For example:

> Morphine, heroin and codeine are all converted to morphine-3-glucuronide. In the case of morphine, this is a result of direct conjugation with glucuronide. In the instance of heroin and codeine, conjugation with glucuronic acid is preceded by phase I biotransformation – hydrolysis or deacetylation – with heroin and demethylation involving oxidation by cytochrome P450 isoenzymes with codeine.

## 7.3   The cytochrome P450 enzyme system

The liver is the organ with the highest concentration of enzymes catalysing biotransformation reactions. These enzymes are also located in the skin, lungs, nasal mucosa (mucosa of the nose), eyes and gastrointestinal tract.

In the liver and in most other organs, they are located in the cells, primarily in the endoplasmic reticulum (microsomes) or in the soluble fraction of the cytoplasm, with a smaller concentration in the mitochondria, nuclei and lysosomes.

Amongst the phase I biotransformation enzymes, the cytochrome P450 system is responsible for most oxidation reactions and is probably the most versatile, detoxifying more xenobiotics than any other enzyme system.

In humans, about 40 different microsomal and mitochondrial P450 enzymes play a key role in catalysing reactions in the following areas:

- the metabolism of drugs, environmental pollutants and other xenobiotics;
- the biosynthesis of steroid hormones;
- the oxidation of unsaturated fatty acids to intracellular messengers, and
- metabolism of fat soluble vitamins.

The liver microsomal P450 enzymes involved in xenobiotic biotransformation belong to three main P450 gene families: CYP 1, CYP 2 and CYP 3. The level and activity of each P450 enzyme varies from individual to individual due to genetic and environmental factors.

It is important to remember that the activity of the CYP isoenzymes can be altered by several agents. For example, there are many drugs that would increase the activity of the isoenzymes and these are called enzyme inducers. Similarly some xenobiotics can inhibit the activity of CYP450 isoenzymes and these are called enzyme inhibitors. The induction of CYP450 isoenzymes by drugs such as phenobarbital (a barbiturate used primarily in the treatment of epilepsy) or rifampicin (an antibiotic used in the treatment of tuberculosis) can prevent the effectiveness of the oral contraceptive drug ethinyl oestradiol.

## 7.4    Common medical signs, symptoms and terms associated with liver dysfunction

**Jaundice:** is a yellowing of the skin (and whites of eyes) by bilirubin, a bile pigment, frequently caused by a liver problem.

**Ascites:** an accumulation of serous fluid within the inner lining of the abdominal cavity (the peritoneal cavity), which causes a 'bulging' abdomen.

**Hepatic encephalopathy:** A condition which is used to describe the deleterious effects of liver failure on the central nervous system. Features include confusion and dementia and often lead to unresponsiveness (coma). A common cause is alcoholic cirrhosis.

## 8    The kidney

The kidneys are two bean-shaped organs about the size of a fist lying below the rib cage. Though small in size (about 0.5% of the body weight), the kidneys receive approximately

20% of the blood that is pumped out from the heart via the renal arteries. The main parts of the kidney are an outer lightly coloured cortex and an inner darker medulla (Figure 12). The renal (kidney) pelvis is the funnel which collects the urine from nephrons and enables the urine to flow to the ureters. The ureters are the tubes that carry the urine from the kidneys to the urinary bladder.

**Figure 12** Diagram of the kidney. Not to scale.

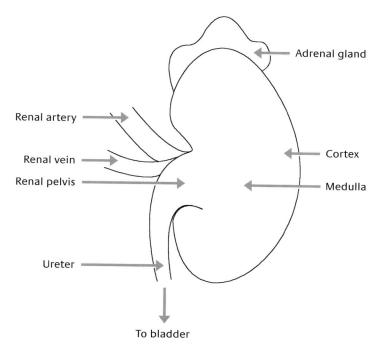

The blood brought to the kidneys by the arteries is filtered under pressure by a part of the basic functional unit of the kidney – the nephron (Figure 13). There are approximately one million nephrons and each nephron is a thin long convoluted tube, surrounded by capillaries, which is closed at one end, where the filtering takes place. The filtered fluid is then absorbed from within the nephron, according to the needs of the body. The cells of the tubules also have the ability to secrete substances into the lumen of the tubule of the nephron to be excreted from the body, in the urine. These are usually unwanted substances and include many toxins and drugs.

The kidney is one of the most important organs through which the body can get rid of waste products and unwanted substances. The blood supply and blood vessels and the structure of the kidney enable the entire blood volume of an individual to be filtered 20–25 times a day. The 'cleaned' blood is returned to the circulation by the renal veins.

Essentially, three basic processes take place in the nephron: filtration, absorption or reabsorption, and secretion or excretion.

**Figure 13** Diagram of the nephron. Not to scale.

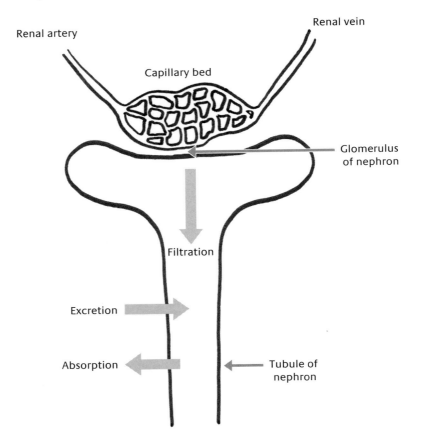

The principal function of the kidney is to produce urine which is excreted from the body and ensures the maintenance of the correct chemical environment (milieu interior) for body cells: water balance, electrolyte balance and the pH of the blood. It has other functions such as producing substances necessary for the formation of red blood cells (erythropoietin), converting vitamin D to an active form which promotes the absorption of calcium from the intestine, and also producing some hormones associated with the regulation of blood pressure.

Urine normally contains surplus water and electrolytes, waste products such as urea, which is formed from the amino acids, uric acid, which is produced from nucleic acids and purines, and creatinine from muscle. Urine also gets rid of excess amounts of acids or alkalis that have either been ingested or are formed following metabolic processes.

It is important to note that most toxic substances and even beneficial substances such as drugs that are used in treatment are eliminated in the urine and the measurement of the relevant constituents can confirm either the use of drug(s) or the exposure to toxic compounds. Thus examination and analysis of the urine is an important investigation in toxicology and acts as a biomarker of exposure. The amounts excreted in the urine may also be an indicator of the severity of exposure to a toxic substance.

## 8.1   Common symptoms associated with disease of the kidneys

**Anuria:** is the complete suppression of urinary secretion by the kidneys.

**Uraemia:** is, in current usage, the entire constellation of signs and symptoms of chronic renal failure including nausea, vomiting anorexia, a metallic taste in the mouth, a uraemic odour of the breath, pruritus, uraemic frost on the skin, neuromuscular disorders, pain and twitching in the muscles, hypertension, oedema, mental confusion and acid base and electrolyte imbalances.

**Dysuria:** is painful or difficult urination.

**Polyuria:** is the passage of a large volume of urine in a given period. This may be a characteristic of diabetes – both diabetes mellitus and diabetes insipidus (see section 9 on hormones).

**Oedema:** is the presence of abnormally large amounts of fluid in the intercellular tissue spaces of the body, usually applied to demonstrable accumulation of excessive fluid in the subcutaneous tissues. Oedema may be localised, due to venous or lymphatic obstruction or to increased vascular permeability, or it may be systemic due to heart failure or renal disease. Collections of oedema fluid are designated according to the site, for example ascites (peritoneal cavity), hydrothorax (pleural cavity) and hydropericardium (pericardial sac).

**Haematuria:** is the presence of blood in the urine.

**Proteinuria:** is the presence of proteins in the urine.

## 9   The endocrine system and the production of hormones

The activities of the organs of the body are primarily controlled by nerve impulses. The other important mode of control of activity is by hormones. These are chemical substances produced by endocrine glands. They enter the blood stream directly following secretions by the glands and are brought to all parts of the body by the cardiovascular system. Most organs are under the influence of both nerve impulses and hormones.

The word 'hormone' is derived from the Greek word *hormao*, which means to excite. A hormone is a naturally occurring substance secreted by specialised cells that affects the metabolism or behaviour of other cells possessing functional receptors for the hormone. Hormones may be hydrophilic, like insulin (from the pancreas), in which case the receptors are on the cell surface, or lipophilic, like steroids (from the adrenal cortex), where the receptor can be intracellular. Thus hormones are substances which circulate in the blood and bring about an effect on distant organs.

The endocrine glands are:
- pituitary
- thyroid
- parathyroid glands
- adrenal glands
- ovaries in the female
- testes in the male
- placenta during pregnancy
- pancreas, which is both exocrine and endocrine (secretions of exocrine glands reach the blood stream through ducts whilst those of endocrine glands reach the blood stream directly).

## 9.1    Pituitary gland

The pituitary gland lies in a bony cavity in the skull called the pituitary fossa. The posterior part of the pituitary is suspended by a structure called the pituitary stalk from a part of the brain called the hypothalamus. The gland has two parts: the anterior pituitary or adenohypophysis, and the posterior pituitary or neurohypophysis (Figure 14). Whilst the posterior pituitary has neural or nerve connections with the brain, the anterior pituitary has vascular connections with the brain.

### 9.1.1 The posterior pituitary

The **posterior pituitary** is composed mainly of nervous tissue descending from the hypothalamus and produces two hormones:

- the antidiuretic hormone (vasopressin), and
- oxytocic hormone (oxytocin).

### *The antidiuretic hormone (ADH)*
The antidiuretic hormone (ADH) is involved intimately with water balance as it controls or regulates the amount of water that is reabsorbed in the kidney. Large doses of ADH cause high blood pressure or hypertension as it tends to cause vasoconstriction or contraction (narrowing) of blood vessels. The amount of ADH secreted is controlled by the amount of water in the blood. If the body is short of water, more ADH will be secreted and more water will be reabsorbed by the kidney tubules and less urine will be formed.

The posterior pituitary may fail to produce ADH in which case the condition is called diabetes insipidus, as excessive amounts of urine are formed and lost from the body and the patients are always very thirsty.

### The oxytocic hormone

The oxytocic hormone is only important during pregnancy. It causes contraction of the pregnant uterus and facilitates the ejection of milk during lactation.

**Figure 14** Diagram of the pituitary gland and its hormones. Not to scale.

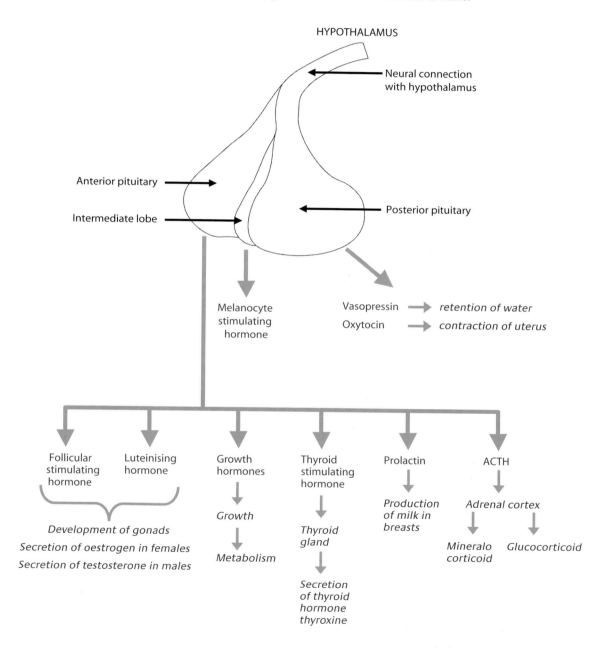

### 9.1.2  The anterior pituitary

The hormones released by the anterior pituitary gland are:
- growth hormone;
- thyrotrophic hormone;
- adrenocorticotrophic hormone; and
- gonadotrophic hormones.

***Growth hormone***

This hormone stimulates the growth of bone and muscle tissue during childhood. If there is excessive production of this hormone before puberty (when the long bones fuse with the growing ends or epiphyses and no further increase in growth can occur), gigantism results. Insufficient production causes dwarfism. Increased production after puberty leads to increase in size of facial bones and bones of the hands and feet – a condition called acromegaly.

## 9.2   Thyroid stimulating hormone and the thyroid gland

The thyroid stimulating hormone acts on the thyroid gland in the neck and stimulates the release of the thyroid hormones – thyroxine and tri-iodothyronine. The thyroid hormone stimulates metabolism by acting on the cells to speed up the rate at which food is used up and converted to heat and energy. The thyroid gland is unique in that it stores its hormones as a colloid in small vesicles in the gland. The other glands store their secretions in the cells themselves. The formation of the thyroid hormone requires iodine which has to be in the diet. In regions where populations may encounter a deficiency of iodine in their diets, iodised salt has helped in the prevention of thyroid disease – particularly the enlargement of the thyroid gland: goitre formation. Deficiency of the thyroid hormone (also called hypothyroidism) in a child causes cretinism where the development of the nervous system is affected and the child is mentally retarded. In an adult, deficiency of thyroid hormone causes myxoedema where the body temperature is low, the heart rate is slow, brain activity is sluggish and there is deposition of fluid-like material under the skin. The face and eyelids become puffy.

If there is increased production of thyroid hormone (hyperthyroidism), metabolism is stimulated and more heat is produced, the heart beats faster, and the heart excitability is increased, which may give rise to disorders of heart rhythm (cardiac arrhythmias). In this situation, which is called thyrotoxicosis, the person is irritable, anxious and nervous. They lose weight though the appetite is good. They often have protrusion of the eye balls (exophthalmos).

In addition, the thyroid gland produces calcitonin which is important in the regulation of calcium balance.

## 9.3   Parathyroid

Parathyroid glands are adjacent to the thyroid gland but are not controlled by the secretions of the anterior pituitary gland. There are four parathyroid glands, two on either side of the thyroid. The hormones from the parathyroid gland control the calcium levels in the blood. Another factor affecting the blood calcium level is calcitonin, which as stated above, is a secretion of the thyroid gland. Calcitonin acts by trapping calcium in the bones. Another important factor determining the level of blood calcium is vitamin D.

With increased activity of the parathyroids (hyperparathyroidism), the plasma level of calcium increases to about 20 mg calcium per 100 ml of blood from a normal of 5.5 mg of calcium per 100 ml of blood. This calcium comes from the bone and the kidney gets rid of it from the body. Thus the bones become thin and fragile and likely to fracture more easily than normal bones with sufficient calcium.

With decreased production of parathyroid hormone (hypoparathyroidism), the blood calcium level falls, which causes increased excitability of the nerves and of the neuromuscular junctions leading to a condition called tetany (this has to be distinguished from the disease tetanus which follows infection with a bacillus *Clostridium tetani*). In tetany, there is spasm of the hands and feet (carpo-pedal spasms). Increased excitability of the nerve cells in the brain may lead to convulsions.

## 9.3  Adrenocorticotrophic hormone (ACTH) and the adrenal gland

The adrenal glands are located on the top of each kidney (see Figure 12). Each adrenal gland consists of a central medulla and an outer cortex.

The adrenal medulla releases the hormones adrenaline and noradrenaline (epinephrine and nor-epinephrine) in response to nerve stimuli that enter the medulla from the sympathetic nervous system. Thus the adrenal medulla is an integral part of the sympathetic nervous system and is intimately involved in the fight or flight responses to stress, where increased sympathetic activity is life saving. It is common to state that a person should have sufficient adrenaline to perform well. The secretions of the hormones from the adrenal medulla are not under the control of the anterior pituitary hormone ACTH.

The adrenal cortex has three layers and each layer produces a different hormone and at least two of the layers are controlled by ACTH from the anterior pituitary gland.

The outer layer – the zona glomerulosa – produces aldosterone, which is necessary for reabsorption of sodium in the kidney. An excess of aldosterone causes salt and water retention. The secretion of aldosterone is considered to be regulated by a hormone secreted by the kidney – renin.

The inner two layers of the adrenal cortex – the zona fasciculata and the zona reticularis – produce hormones collectively known as corticosteroids. The main corticosteroid secreted is cortisol (hydrocortisone). The corticosteroids have several actions:

- favour the utilisation of proteins for the production of heat and energy in preference to the use of carbohydrates;

- anti-allergy;
- anti-inflammatory, and
- some aldosterone-like effects – causes retention of sodium and of water and loss of potassium. The salt and water retention may lead to oedema and/or high blood pressure (hypertension).

Cortisol tends to reduce the utilisation of carbohydrates for energy, thus the blood sugar level often increases (a diabetogenic effect). When body proteins are broken down, wound healing is impaired and the effect on suppression of immune or inflammatory response can lead to 'masking' of infections (which may cause delays in diagnosis) and also an increased susceptibility to infections.

Over-production of the adrenal cortex hormone leads to Cushing's syndrome, which is characterised by 'moon face', due to redistribution of fat and swelling of the face. Redistribution of body fat leads to 'an egg on matchsticks' appearance: an expanded abdomen and chest with 'skinny' limbs, particularly lower limbs, diabetes and increased blood pressure. The skin tends to bruise easily and purple striae appear on the skin and females develop hirsutism. There may also be psychological changes.

Changes similar to Cushing's Syndrome follow treatment with corticosteroids over a period of time for several common disease states. An excessive production of aldosterone leads to Conn's disease, which is associated with muscular weakness, increased loss of potassium and water in the urine.

Decreased activity of the adrenal gland leads to Addison's Disease. This was common following tuberculosis affecting the adrenal gland when both the medulla and cortex were affected. In Addison's disease, sodium and water are lost from the body and this causes a lowering of blood pressure, muscle weakness, nausea and vomiting. The production of catecholamines (e.g. adrenaline and noradrenaline) is affected and there is increased production of melanin instead. This leads to increased pigmentation, particularly of exposed parts. Episodes of low blood sugar may occur as adrenaline plays an important role in mobilising glucose, particularly in times of stress.

## 10    Immunology

Immunology is the study of the physiological responses by which the body destroys or neutralises foreign matter or xenobiotics, living and non-living, as well as cells of its own that have become altered in certain ways. The ability of the immune response to protect us against bacteria, fungi, viruses and other parasites and other foreign matter is one of the most important defence mechanisms of the human body.

This immune response – the process by which xenobiotics are destroyed or neutralised – is therefore essential for a healthy disease-free life. The immune response can also destroy cancer cells that arise in the body and also worn out or damaged cells such as old red blood cells or erythrocytes.

Immune responses can be broadly classified into:

1. Non-specific immune responses, which recognise in a non-selective manner all foreign substances.
2. Specific immune responses against substances that are specifically identified and then attacked.

Bacteria have the ability to cause damage at their sites of invasion or can release into the body fluids (extracellular fluids of which blood is the most important) toxins that are carried to other parts of the body to cause damage to cells.

The body also needs protection against viruses, which are essentially nucleic acids surrounded by a protein coat. Unlike bacteria, which have their own metabolic processes and can multiply independent of other cells, viruses lack the enzyme processes and other cell constituents such as ribosomes for their own metabolism and energy production. Therefore, viruses can only multiply whilst living inside other cells whose biochemical apparatus they make use of. The nucleic acids in the viruses cause the production/manufacture of proteins required for the viruses to multiply and also the energy to multiply.

The cells and associated components that carry out immune responses are collectively called the immune system. Though called a system, it has no anatomical continuity but consists of diverse collections of cells found both in the blood and tissues (cells) throughout the body.

Cells mediating the immune response are:

1. White blood cells or leucocytes, including neutrophils, basophils, eosinophils, monocytes and lymphocytes. The lymphocytes are grouped into B cells and T cells (cytotoxic T cells, helper T cells, suppressor T cells etc.). White blood cells can leave the circulation or blood (unlike the red blood cells) and enter tissues and function in the tissues.
2. Plasma cells found in peripheral lymph organs. Plasma cells differentiate from lymphocytes in the tissue and are not found in the blood as the name suggests.
3. Macrophages present in almost all tissues and organs are large cells but their structure may vary from tissue to tissue. They are derived from monocytes (white blood cells) that leave the blood vessels to enter the tissues. As their main function is to engulf foreign material, they are strategically located at sites where entry of foreign substances or organisms is likely to take place.
4. Mast cells are also found in all tissues and organs. Mast cells differentiate from basophils that have left the blood vessels and a characteristic feature is that they usually contain large numbers of secretory vesicles and they secrete mainly locally acting chemical messengers e.g. histamine. These cells are involved in allergic responses such as hypersensitivity reactions.

## 10.1  Inflammation

This is the local reaction of the body to injury or infection which essentially destroys or inactivates the foreign invaders and prepares the body to repair any injury caused. The main role is by phagocytes which engulf the foreign material by a process called phagocytosis. Once inside the phagocyte, the foreign substance is destroyed. The important phagocytes are the neutrophils, monocytes and macrophages.

The usual clinical manifestations of inflammation are redness, swelling, heat and pain, which are produced by a variety of chemical messengers or mediators. The better known of these mediators are the kinins, histamine, complement and eicosanoids. The kinins are produced from the plasma protein kininogen whilst histamine is released from mast cells.

Two important mediators – interleukin 1 (IL1) and tumour necrosis factor are protein in nature and are released by monocytes and macrophages during an inflammatory response.

Complement kills microbes without prior phagocytosis. Complement is always present in the blood albeit in an inactive form most of the time. Activation of complement in response to an infection or tissue injury generates active molecules from inactive precursors and the complement system is comprised of at least 20 distinct proteins. Complement also stimulates the secretion of histamine from mast cells and effectively increases the blood flow to the injured area and facilitates the movement of phagocytes such as the neutrophils to the injured area from within the blood vessels.

Lymphocytes also circulate in the blood but tend to gather in large numbers in groups of organs and tissues called lymphoid organs such as bone marrow and the thymus gland (gland found in the chest which tends to atrophy or becomes very small in size after puberty), lymph nodes, spleen and tonsils. These cells also concentrate in the lining of the intestine, and those of the respiratory, genital and urinary tracts.

The lymphatic system is a network of lymphatic vessels and lymph nodes found along these vessels, through which lymph, a fluid derived from interstitial fluid, flows. It constitutes a route by which interstitial fluid can reach the blood vessels or the cardiovascular system. This movement of interstitial fluid as lymph to the cardiovascular system is very important because the amount of fluid filtered out of all the blood vessel capillaries (excepting those of the kidney) exceeds that which is reabsorbed by approximately four litres each day. These four litres are returned to the blood via the lymphatic system. In the process, the small amount of protein that usually leaks out of the capillaries is also brought back into the circulation by the lymphatic system.

Also important is that the lymph node cells encounter the materials that start off their response, that is, the immune response via the lymph flowing through them. Each lymph node is a honeycomb of sinuses (enlargements or sac like dilations containing lymph) lined by macrophages with large clusters of lymphocytes between the sinuses. The spleen is the largest of the organs containing lymphoid tissue which lies on the left side of the abdominal cavity between the stomach and the diaphragm (the large muscle that is essential for breathing and separates the thoracic cavity from the abdominal cavity).

The other structures with large collections of lymphoid tissue are the tonsils, which are small rounded structures in the throat which often get inflamed in children resulting in the common condition called tonsillitis. There are multiple populations and sub-populations of lymphocytes termed B lymphocytes, T lymphocytes, cytotoxic, helper and suppressor T cells.

There are two broad categories of specific immune responses. Firstly, a lymphocyte is programmed to recognise a specific antigen. Antigen is a foreign substance that triggers a specific immune response and is not an anatomical description but is a functional description. The ability of lymphocytes to distinguish one antigen from another is the basis of specific immune responses. Recognition of an antigen implies that antigen gets bound to the lymphocyte which has receptors for that antigen.

Once the lymphocyte has attached itself to the antigen, it divides into different types of cells, and this takes place at the site where the antigen has attached itself to the lymphocyte. Some of the divided cells will either set upon to attack the antigens, whilst others may influence both the activation and function of these 'attack cells'.

The activated cells attack all the antigens that initiated the immune response. The manner in which lymphocytes attack the 'invaders' is by two methods: antibody-mediated or humoral- and cell-mediated.

Antibodies are proteins that are both present in the plasma membranes of B cells and are also secreted by them. These antibodies travel along the blood stream to all parts of the body, combine with the antigens and direct an attack by phagocytes and complement that eliminates the antigen or the cells bearing them. Antibodies belong to a group of proteins called immunoglobulins.

In cell-mediated immunity, the T lymphocytes and natural killer cells travel to the location of cells bearing on their surface antigens that initiated the immune response, and directly kill them.

Two broad generalisations can be made. Antibody-mediated responses carried out by B lymphocytes have a large range of targets and are the major defence against bacteria, viruses and other microbes and against toxic molecules. Cell-mediated killing by T lymphocytes and natural killer cells is against a more limited number of targets, specifically the body's own cells that have become cancerous or infected with viruses. The helper cells activate both humoral- and cell-mediated immune responses. The helper cells are essential for the production of antibodies except in the case of a small number of antigens. Suppressor T cells inhibit the function of both B cells and cytotoxic T cells.

## 11    Further reading

Ganong WF. (2003) *Review of Medical Physiology*. 21st edition. McGraw Hill Medical, New York.

Green JH. (1976) *An Introduction to Human Physiology*. 4th edition. Oxford University Press, London.

Haslett C, Chilvers ER, Hunter JA, Boon NA. (2002) *Davidson's Principles and Practice of Medicine*. 19th edition. Churchill Livingstone, Edinburgh.

Merkle CJ. (2005) *Handbook of Pathophysiology*. 2nd edition. Lippincott, Williams and Wilkins, Philadelphia, PA.

# Glossary and Abbreviations

**absorption** 1. The entry of a substance into the human body usually via skin, lungs or gastro-intestinal tract. 2. Take up of a gas by a solid or liquid, or the take up of a liquid by a solid. It differs from adsorption in that the absorbed substance permeates the bulk of the absorbing substance.

**Acceptable Daily Intake (ADI)** Estimate of the amount of a substance in food or drinking water, expressed on a body mass basis (usually mg/kg body weight), which can be ingested daily over a lifetime by humans without appreciable health risk. ADI is normally used for food additives (tolerable daily intake is used for contaminants).

**acidosis** Pathological condition in which the hydrogen ion concentration of body fluids is above normal and hence the pH of blood falls below the normal range (7.4).

**acrocyanosis** Bluish discolouration of the extremities – hands and feet – due to poor oxygen supply.

**acrodynia** Form of mercury poisoning, usually seen in children. Symptoms include pain, pink discolouration of extremities (hands and feet), itching and peeling of the skin (desquamation), and may be accompanied by irritation.

**ACTS** Advisory Committee on Toxic Substances, Health and Safety Executive.

**acute** Occurring over a short time.

**acute effect** Effect of short duration (hours or a few days) immediately following exposure.

**acute exposure** Contact with a substance that occurs only once (or for a short period usually under 24 hours).

**additive effect** A biological response to the exposure to multiple substances that equals the sum of responses to all the individual substances under the same conditions.

**ADI** *See Acceptable Daily Intake.*

**ADI "not specified" No acceptable daily intake allocated:**
Terminology used by JECFA in situations where an ADI is not established for a substance under consideration because (a) insufficient safety information is available, (b) no information is available on its food use, (c) specifications for identity and purity have not been developed.

**ADMS** Atmospheric Dispersion Modelling System: Commercially available short-range dispersion model developed in the UK.

**adsorption** The physical or chemical binding of gases or liquids onto solid particles. *See also absorption.*

**adverse health effect** A change in morphology, physiology, growth, development or lifespan of an organism which results in impairment of functional capacity or impairment of capacity to compensate for additional stress or increase in susceptibility to the harmful effects of other environmental influences.

**aerobic**  Requiring oxygen to survive. Usually applied to bacteria which cannot survive or multiply without oxygen.

**ALARP**  As Low As Reasonably Practicable

**alkalosis**  Pathological condition in which the hydrogen ion concentration of body fluids is below normal and hence the pH of blood rises above the normal range (usually a pH above 7.4).

**allergen**  A substance capable of producing a specific immunological response (restricted mainly to immediate hypersensitivity or anaphylactic reactions).

**alopecia**  A general term for loss of hair.

**ambient**  Surrounding (for example ambient air, water, sediment or soil). Refers to the environment to which an individual may be exposed.

**anaemia**  Anaemia is used usually to indicate a reduction in haemoglobin in the blood.

**amnesia**  Loss of memory.

**anaerobic**  Capable of existing (living) in the absence of oxygen.

**analgesia**  Usually medications used to relieve pain or reduce the sensitivity to pain.

**anaphylaxis**  Immediate, often life threatening hypersensitivity (allergic) reaction to an antigen (a substance that induces a specific immunological response). *See antigens.*

**aneugenic**  Inducing aneuploidy. *See aneuploidy.*

**aneuploid**  A normal human cell has 23 pairs of chromosomes: a cell or organism with missing or extra chromosomes is known as an aneuploid.

**aneuploidy**  The circumstances in which the total number of chromosomes within a cell is not an exact multiple of the normal haploid (*see polyploidy*) number. Chromosomes may be lost or gained during cell division.

**agonist**  1. A substance that tends to increase the action of another. 2. A drug or other substance having a specific cellular affinity that produces a predictable biological reaction.

**agonistic effect**  A positive biological response following the action of a substance at a specific site.

**anhydrous**  A chemical substance without water.

**anorexia**  Loss of appetite. (NB *Anorexia nervosa* is the term used to describe an eating disorder.)

**anosmia**  Loss of sense of smell.

**anoxia**  Strictly this is the total absence of oxygen but anoxia is sometimes used to mean decreased oxygen supply in tissues – i.e. hypoxia.

**antagonist effect**  A negative biological response following the blocking of the action of a substance at a specific site.

**antagonistic effect**  A biological response to exposure to multiple substances which is **less** than would be expected if the known effects of the individual substances were added together.

**antidote** A general term for a substance to counteract a poison's toxic effects.

**anuria** No output of urine in a 24-hour period.

**aplastic anaemia** Type of anaemia where the bone marrow fails to produce an adequate number of all blood cells and platelets.

**apnoea** Temporary cessation of breathing.

**aqueous** Water based.

**ARDS** Acute Respiratory Distress Syndrome.

**areflexia** Absence of reflexes – usually reflexes assessed by examination of the nervous system.

**ARF**  1. Acute Renal Failure 2. Acute Respiratory Failure

**arrhythmia** Any variation from the normal rhythm of the heartbeat.

**asbestosis** Chronic fibrotic lung disease caused by inhaling airborne asbestos fibres.

**aspiration** When a liquid or object is inhaled into the lungs. A common cause is inhaling (aspirating) acid or vomit from the stomach.

**AST**  Aspartate aminotransferase: an enzyme normally present in the liver; its level in blood provides a test of liver function (formerly known as glutamic oxaloacetic transaminase).

**asymptomatic** A subject without any complaints (symptoms).

**asystole** Absence of contraction of the heart muscle to produce a heartbeat.

**ataxia** Loss of co-ordination of parts of the body. It affects the parts of the nervous system that control movement and balance leading to unstable posture or gait.

**atrial fibrillation** A condition in which the atria (the two upper chambers of the heart) contract at a very high rate and in an irregular way.

**atrophy** Decrease in size or wasting away of a body part or tissue.

**ATSDR** Agency for Toxic Substances and Disease Registry, U.S. Department of Health and Human Services.

**BaP**  Benzo(a)pyrene

**bioavailability** A term referring to the proportion of a substance which reaches the systemic circulation unchanged after a particular route of administration.

**biologic indicators** A species or other biological end-point used as a quantifiable proxy to measure a condition of interest.

**biological uptake** The transfer of substances from the environment to plants, animals, and humans.

**biological monitoring / biomonitoring** Scientific technique used to assess human exposure to chemicals using biological samples.

**biological sample** A tissue or fluid sample taken from a person (or animal), e.g. urine, blood, hair etc.

**biomarker**  Observable change (not necessarily pathological) in an organism related to a specific exposure or effect.

**biota**  All living organisms as a totality.

**biotransformation**  Chemical alteration of a substance within the body, as by the action of enzymes. This process usually leads to less harmful products or those that could be eliminated from the body more easily than the parent substance. Sometimes, it may result in a more active or harmful product.

**BMGV**  Biological Monitoring Guidance Values.

**body**  Total amount of substance of a chemical present in a biological sample at a given time.

**brady-**  Prefix meaning slow, e.g. bradycardia – slow heart rate.

**bradycardia**  Slow heart rate.

**bronchospasm**  Narrowing of the small bronchi (bronchioles) by muscular contraction.

**bundle branch block**  Interruption of conduction of cardiac impulses from the upper chambers of the heart, the atria, to the lower chambers of the heart, the ventricles, which usually results in a slow heart rate.

**cancer**  A synonym for a malignant neoplasm, that is a tumour that grows progressively, invades local tissue and spreads to distant sites. *See also tumour.*

**cancer risk**  Probability that cancer will be produced by exposure, e.g. to a hazardous chemical.

**carboxyhaemoglobin (COHb)**  Complex formed between carbon monoxide and haemoglobin in the blood. Haemoglobin has a much higher affinity for carbon monoxide than oxygen; hence the amount of oxygen in the blood is greatly reduced. *See haemoglobin.*

**carcinogen**  The causal agents which induce tumours.

**carcinogenic**  Liable to cause cancer.

**cardiac**  Referring to the heart.

**CAS number**  Number assigned by the Chemical Abstract Service (CAS, a division of the American Chemical Society) to a specific chemical. CAS numbers are assigned sequentially and serve as a concise, unique means of identification. The numbers have no chemical significance.

**case**  A medical or epidemiologic evaluation of one person or a small group of people to gather information about specific health conditions and past exposures.

**case-control study**  An epidemiological study where a comparison is made between the proportion of cases (individuals with disease) that have been exposed to a particular hazard (e.g. a chemical) and the proportion of controls (individuals without disease) that have been exposed to the hazard.

**catecholamine**  Group of compounds including epinephrine (adrenaline) and norepinephrine (noradrenaline) released from the adrenal glands in response to stress. Typical effects produced are an increase in heart rate, blood pressure, breathing rate etc.

**CBR**  Refers to Chemical, Biological or Radiological.

**CBRN** Refers to Chemical, Biological, Radiological and Nuclear.

**CCA**   Civil Contingencies Act 2004 – the legislation that defines UK emergency planning and response and sets expectations for civil protection.

**CCDC** Consultant in Communicable Disease Control – specialist doctor employed by the Health Protection Agency.

**Central Nervous System (CNS)**  The part of the nervous system that consists of the brain and the spinal cord.

**CfI**   Centre for Infections, Health Protection Agency.

**CHaPD** Chemical Hazards and Poisons Division, Health Protection Agency.

**CHEMDATA**  Emergency response computer database available from the National Chemicals Emergency Centre (part of the AEA Group) used by the fire service, and other emergency services in the UK and worldwide for chemical information.

**CHEMET**   A service from the Meteorological Office, providing information on weather conditions as they affect an incident involving hazardous chemicals (e.g. anticipated behaviour of any plume). CHEMETs are available on request by the emergency services.

**CHEMSAFE** Chemical Industry Scheme for Assistance in Freight Emergencies.

**CHIP**  HSE's Chemicals (Hazard Information and Packaging) Regulations.

**chromatid**  One of the paired and parallel strands of a duplicated chromosome joined by a central centromere.

**chromosomal aberrations**  Collective term for particular types of chromosome damage induced after exposure to exogenous chemicals or physical agents that damage the DNA. *See clastogen.*

**chromosome**  In simple organisms such as bacteria and some viruses, the chromosome consists of a single circular molecule of DNA containing the entire genetic material of the cell. In the cells of more complex organisms, such as animals and plants, the chromosomes are thread-like structures, composed mainly of DNA, which are present in the nuclei of every cell. They occur in pairs, the numbers varying from one to more than 100 per nucleus in different species. Normal somatic cells in humans have 23 pairs of chromosomes, each consisting of linear sequences of DNA which are known as genes.

**chronic effect**  A prolonged health effect that occurs due to an exposure, and tends to persist for a long time even after cessation of exposure.

**chronic exposure**  Continued exposure occurring over an extended period of time, or a significant fraction of the life time of a human or test animal.

**CIMAH** Control of Industrial Major Accident Hazards Regulations (now replaced by *COMAH*).

**CIMAH/COMAH sites**  Industrial sites that are subject to the Control of Industrial Major Accident Hazards Regulations 1984. From February 1999, these were replaced by the Control of Major Accident Hazards Regulations.

**clastogen**  An agent that produces chromosome breaks and/or consequent gain, loss or rearrangement of pieces of chromosomes. Clastogens may be viruses or physical agents as well as chemicals.

**clastogenicity**  Inducing chromosome breaks and other structural aberrations.

**CLAW**  Control of Lead at Work Act 1998.

**CLEA**  Contaminated Land Exposure Assessment model.

**cluster investigation**  A method of sampling where there is review of an unusual number, real or perceived, of health events (for example, reports of cancer) grouped together in time and location. Cluster investigations may be designed to confirm case reports; determine whether they represent an unusual disease occurrence; and, suggest hypotheses regarding possible causes and contributing environmental factors for potential further investigation.

**CMO**  Chief Medical Officer.

**CNS depression**  Decrease in function of the central nervous system resulting in a state that can range from drowsiness to coma.

**CO**    Carbon monoxide.

**COC**  Committee on Carcinogenicity of Chemicals in Food, Consumer Products and the Environment.

**COM**  Committee on Mutagenicity of Chemicals in Food, Consumer Products and the Environment.

**COMAH**  Control of Major Accident Hazards Regulations. *See also CIMAH/COMAH sites.*

**COMEAP**  Committee on Medical Effects of Air Pollution.

**concentration**  The amount of a substance present in a certain amount of soil, water, air, food, blood, hair, urine, breath, or any other media.

**congener**  Substance which by structure, function or origin is similar to another.

**conjunctivitis**  Inflammation of the conjunctiva, the mucous membrane covering the white of the eye and the inner lining of the eyelids.

**contaminant**  A substance that is either present in an environment where it does not belong or is present at levels that might cause harmful (adverse) health effects.

**convulsions**  Violent involuntary contraction of muscles.

**coordination**  The harmonious integration of the expertise of all the agencies involved, with the object of effectively and efficiently bringing the incident to a successful conclusion.

**COSHH**  Control of Substances Hazardous to Health Regulations.

**COT**  Committee on Toxicity of Chemicals in Food, Consumer Products and the Environment (non-food).

**cyanosis**  Bluish discolouration of skin, mucous membranes (lips), finger nails and other tissues due to deoxygenated haemoglobin (i.e. haemoglobin without oxygen bound to it).

**cytochrome C oxidase** An enzyme necessary for the cells to utilise oxygen. It is the terminal enzyme in the electron transport chain in mitochondria.

**delayed health effect** A disease or an injury that happens as a result of exposures that have occurred in the past.

**dermal** Referring to the skin. For example, dermal absorption means passing through the skin.

**dermal contact** Contact with the skin.

**dermatitis** Inflammatory disorder of the skin.

**descriptive epidemiology** The study of the amount and distribution of a disease in a specified population by person, place, and time.

**detection limit** The lowest concentration of a chemical that can reliably be detected/measured from a zero concentration.

**dilated pupils** Large pupils; mydriasis.

**dioxin** Dioxins are members of a large group of substances with similar structure (chemically they are referred to as polychlorinated dibenzo-p-dioxins). They are not produced intentionally but very small amounts are produced in combustion processes and as a by-product in certain industrial processes. They have similar types of toxicity but vary markedly in their potency. The most potent is the 2,3,7,8-tetrachloro derivative, often referred to as TCDD. This is extremely toxic. The toxicity of other dioxins is expressed relative to TCDD. In some cases this is several orders of magnitude less than TCDD.

**diplopia** Double vision.

**disease prevention** Measures used to prevent a disease or reduce its severity.

**disease registry** A system of ongoing registration of all cases of a particular disease or health condition in a defined population.

**diuresis** Increased formation and passage of urine.

**DNA** Deoxyribonucleic acid. The carrier for genetic information for all living organisms except the group of RNA viruses. Each of the 46 chromosomes in normal human cells consists of 2 strands of DNA containing up to 100,000 nucleotides, specific sequences of which make up genes. DNA itself is composed of two interwound chains of linked nucleotides.

**dose (for chemicals that are not radioactive)** Total amount of a substance administered to, taken or absorbed by an organism (latter may be referred to as absorbed dose).

**dose-response relationship** The relationship between the dose of a substance and the resulting changes in body function or health (response), usually plotted as a graph, with the dose on the x axis and the response on the y axis.

**dys-** Prefix meaning difficult, painful, abnormal.

**dysarthria** Difficulty in speaking caused either by a disturbance of the speech centre in the brain or the muscles involved in speech.

**dyskinesia** Difficulty in performing voluntary movement.

**dysphagia** Difficulty in swallowing.

**dysphonia** General term covering disorders of voice including hoarseness.

**dyspnoea** Difficulty in breathing or shortness of breath.

**dystonic movements** Neurological movement disorder caused by prolonged, repetitive muscle contractions that may cause twisting, jerking or repetitive movements.

**dysuria** Painful urination.

**EA** Environment Agency.

**EC** European Commission.

**EC Directive** Directive to member states of the European Union to draw up national legislation to implement the content of the Directive.

**ECG** Electrocardiogram: instrument that measures and records the electrical activity of the heart.

**ECG changes** Changes in cardiac rhythm, rate or electrical activity shown on an electro-cardiograph.

**eczema** General term for a range of inflammatory skin conditions whose characteristic signs may include dryness, redness, itching, oozing blisters, crusts and scabs.

**EEG** Electroencephalogram: an instrument that measures and records the electrical activity of the brain.

**embolism** Sudden blocking of a blood vessel or vein by a clot or foreign body from a site distant to the site of blockage.

**emesis** Vomiting.

**encephalitis** Inflammation of the brain.

**encephalopathy** Disease states which manifest as altered functions of the brain. May be seen with liver failure (hepatic encephalopathy in alcoholics) and in kidney failure.

**endarteritis obliterans** A disease of arteries, usually of the legs, which causes a marked decrease of blood supply to the muscles in the leg and causes pain during walking; referred to as claudication.

**Environmental Health Officer (EHO)** A professional officer responsible for assisting people to attain environmental conditions that are conducive to good health. Most EHOs work for local authorities and are concerned with administration, inspection, education and law enforcement.

**environmental media** Soil, water, air, biota (plants and animals), or any other parts of the environment that can contain contaminants.

**EPA** Environmental Protection Act (UK).

**epidemiology** The study of the distribution and determinants of disease or health status in a population.

**epistaxis** Bleeding from the nose.

**erythema**  Reddening of the skin due to congestion of blood or increased blood flow to the skin.

**erythrocyte superoxidase dismutase**  An enzyme present in red blood cells involved in the reduction of superoxide radicals to hydrogen peroxide. It acts as an antioxidant protecting against the harmful effects of the active oxygen species.

**euphoria**  Exaggerated feeling of well being.

**exposure**  The process by which a substance becomes available for absorption by a population by any route, e.g. swallowing, breathing, or contact with the skin or eyes. Exposure may be short-term (acute exposure), of intermediate duration, or long-term (chronic exposure).

**exposure assessment**  The process of finding out how people come into contact with a hazardous substance, how often and for how long they are in contact with the substance, and the amount with which they are in contact.

**exposure investigation**  The collection and analysis of site-specific information and biologic tests (when appropriate) to determine whether people have been exposed to hazardous substances.

**exposure pathway**  The route a substance takes from its source (where it began) to its end point (where it ends), and how people can come into contact with (or be exposed to) it. An exposure pathway has five parts: a source of contamination (such as an abandoned business); an environmental media and transport mechanism (such as movement through groundwater); a point of exposure (such as a private well); a route of exposure (eating, drinking, breathing, or touching), and a receptor population (people potentially or actually exposed). When all five parts are present, the exposure pathway is termed a completed exposure pathway.

**exposure registry**  A system of ongoing follow up of people who have had documented environmental exposures.

**exposure-dose reconstruction**  A method of estimating the amount of people's past exposure to hazardous substances. Computer and approximation methods are used when past information is limited, not available, or missing.

**extrapyramidal symptoms (EPS)**  Excess involuntary movements.

**fasciculations**  Visible twitching of muscles – distinct from muscle spasms.

**furans**  Dioxins and furans are chlorinated aromatic hydrocarbon species.

**G6PD**  Glucose 6 phosphate dehydrogenase – an enzyme present in red blood cells.

**gene**  The functional unit of inheritance; a specific sequence of nucleotides along the DNA molecule forming part of a chromosome.

**Good Agricultural Practice**  Good agricultural practice is the recommended usage of a pesticide which is necessary and essential for the control of a pest under all practical conditions bearing in mind any toxicological hazards involved.

**haem-**  Prefix referring to blood.

**haematemesis**  Vomiting of blood.

**haematoma**  Localised accumulation of blood, usually clotted, in an organ, space, or tissue, due to a failure of the wall of a blood vessel.

**haematuria**  Presence of blood in the urine.

**haemoglobin**  Oxygen-carrying substance in red blood cells.

**haemolysis**  Breakdown of red blood cells usually due to disruption of red blood cell membrane which releases haemoglobin into the plasma.

**haemoptysis**  Coughing up of blood.

**haemorrhage**  Bleeding.

**hazard**  Set of inherent properties of a substance, mixture of substances, or a process involving substances that make it capable of causing adverse effects to organisms or the environment, depending on the extent of exposure.

**hazard identification**  A process by which potential hazards are identified.

**Hazardous Substance Release and Health Effects Database (HazDat)**  The scientific and administrative database system developed by ATSDR (*see ATSDR*) to manage data collection, retrieval, and analysis of site-specific information on hazardous substances, community health concerns, and public health activities.

**HAZCHEM**  Hazardous chemical label.

**HAZMAT**  Incidents involving hazardous materials.

**head space analysis**  Chemical analysis of vapour given off by a liquid mixture.

**health investigation**  The collection and evaluation of information about the health of community residents. This information is used to describe or count the occurrence of a disease, symptom, or clinical measure and to assist in investigating the possible association between the occurrence and exposure to hazardous substances.

**heart block**  Interruption of conduction of cardiac impulses which usually causes the slowing of the heart.

**hepatic**  Referring to the liver.

**hepatitis**  Inflammation of the liver cells.

**HMEI**  Hypothetic Maximally Exposed Individual.

**HPA**  Health Protection Agency.

**HSE**  The Health and Safety Executive. Government body in the UK with responsibility for enforcing health and safety legislation and investigation of work-related accidents.

**hyper-**  Prefix meaning above, more than normal, excessive.

**hyperactivity**  Increased activity in an individual or of a biological system.

**hyperacussis**  Heightened sense of hearing.

**hyperaesthesia**  Increased sensitivity to touch and other sensory stimuli.

**hypercalcaemia**  Abnormally increased concentration of calcium in the blood.

**hypercapnia**  Excess of carbon dioxide in the blood.

**hyperglycaemia** Abnormally increased concentration of glucose (sugar) in the blood.

**hyperkalaemia** Abnormally increased concentration of potassium ions in the blood.

**hyperkeratosis** Thickening of the outer layer (epidermis) of the skin.

**hypernatraemia** Abnormally increased concentration of sodium ions in the blood.

**hyperpigmentation** Increased pigmentation.

**hyperpyrexia** High body temperature commonly called fever.

**hyperreflexia** Increased reflexes.

**hypersalivation** Increased salivation/drooling.

**hypertension**  High blood pressure. Usually refers to the systemic circulation – i.e. arteries and arterioles from the aorta. May be used to refer to a particular circulation, e.g. pulmonary hypertension (increased blood pressure in the pulmonary circulation) or portal hypertension (increased pressure in portal circulation to liver).

**hypertonia** Increased muscle tone.

**hyperventilation** Increased breathing rate.

**hypo-** Prefix meaning below, less than normal.

**hypocalcaemia** Abnormally decreased concentration of calcium ions in the blood.

**hypoglycaemia** Abnormally decreased concentration of glucose in the blood.

**hypokalaemia** Abnormally decreased concentration of potassium ions in the blood.

**hyponatraemia** Abnormally decreased concentration of sodium ions in the blood.

**hyporeflexia** Decreased muscle reflexes.

**hypotension** Low blood pressure.

**hypothermia** Low body temperature.

**hypotonia** Decreased muscle tone.

**hypoventilation** Reduced rate or depth of breathing.

**hypoxia** Decreased oxygen content in the body tissues.

**IARC** International Agency for Research on Cancer.

**ICSC** International Chemical Safety Card.

**ICU** Intensive Care Unit.

**IDLH** Immediately Dangerous to Life and Health.

***in vitro*** A Latin term used to describe effects in biological material outside the living animal. Literally 'in glass'. Used to refer to studies in a laboratory involving isolated organs, tissues or cells.

***in vivo*** A Latin term used to describe effects in living animals. Literally 'in life'. Refers to studies carried out on a living organism.

**incidence**  The number of new cases of disease in a defined population over a specific time period.

**ingestion**  The act of swallowing something through eating, drinking, or mouthing objects. A hazardous substance can enter the body this way.

**inhalation**  The act of breathing in. A hazardous substance can enter the body this way.

**insomnia**  Inability to sleep.

**IPCS**  International Programme on Chemical Safety.

**irritable**  Abnormally sensitive to stimuli.

**ischaemia**  Local deficiency of blood supply and hence oxygen to an organ or tissues, usually due to constriction of the blood vessels or to obstruction.

**ISO 14001**  International (ISO) Standard for Environmental Management Systems.

**ISO 9001**  International (ISO) Standard for Quality Management Systems.

**I-TEQ**  International Toxic Equivalent Quotient (used for dioxins and furans).

**jaundice**  Pathological condition characterised by deposition of bile pigment in the skin and mucous membranes, including the conjunctivae, resulting in yellow appearance of the patient.

**JECFA**  Joint FAO/WHO Expert Committee on Food Additives.

**lacrimator**  Substance that irritates the eyes and causes tearing.

**$LD_{50}$**  The dose of a toxic compound that causes death in 50% of a group of experimental animals to which it is exposed. It can be used in the assessment of the acute toxicity of a compound but is being superseded by more refined methods.

**$L_{den}$**  Day-evening-night level in decibels as an indicator for "annoyance".

**LDL:HDL cholesterol**  Ratio of low density lipoprotein cholesterol to high density lipoprotein cholesterol.

**lead time**  The period of time from the exposure to the development of adverse health effects.

**leucocytosis**  Increased number of white blood cells in the blood.

**leucopaenia**  Decreased number of white blood cells in the blood.

**LFT**  Liver Function Test.

**limit of detection**  The lowest concentration that can be measured.

**lindane gamma**  Gamma hexachlorocyclohexane, a pesticide.

**lipophilic**  Having affinity for lipids (fatty compounds). Dissolves much more readily in lipids than water.

**LOAEL**  Lowest Observed Adverse Effects Level.

**LTEL**  Long Term Exposure Limit.

**malaise**  Vague feeling of lethargy and fatigue.

**Maximum Residual Level**  *See MRL.*

**MSDS** Material Safety Data Sheet.

**meiosis** Process of "reductive" cell division, occurring in the production of gametes, by means of which each daughter nucleus receives half the number of chromosomes characteristic of the somatic cells of the species.

**MEK** Methylethylketone.

**MELs** Maximum Exposure Limit – this is an obsolete term and has been superceded by WELs.

**melaena** Black stools due to blood pigments or altered blood.

**metabolism** The conversion or breakdown of a substance from one form to another by a living organism which usually results in the production of a less toxic substance or a substance that could be eliminated from the body more easily. The products of a metabolic process are metabolites.

**metabolite** Any product of metabolism.

**methaemoglobinaemia** Presence of methaemoglobin (altered haemoglobin) in the blood.

**MetHb** methaemoglobin.

**mg/cm²** milligram per square centimetre (of a surface).

**mg/kg** milligram per kilogram.

**mg/m³** milligram per cubic metre; a measure of the concentration of a chemical in a known volume (a cubic metre) of air, soil, or water.

**MIC** Methyl isocyanate.

**micronuclei** Isolated or broken chromosome fragments which are not expelled when the nucleus is lost during cell division, but remain in the body of the cell forming micronuclei. Centromere positive micronuclei contain DNA and/or protein material derived from the centromere. The presence of centromere positive micronuclei following exposure to chemicals can be used to evaluate the aneugenic potential of chemicals.

**miosis** Constricted pupils (the size of the pupil is less than 2 mm).

**mitochondria** Rod-shaped constituents of a cell involved in cell respiration producing energy for the organism. Referred to as the 'power house' of cells.

**mitotic index** A measure of the rate of proliferation of cells and is the ratio between number of cells dividing (mitotic cells) to cells that are not dividing.

**ml** millilitre.

**mm** millimetre.

**mmol** millimole.

**morbidity** State of being ill or diseased. Morbidity is the occurrence of a disease or condition that alters health and quality of life.

**MRL** Maximum Residue Limit. The maximum concentration of residue (expressed as milligrams of residue per kilogram of food/animal feeding stuff) resulting from, for example, the use of a pesticide, likely to occur in or on food and feeding stuffs after the use of pesticides according to Good Agricultural Practice (GAP). *See Good Agricultural Practice.*

**MRL "not specified"** Maximum Residue Limit not specified. Available data on the identity and concentration of residues of the veterinary drug in animal tissues indicate a large margin of safety for consumption of residues in food when the drug is used according to good practice in the use of veterinary drugs. For that reason, and for the reasons stated in the individual evaluation, the Committee referred to above (*see MRL*) has concluded that the presence of drug residues in the named animal product does not present a health concern and that there is no need to specify a numerical MRL.

**mucosa** Surface membrane lining the nose, respiratory tract and other cavities of the body.

**mutagen** A substance that causes mutations (alterations or loss of genes or chromosomes).

**mutagenic** The ability of a substance to increase the occurrence of mutations.

**mutation** A permanent change in the amount or structure of the genetic material in an organism or cell which can result in a change in phenotypic characteristics. The alteration may involve a single gene, a block of genes, or a whole chromosome. Mutations involving single genes may be a consequence of effects on single DNA bases (point mutations) or of large changes, including deletions, within the gene. Changes in whole chromosomes may be numerical or structural. A mutation in germ cells of sexually reproducing organisms may be transmitted to the offspring, whereas a mutation that occurs in somatic cells may be transferred only to the descendant daughter cells.

**mydriasis** Dilated pupils.

**myo-** Prefix referring to muscle.

**myocardial infarction** Area of *necrosis* (death of heart muscle cells) resulting from inadequate blood supply to the heart muscle (i.e. heart attack).

**myocarditis** Inflammation of the heart muscle.

**myocardium** Heart muscle.

**NAMAS** National Accreditation of Measurement and Sampling: accreditation given to laboratories from *UK Accreditation Service, UKAS.*

**NAME** Nuclear Accident ModEl. Long-range dispersion model run by the UK Meteorological Service.

**ND** Not detected.

**necrosis** Localised death of tissues or cells.

**neoplasm** *See tumour.*

**neoplastic** Pertaining to or like a neoplasm.

**neuroleptic** Describing the effect on cognition and behaviour of antipsychotic drugs.

**neuropathy** Any disease of the central or peripheral nervous system.

**NFAR** No further action required.

**ng**    nanogram (1 billionth of a gram).

**NIOSH**  National Institute for Occupational Safety and Health.

**NOAEL**  No observed adverse effect level. The highest administered dose at which no adverse effects are observed.

**NOx**  Oxides of nitrogen, NO and $NO_2$ are commonly referred to as NOx.

**NPIS**  National Poisons Information Service.

**nucleotide**  The 'building block' of nucleic acids such as the DNA molecule. A nucleotide consists of one of four bases – adenine, guanine, cytosine, or thymine – attached to a phosphate-sugar group. In DNA the sugar group is deoxyribose, while in RNA (a DNA related molecule that helps to translate genetic information into proteins) the sugar group is ribose, and the base uracil substitutes for thymidine. Each group of three nucleotides in a gene is known as a codon. A nucleic acid is a long chain of nucleotides joined together and therefore is sometimes referred to as a 'polynucleotide'.

**nystagmus**  Involuntary, rapid, repetitive to and fro movement of the eyes.

**Occupational Exposure Limit (OEL)**  The concentration in air of a chemical in the workplace that is thought to be safe. This means that most workers can be exposed at the given concentration or lower without harmful effects for specified periods.

**oedema**  Presence of abnormally large amounts of fluid in intercellular spaces of body tissues causing swelling.

**oedema, cerebral**  Swelling due to excessive fluid in the brain.

**oedema, pulmonary**  Accumulation of fluid in the lungs – occurs in the small air sacs or alveoli.

**OES**    Occupational Exposure Standard.

**oliguria**  Excretion of a reduced amount of urine (less than 400 ml per day in adults).

**organoleptic properties**  Properties relating to taste and odour.

**OSHA**  Occupational Safety and Health Administration (USA).

**PAH**    Polycyclic aromatic hydrocarbon.

**palpitation(s)**  Sensation of rapid or irregular heartbeat felt by a subject – also refers to undue awareness of the heart beat.

**papilloedema**  Oedema of the optic disc – usually indicates raised pressure within the skull, for example with a brain tumour.

**paraesthesia**  Number of abnormal sensations anywhere in the body but usually in limbs, e.g. tingling, pricking, burning, pins and needles, partial numbness.

**Patient Group Directions (PGDs)**  Documents that make it legal for medicines to be given to groups of patients, e.g. in a mass casualty situation, without individual prescriptions having to be written for each patient. They can also be used to empower staff other than doctors legally to give the medicines in question.

**PBB**    Polybrominated biphenyls.

**PCB**    Polychlorinated biphenyl.

**peripheral neuropathy**  Any disease of the peripheral nerves.

**pH**    Acidity/alkalinity scale.

**photophobia**  Abnormal intolerance to light of the eyes.

**pica**    A craving to eat non-food items, such as dirt, paint chips, and clay.  Some children exhibit pica-related behaviour.

**plumbosolvency**  Solvency of lead in water.

**PM**    Particulate matter.

**PM$_{10}$**    Particulate matter between 2.5 and 10 μm in diameter.

**PM$_{2.5}$**    Particulate matter less than 2.5 μm in diameter.

**pneum-**  Referring to the lungs.

**pneumonitis**  Inflammation of the lungs.

**point of exposure**  The place where someone can come into contact with a substance present in the environment.

**point source emission**  Single emission source in a defined location.

**polydypsia**  Excessive intake of water (increased thirst), a common symptom of diabetes.

**polyneuropathy**  Any disease which involves several nerves.

**polyploidy**  Having three or more times the haploid (single set of unpaired chromosomes as found in germ cells) number of chromosomes. Somatic cells from animals generally contain a diploid set of chromosomes, with pairs of equivalent chromosomes, so that twice the haploid number is present.

**polyuria**  Passage of a large volume of urine.

**population**  A group or number of people living within a specified area or sharing similar characteristics (such as occupation or age).

**portal vein**  A vein in the liver that receives many tributaries, including the splenic vein from the spleen and pancreas, the gastric vein from the stomach, the mesenteric vein from the small and large intestines, and the rectal vein from the rectum and anus.

**ppb**    parts per billion.

**PPE**    Personal Protective Equipment.

**ppm**    parts per million.

**ppt**    parts per trillion.

**prevalence**  The number of people with a condition (e.g. disease or symptom) at any one time related to the size of the population.

**prevalence survey**  The measure of the current level of disease(s), symptoms or exposures. This is often carried out using a questionnaire that collects self-reported information from a defined population.

**proteinuria**  Excretion of excessive amounts of protein (derived from blood plasma or kidney tubules) in the urine.

**prothrombin time**  A laboratory measurement of the time taken for blood to clot.

**proximal**  Nearest to the head.

**psychosis**  Any major mental disorder characterised by derangement of the personality and loss of contact with reality.

**PTSD**  Post Traumatic Stress Disorder.

**pupils constricted**  Small pupils.

**pupils fixed**  Condition when pupils do not react to light – i.e. constrict when a light is directed to the pupil.

**PVC**  Poly Vinyl Chloride.

**pyrexia**  Fever, high temperature.

**QRA**  Quantitative Risk Assessment.

**REACH**  Registration, Evaluation, Authorisation and Restriction of Chemical substances

**reference dose (RfD)**  A US Environmental Protection Agency term used for an estimate (with uncertainty spanning perhaps an order of magnitude) of a daily exposure to the human population (including sensitive subgroups) that is likely to be without appreciable risk of deleterious effects during a lifetime.

**renal**  Referring to the kidneys.

**rhabdomyolysis**  Breakdown of muscle tissue resulting in release of myoglobin into the bloodstream.

**rhinorrhoea**  Discharge from the nose.

**risk**  Possibility that a harmful event (death, injury or loss) arising from exposure to a chemical or physical agent that may occur under specific conditions.

**risk assessment**  Identification and quantification of the risk resulting from a specific use or occurrence of a chemical or physical agent, taking into account possible harmful effects on individual people or society of using the chemical or physical agent in the amount and manner proposed and all the possible routes of exposure. Quantification ideally requires the establishment of dose-effect and dose-response relationships in likely target individuals and populations.

**risk communication**  Interpretation and communication of risk assessments in terms that are comprehensible to the general public or to others without specialist knowledge.

**risk reduction**  Actions that can decrease the likelihood that individuals, groups, or communities will experience disease or other adverse health conditions.

**route of exposure**  The way people come into contact with a hazardous substance.  Three common routes of exposure are breathing (inhalation), eating or drinking (ingestion), or contact with the skin (dermal contact).

**safety factor**  *See uncertainty factor.*

**sample**  1. In statistics, a group of individuals often taken at random from a population for research purposes.  2. One or more items taken from a population or a process and intended to provide information on the population or process.  3. Portion of material selected from a larger quantity in some manner chosen so that the portion is representative of the whole.

**sample size**  The number of units chosen from a population or an environment.

**SGOT**  *See AST.*

**sinus tachycardia**  Increased but regular heart rate.

**sister chromosome exchange (SCE)**  Exchange of genetic material between 2 sub-units of a replicated chromosome.

**'SLUDGE'**  Acronym used to describe the clinical effects of acute organophosphorous intoxication: Salivation, Lacrimation, Urination, Defaecation and Gastric Emesis.

**SNARL**  Suggested No Adverse Effect Level. Maximum dose or concentration that on current understanding is likely to be tolerated by an exposed organism without producing any harm.

**solvent**  A liquid capable of dissolving or dispersing another substance (for example, acetone or mineral spirits).

**somatic**  1. Pertaining to the body as opposed to the mind.  2. Pertaining to non-reproductive cells or tissues.  3. Pertaining to the framework of the body as opposed to the viscera.

**SOx**  Oxides of sulphur, SO and $SO_2$, are commonly referred to as SOx.

**stakeholders**  Those with a personal or professional interest in a particular issue.

**statistics**  A branch of mathematics that deals with collecting, reviewing, summarising, and interpreting data or information. Statistics are used to determine whether differences between study groups are meaningful.

**STEL**  Short Term Exposure Limit.

**synergism**  Pharmacological or toxicological interaction in which the combined biological effect of two or more substances is greater than expected on the basis of the simple summation of the pharmacological toxic effects of each of the individual substances.

**synergistic effect**  Biological effect following exposure simultaneously to two or more substances that is greater than the simple sum of the effects that occur following exposure to the substances separately.

**tachy-** A prefix meaning rapid.

**tachypnoea**  Increased frequency of respiration (breathing).

**TDI**  Tolerable Daily Intake. An estimate of the amount of contaminant, expressed on a body weight basis (e.g. mg/kg bodyweight), that can be ingested daily over a lifetime without appreciable health risk.

**temporary ADI**  Used by JECFA when data are sufficient to conclude that use of the substance is safe over the relatively short period of time required to generate and evaluate further safety data, but are insufficient to conclude that use of the substance is safe over a lifetime. A higher-than-normal safety factor is used when establishing a temporary

ADI and an expiration date is established by which time appropriate data to resolve the safety issue should be submitted to JECFA. The temporary ADI is listed in units of mg per kg of body weight.

**temporary MRL**  Temporary Maximum Residue Limit. Used by JECFA when a temporary ADI has been established and/or when it has been found necessary to provide time to generate and evaluate further data on the nature and quantification of residues. Temporary MRLs are expressed in terms of mg residue per kg food.

**TEQ**  Toxic equivalent quotient. *See also I-TEQ.*

**teratogen**  A substance which, when administered to a pregnant woman or animal, can cause congenital malformations (structural defects) in the baby or offspring.

**THOR** The Health and Occupational Reporting activity, Centre of Occupational and Environmental Health, University of Manchester.

**time weighted average**  Concentration of a hazardous substance, usually in air, averaged over a specified period of time. For example, for occupational exposures it is usually averaged over 8 hours.

**tinnitus**  Ringing in the ears.

**TOXBASE**  Online information resource developed by the National Poisons Information Service (NPIS).

**toxic agent**  Chemical or physical (for example, radiation) agents that, under certain circumstances of exposure, can cause harmful effects to living organisms.

**toxicant**  Synonym for toxic agent/substance.

**toxicity**  Ability of a substance to cause damage to living tissue.

**toxicology**  The study of the harmful effects of substances on humans or animals.

**toxin**  Toxic substance produced by a biological organism such as a microbe, animal or plant.

**TOXNET**  US National Library of Medicine toxicology data service.

**TREMCARD**  Transport Emergency Cards.

**triage**  Process of assessment and allocation of priorities by the medical or ambulance staff at the site or casualty clearing station prior to evacuation. Triage may be repeated at intervals and on arrival at a receiving hospital.

**tumour**  A mass of abnormal, disorganised cells arising from pre-existing tissue which are characterised by excessive and uncoordinated proliferation and by abnormal differentiation.

**Benign tumours** show a close morphological resemblance to their tissue of origin, grow in a slow expansile fashion and form circumscribed and (usually) encapsulated masses. They may stop growing and they may regress. Benign tumours do not infiltrate through local tissue and they do not metastasise. They are rarely fatal.

**Malignant tumours** resemble their parent tissues less closely and are composed of increasingly abnormal cells in terms of their form and function. Well-differentiated examples still retain recognisable features of their tissue of origin but these characteristics are progressively lost in moderately and poorly differentiated malignancies; undifferentiated or anaplastic tumours are composed of cells which resemble no known normal tissues. Most malignant tumours grow rapidly, spread progressively through adjacent tissues and metastasise to distant sites.

**TWA**  Time Weighted Average.

**uncertainty factor**  Value used in extrapolation from experimental animals to man (assuming that man may be more sensitive), or from selected individuals to the general population. For example a value applied to the NOAEL to derive an ADI or a TDI. The value depends on the size and type of population to be protected and the quality of the toxicological information available. (In the past the term safety factor was used rather than uncertainty factor.)

**-uria**  Suffix referring to urine.

**urinary incontinence**  Inability to control urination.

**urinary retention**  Inability to pass urine despite a full bladder.

**urticaria**  Vascular reaction of the skin marked by the transient appearance of smooth, slightly elevated patches (wheals, hives) that are redder or paler than the surrounding skin and often associated with severe itching.

**ventricular fibrillation**  A life-threatening disturbance of cardiac rhythm which leads to ineffective pumping of blood from the heart and can cause death.

**ventricular tachycardia**  A type of *arrhythmia* in which the heart beats at an abnormally fast rate and which may lead to potentially lethal ventricular fibrillation if untreated or prolonged.

**vertigo**  Dizziness associated with sensation of movement or spinning. May be associated with height reached whilst walking or climbing.

**VOC**  Volatile Organic Compound. An organic compound that evaporates readily into the air. VOCs include substances such as benzene, toluene, methylene chloride, and methyl chloroform.

**vulnerable populations**  People who might be more sensitive or susceptible to exposure to hazardous substances because of factors such as age, occupation, sex, or behaviours (for example, cigarette smoking). Children, pregnant women, and older people are often considered vulnerable populations.

**WEL**  Work place Exposure Limit.

**WHO**  World Health Organization, United Nations.

## Sources

The explanations used in this glossary are derived from many sources, including:

- ATSDR *Glossary of terms*. Agency for Toxic Substances and Disease Registry, U.S. Department of Health and Human Services (accessed 2006) www.atsdr.cdc.gov

- IPCS *JECFA glossary of terms*. International Programme on Chemical Safety, World Health Organization (accessed 2006) www.who.int/ipcs

- SIS *Glossary for Chemists of Terms Used in Toxicology*. Specialized Information Services, United States National Library of Medicine (accessed 2008)  www.sis.nlm.nih.gov

# Index

**A**

abamectin 198
absorbed dose, definition 12
absorption routes for toxins in the body 8
Acceptable Daily Intake (ADI) for food
    additives 158–9
acetylcholine (ACh) neurotransmitter
    22–4, 196–7, 224–5
acetylcholinesterase (AChE) 22–4, 196–7,
    224–5
acids 6
ACOEM (American College of
    Occupational and Environmental
    Medicine) 119
acrylamide 23, 160
acrylonitrile 7
acute incidents, human biomonitoring
    studies 54–5
acute respiratory failure 29
adenosine triphosphate (ATP) 30
administered dose, definition 12
adrenaline overdose 25
agranulocytosis 30
air pollution (UK) and health 122–9
    air quality standards 128–9
    carbon monoxide 125, 127
    carcinogenic outdoor air pollutants 127
    Clean Air Act (1956) 122
    effects on life expectancy 123
    growing awareness of health risks
        122–3
    history 122
    indoor air pollutants 127–8
    international air pollution control 129
    London smogs 122–3
    metal particles 124
    nano-particles (ultrafine particles) 125
    nitrogen dioxide 123, 125, 126
    nitrogen oxides (NOx) 123, 125, 126
    organic compounds 124, 127
    ozone 123, 125–6
    particulate matter (PM) 123–5
    photochemical smog 123
    pollutant gases 125–8

    smogs 122–3
    sulphur dioxide 125, 126
    sulphur dioxide effects (case study) 95
    air quality guidelines (WHO) 68, 129
ALARP (as low as reasonably practicable)
    risk reduction 118
ALARP (as low as reasonably practicable)
    exposure 36
alcohol, effects 7, 26, 27, 28
alcohol dehydrogenase, effects of genetic
    polymorphism 93
aldrin 195–6
alkalis 6
allergic reactions 7, 31–2, 34
alternative medicines see traditional
    medicines
aluminium toxicity 186–7
alveoli, target for toxic substances 28–9
Alzheimer's disease 186
Ames test 40–1
aminopyrine 32
anaesthetics 7, 27
anaphylaxis 31
aneugenicity (numerical chromosome
    aberrations) testing 40, 41–2
aniline dyes 32
anthrax, US postal incident (2001) 231
anticholinesterase insecticides 196–7
antidotes, list of those available 81
aplastic anaemia 30
arsenic toxicity 184–5
arterial system
    abnormal function 26
    normal function see Appendix
    targets for toxic agents 25, 26
arteries see arterial system
asbestos 7, 29
aspartame 159
asphyxiants (simple and chemical types)
    6
aspirin 205
atropine 23, 25, 27, 34, 81
ATSDR (Agency for Toxic Substances and
    Disease Registry) 67

autoimmunity 31–2
avermectin 198
AVPU assessment 79

**B**
benzene 7, 127
bilirubin 28
biochemical toxicology 19, 21–2
biological monitoring guidance values
    (BMGV) 118
biological weapons 219
biomarkers see human biomonitoring
biomonitoring see human biomonitoring
bladder, target organ 32
blood cells, target of toxic substances 30
bone marrow, target of toxic substances
    30
botulinum toxin 222, 223, 225
botulism (caused by botulinum toxin)
    24, 225
brain, target organ 20, 22
brainstem, target organ 28–9
breast cancer 196, 210
breast-feeding, traditional medicines to
    avoid 212
1,3-butadiene 127

**C**
cadmium, half-life in parts of the body 15
carbamate insecticides 24, 27, 196–7
carbon dioxide 6
carbon disulphide 7, 23
carbon monoxide (CO), in air pollution
    125, 127
carbon monoxide (CO) poisoning 6, 30,
    164–72
    binding to haemoglobin 167–8, 169
    binding to myoglobin 169
    characteristics of CO 164
    chronic illness 164
    CO monitors and alarms 172
    deaths and ill-health caused by 164
    effects during pregnancy 170, 171
    effects of acute poisoning 165–6
    effects of chronic poisoning 164, 165,
        166–7
    effects on cardiovascular disease
        patients 170, 171

effects on children 170, 172
effects on older patients 170
effects on the developing foetus 170
formation of carboxyhaemoglobin
    (COHb) 167–8, 169
need for public education 172
sources of CO 164–5
toxic effects in the body 167–70
treatment 171
vulnerable population groups 170–1
carbon tetrachloride 7, 27, 28
carcinogenicity studies 45–6 see also
    mutagenicity studies
carcinogens 7
    outdoor air pollutants 127
    vinyl chloride monomer 113
carcinoma of the bronchus 29
cardiotoxins 7
cardiovascular system
    heart as target organ 25
    normal function 24–5
    targets for toxic agents 25
cell-mediated hypersensitivity 23
central nervous system
    abnormal function 22
    brain 20, 22
    normal function 22
    target organs 20
Chemfinder, website 18
Chemical Abstract Service (CAS)
    chemical identification numbers
        4–5, 63
    website 18
Chemical, Biological, Radiological and
    Nuclear weapons (CBRN) 219
Chemical Hazards and Poisons Division
    (CHaPD) of HPA 82
chemical identification, numerical
    systems 63
Chemical Incident Plan (emergency
    departments) 82–3
chemical incidents see medical
    management of chemical incidents
chemical warfare agents 34, 217–33
    agents affecting tissue respiration
        (cyanides) 226–7, 228
    chemical and biological weapons
        (CBW) spectrum 221–2

Chemical, Biological, Radiological and Nuclear Weapons (CBRN) 219
classification 219, 224–8
definition 218–19
definition of hazard 220–1
definition of threat 220–1
differences between military and civilian exposures 220, 221
disabling and knockdown agents 224
emergency medical management of casualties 227–31
expressions of toxicity 222, 223–4
First World War 217, 219–20
Hazmat response 228–30, 233
historical development and use of chemical weapons 219–20
latency of action 222
lessons from recent urban terrorist incidents 231–3
life support for CW agent casualties (TOXALS) 231
lung damaging agents (pulmonary oedemagens) 225
medical management of chemical incidents 219
methods of release 218–19
nerve agents 224–5
pathophysiological effects 223–4
persistency 222
properties 222–4
radiological agents 219
ratio of dead to wounded 220
toxidromes 77
toxins 222
transmissibility 222
treatment for chemical casualties 231
use in civilian settings 217–18
vesicant agents 225–6, 227
chemicals
  numbers with reliable toxicology information 4–5
  potential means of harmful exposure 5
  safety in manufacture, storage and use 4–5
  types of environmental contamination 5
children, susceptibility to environmental

hazards 89–92 see also specific hazards
chlorine 110–11, 224, 225
chloroform 7
chlorpyrifos 197
cholinergic nervous system 22–4
chromium 7, 187–9
chromosomes
  aneugenicity testing 40, 41–2
  clastogenicity testing 40, 41–2
chronic exposure, human biomonitoring studies 54–5
chronic respiratory failure 29
clastogenicity (structural chromosome aberrations) testing 40, 41–2
Claviceps purpurea (ergot fungus) 26
clinical toxicology 3
Clostridium botulinum (cause of botulism) 222, 225
Clostridium welchii (cause of gas gangrene) 34
colophony 7
Committee on Carcinogenicity (CoC) 67
Committee on Medical Effects of Air Pollution (COMEAP) 68
Committee on Mutagenicity (CoM) 67
Compendium of Chemical Hazards (HPS) 65
contaminated land assessment 130–9
  assessment criteria 130, 135, 136–9
  bioaccessibility testing 134–6
  chemical analysis of sample 134
  CLEA model 68, 98, 137–8
  contaminant levels compared to risk assessment criteria 139
  definition of 'contaminated land' 131
  Environment Act (1995) 131
  Environmental Protection Act (1990) 131
  environmental sampling 132–4
  exposure assessment models 136–8
  geology of the site 131–2
  Health Criteria Values (HCVs) 135, 136–7
  industries associated with land contamination 131
  land-use history of the site 131–2
  naturally-occurring hazardous

substances 131
nature of land contamination 131
options appraisal for contaminated
    land 139
quality of analytical data 136
site investigation 132–6
site-specific assessment criteria (SSAC)
    137–9
Soil Guideline Values (SGVs) 130,
    136–7, 138–9
source-pathway-receptor model 137
statistical treatment of analytical data
    138–9
tolerable daily soil intake (TDSI) 135
Tox Reports 135, 136
toxicological information 136
Contaminated Land Exposure
    Assessment (CLEA) model 68, 98,
    137–8
copper toxicity 189–90
corrosives 6
coumarins 199
Cryptosporidium, water safety
    requirements 146
cyanides (agents affecting tissue
    respiration) 30, 81, 226–7, 228
cyanogens 224, 226–7
CYP2C8 enzyme 10
CYP2C9 enzyme 10
cypermethrin 197
cytochrome P450 enzymes 10, 93
cytochrome system in mitochondria 30
cytochromes 6

**D**
danger see risk
DDT (dichloro-diphenyl-trichloroethane)
    195–6, 210
deadly nightshade (Atropa belladonna)
    25, 34 see also atropine
deltamethrin 197
dermal exposure to toxic agents 8, 9
Derris 198
diazinon 197
dibromodichloropropane 7
2,4-dichlorophenoxyacetic acid (2,4-D)
    199
dichlorvos 196

dicobalt edentate 81
dieldrin 195–6
digoxin 205
dimethyl sulphate 7
dioxins 31, 160–1
diquat 198–9
disabling agents 224
distribution of toxins in the body 8
disulfoton 197
dosage, margin of safety 13–14
dosage terminology 12
dose 12
    and exposure 3
    and toxicity 3, 12
    target dose 12
dose-response assessment (risk
    assessment model) 17
dose-response curve 13–14
drinking water quality 144–54
    Cryptosporidium safety requirements
        146
    Drinking Water Inspectorate (DWI)
        144–51
    private water supplies 145
    public water supplies 145
    regulatory framework 145–6
    standards of water quality 145–6
    supply of wholesome water 145–6
    testing and reporting 146
    water safety 146
    WHO drinking water quality guidelines
        68–9, 146
drinking water quality incidents 146–54
    definition of an incident 148
    DWI notification requirements 146–7
    examples of chemical contamination
        incidents 151–4
    investigation of incidents 147–8
    learning needs in the water industry
        154
    notification requirements 146–7
    numbers reported to DWI 150–1
    outcome of investigations 149–50
    supply of unfit water 149
drugs
    derived from recombinant DNA 31
    hepatotoxicity 28
dysrhythmias (heart) 25

**E**

EC
  Air Quality Directives 129
  REACH agency 119
EC number (chemical identifier) 63
ECETOC (European Centre for
    Ecotoxicology and Toxicology of
    Chemicals) 67
eczema 34
effective dose (ED) 13–14
EH40 list of exposure limits 117–18
elderly people
  susceptibility to environmental hazards
    92
  traditional medicines to avoid 213
emergency departments see medical
    management of chemical incidents
endosulfan 195
endrin 195–6
Environment Act (1995) 131
Environment Agency, Contaminated
    Land Exposure Assessment (CLEA)
    68, 98, 137–8
environmental contamination, types of 5
environmental epidemiology, use of
    human biomarkers 53
Environmental Protection Act (1990) 131
environmental toxicology 3
enzymes
  inducers 10
  inhibitors 10
  see also cytochromes
epithelial system
  abnormal function 33–4
  eyes 33–4
  normal function 33
  skin 8, 9, 33, 34
  target organs 33–4
ergotamine poisoning 26
ethanol 4, 7
ethical issues, human biomonitoring
    studies 58
excretion routes for toxins in the body 8
experimental methods see investigation
    of toxic effects
expert help, sources 81, 82
exposure, and toxic effect 3 see also
    routes of exposure

exposure assessment 97–104
  definition 97
  definition of exposure in health studies
    97
  factors affecting exposure 98
  group level estimation 99–100
  individual level estimation 98–9
  pollution data interpolation methods
    103–4
  purpose and uses 97
  risk assessment model 17
  source-pathway-receptor model 98
  use of GIS to integrate data 100–4
exposure dose, definition 12
eyes
  abnormal function 33–4
  absorption of toxic agents 8
  indicator of toxic effects 33–4
  irritancy study methods 37
  target organs 33–4

**F**

familial adenomatous polyposis coli 38
fertility, impaired see reproductive
    system
First World War, use of chemical weapons
    217, 219–20
fish, contaminants in 160–1, 181
flumethrin 197
foetus, susceptibility to environmental
    hazards 89–92
food additives and contaminants 156–61
  Acceptable Daily Intake (ADI) for
    additives 158–9
  acrylamide 160
  aspartame 159
  contaminants in fish 160–1
  examples of additives 157
  examples of contaminants 156
  health-based guidance values 158–9
  independent scientific advisory
    committees 157
  recent issues 159–61
  regulatory limits 158–9
  risk assessment (or safety assessment)
    157–8
  Sudan dyes 159–60
  Tolerable Daily Intake (TDI) for

contaminants 158–9
food poisoning (botulism) 24
free radicals 28
fungicides 198

**G**
gas gangrene 34
gastro-intestinal system
  abnormal function 27
  actions of toxic substances 27
  normal function see Appendix
  target organs 26, 27
gene mutagenicity testing 40–1, 42
genetic polymorphisms
  and susceptibility to environmental
    hazards 92–3
  as biomarkers of susceptibility 52–3
gentamycin 32
Ginkgo biloba 204
GIS (Geographical Information Systems)
  use in exposure assessment 100–4
  use in monitoring and modelling 100–4
Glasgow Coma Scale (GCS) 79, 80
glufosinate 199
glyceryl trinitrate 26
P-glycoproteins (P-gp) 10
glyphosate 199
Guillain Barré syndrome (acute
    idiopathic inflammatory
    polyneuropathy) 23
Guinea Pig Maximisation Test 37

**H**
haematopoietic system
  abnormal function 30
  normal function 30
  target organs 30
  toxins 7
haemoglobin 30
half-life of a xenobiotic agent (foreign
    substance) 15
halogenated hydrocarbons 7
harm
  physiological 15
  psychological 15–16
Haz-map occupational toxicology
    database 119
hazard, definition 15

hazard identification (risk assessment
    model) 16–17
Hazmat response, civilian chemical
    warfare agent incident 228–30, 233
Health and Safety at Work (etc.) Act 1974
    (HASAWA) 109
Health and Safety Commission (HSC) 109
  advisory committee on toxic
    substances (ACTS) 68, 117
Health and Safety Executive (HSE) 18, 109
Health Criteria Values (HCVs) 135, 136–7
health protection, role of toxicology 4–5
heart
  abnormal function 25
  direct and indirect toxic effects 25
  normal function see Appendix
  target organ 25
heavy metal poisoning, antidotes 81
heavy metal toxicity 174–90
  aluminium 186–7
  arsenic 184–5
  chromium 187–9
  concept of ALARP exposure 176
  copper 189–90
  definition of heavy metal 174–5
  general symptoms 175 see also specific
    metals
  lead 176–9
  mercury 181–3
  metal fume fever 180–1
  routes of exposure 175–6
  sources of heavy metals 175
  thallium 185–6
  zinc 179–81
heavy metals 30, 32
  contamination of traditional medicines
    206–7
hepatocytes 27–8
hepatotoxic drugs 28
hepatotoxins 7
herbal medicines see traditional
    medicines
herbicides 198–9
n-hexane 23
history of development of toxicology 3–4
horse chestnut 205
HSDB (Hazardous Substances Data Bank)
    66

human biomonitoring
  biomarkers of clinical disease 53
  biomarkers of effect 51, 52
  biomarkers of exposure and uptake 51, 52
  biomarkers of susceptibility 51, 52–3
  classes of biomarker 51, 52–3
  definition 50, 53
  definition of a biomarker 51
  genetic polymorphisms 52–3
  national programmes 50
  purpose 50
  use of biomarkers 50–1
human biomonitoring studies 50
  activities where biomarkers can be used 54
  acute incidents 54–5
  chronic exposure 54–5
  confounding factors 57
  ethical issues 58
  interpretation and use of biomarkers 53–4
  selection of biomarker 55–7
  study design, conduct and communication 54–7
  toxicodynamics of the chemical of metabolites 57
  toxicokinetics of the chemical or metabolites 55–6
hydralazine 32
hydrogen cyanide 223, 224, 226–7, 228
hydrogen sulphide 6
hypersensitivity 31–2
hypoxia 29

I
imidacloprid 198
immune reaction, interruption of nerve conduction 23
immune system
  abnormal function 31
  direct immunotoxicity 31
  failure 30
  indirect immunotoxicity 31–2
  normal function see Appendix
  targets of toxic substances 31–2
immunostimulation 31
immunosuppression 31

INCHEM (IPCS) 65
information sources see toxicological information
ingestion (oral) of toxic agents 8–9
inhalation of toxic agents 8, 9
injection of toxic agents 8, 9
insecticides
  control of vector-borne diseases 193–4
  target species 194
  toxicity 195–8
International Union of Pure and Applied Chemistry (IUPAC), chemical identification system 63
Internet resources, toxicological information sources 64–7
investigation of toxic effects
  acute toxicity study methods 36–7
  ALARP (as low as reasonably practicable) exposure 36
  animal welfare 35–6, 37
  carcinogenicity studies 45–6 see also mutagenicity studies
  carcinogens 36
  components of a toxicological profile 36
  extrapolation from animal data 36
  LD50 approach 37
  mutagenic substances 36
  mutagenicity studies (potential carcinogenicity) 39–45
  NOAEL (no observed adverse effects level) 36
  non-genotoxic carcinogens 40
  OECD Guidelines 35–6, 37–8, 40, 42–7
  repeated dose toxicity study (28 or 90 day) 38–9
  reproductive toxicity study methods 46–8
  skin and eye irritancy study methods 37
  skin sensitisation study methods 37–8
  threshold for toxic effects 36
  Uncertainty Factors (Assessment Factors) 36
  use of animals 35–6
IRIS (Integrated Risk Information System) (US EPA) 66
irritants 6

**J**
jaundice 28

**K**
kidneys, target organs 32
knock down agents 224
   Moscow terrorist siege (2003) 233

**L**
large intestine, target organ 26, 27
lead 7, 23
   antidotes for poisoning 81
   exposure (case study) 93–4
   legislation 178–9
   toxicity 176–9
lead time for harmful effects 2
lethal concentration 50% (LC50) 13
lethal dose 50% (LD50) 13
leukaemia 30
Lewisite 223, 224
lindane 195
liver
   abnormal function 28
   blood supply 26, 27–8
   cytochrome P450 enzymes 10
   failure 28
   normal function 27–8 see also
      Appendix
   target organ 27–8
LOAEL (lowest observed adverse effect
   level) 14
Local Lymph Node Assay (LNA) 38
LOEL (lowest observed effect level) 14
lung damaging agents (pulmonary
   oedemagens) 225
lungs, target organs 28–9

**M**
Major Incident Plan 82–3
malaria, use of insecticides control
   mosquitoes 193–4, 196, 197
malathion 197
margin of safety (dosage) 13–14
medical management of chemical
   incidents 71–83
   ABCDE approach to patients 79–80
   antidotes 80, 81
   Chemical Hazards and Poisons

      Division (CHaPD) of HPA 82
   Chemical Incident Plan (emergency
      departments) 82–3
   containment 74–5
   decontamination 75–6, 78
   definitive care 78–81
   enhanced elimination techniques 80–1
   gastrointestinal decontamination 78
   Major Incident Plan 82–3
   multiple casualties 74
   National Poisons Information Service
      (NPIS) 82
   planning and preparation 82–3
   recognition of the chemical substance
      73–4
   risks to healthcare staff 72–3
   secondary contamination risk 72–3, 74
   secondary contamination sources 72
   sources of expert help 81, 82
   STEP 1-2-3 system 74
   symptomatic and supportive therapy
      78–80
   Toxbase on-line information resource
      (NPIS) 82
   toxidromes of chemical warfare agents
      77
   treatment prior to decontamination
      76, 78
   see also chemical warfare agents
medical toxicology 3, 20
mercury 7, 81, 181–3
mesothelioma 29
metaldehyde 199
methane 6
methiocarb 199
methyl-isocyanate 225
methylene chloride (paint stripper) 165
methylmercury in fish 160–1, 181
metrifonate 197
mitochondria, target of toxic substances
   29, 30
moluscicides 199
morphine 27, 33
Moscow terrorist siege (2003), knock
   down agent 233
mosquito control, use of insecticides
   193–4, 196, 197
mouth, target organ 26, 27

mucous membranes
    absorption of toxic substances 8, 9
    target organs 33–4
multiple organ dysfunction syndrome 34
mustard gas 30, 34, 223, 224, 225–6, 227
mutagenicity studies (potential
    carcinogenicity) 39–45
mutagens 7
myocytes 25

**N**
1-naphthylamine 7
2-naphthylamine 7
National Chemical Emergency Centre,
    website 18
National Poisons Information Service
    (NPIS) 82
nephrotoxins 7
nerve agents (organophosphates) 224–5
    antidotes 81
nervous system, target organs 20, 22–4
neurotoxins 7, 225
nickel 7
nickel contact dermatitis 32, 34
nicotine and neonicotinoid insecticides
    198
nitrites, vasodilation 26
nitrogen 6
nitrogen dioxide, air pollution 123, 125,
    126
nitrogen oxides (NOx), air pollution 123,
    125, 126
NOAEL (no observed adverse effects
    level) 14, 36
NOEL (no observed effect level) 14
non-genotoxic carcinogens 40
noradrenaline 23
nuclear weapons 219

**O**
occupational toxicology 3, 108–19
    ACOEM (American College of
        Occupational and Environmental
        Medicine) 119
    ALARP (as low as reasonably
        practicable) risk reduction 118
    biological monitoring guidance values
        (BMGV) 118

chlorine exposure example 110–11
Control of Substances Hazardous to
    Health Regulations (COSHH) 115–16,
    117
definition and scope 108–9
EH40 list of exposure limits 117–18
employers' legal obligations 118
European Community REACH agency
    119
Haz-map occupational toxicology
    database 119
Health and Safety at Work (etc.) Act
    1974 (HASAWA) 109
Health and Safety Commission (HSC)
    109
Health and Safety Executive (HSE) 109
hierarchy of control measures 115
history of occupational diseases 109–10
HSC Advisory Committee on Toxic
    Substances (ACTS) 117
identifying occupational disease
    113–14
international resources 119
legal controls and standards 115–16
long-term exposure limits (LTELs) 117
multi-exposure and interactions
    114–15
occupational exposure limits 116–18
risk assessment 113–14, 115
risk management 115–18
short-term exposure limits (STELs) 117
source-pathway-receptor model 114
sources of information 119
substitution of hazardous materials
    115–16
surveillance systems 119
SWORD scheme 119
THOR surveillance system 119
types of adverse effects 110–13
vinyl chloride monomer example
    111–13
workplace exposure limits (WELs)
    116–18
OECD Guidelines, investigation of toxic
    effects 35–6, 37–8, 40, 42–7
oesophagus, target organ 26, 27
oocytes, target of toxic substances 32–3
opioids 29

Orfila, Matteo 4
organic anion transporting polypeptides
    (OATPs) 10
organic solvents 6
organochlorine insecticides 195–6
organophosphate-induced delayed
    polyneuropathy (OPIDP) 197
organophosphates (OP) 29
  antidotes 81
  insecticides 196–7
  nerve agents 224–5
  signs and symptoms of poisoning
    23–4, 27, 33
ovaries, target organs 32–3
ozone
  air pollution 123, 125–6
  pulmonary toxin 7

P
pancytopaenia 30
Paracelsus 3, 4, 15
paracetamol 28
paraquat 29, 198–9
parathion 197
particulate air pollution 123–5
penicillins 31
per-fluoro isobutylene (PFIB) 225
peripheral nervous system
  abnormal function 23–4
  acetylcholine (ACh) neurotransmitter
    22–4
  autonomic nerves 22, 23
  autonomic nervous system 23
  cholinergic nervous system 22–4
  failure of chemical transmission 23
  failure of nerve conduction 23
  motor nerves 22, 23
  muscarinic cholinergic effects 23
  nicotinic cholinergic effects 23
  normal function 22–3
  parasympathetic system 23
  sensory nerves 22, 23
  sympathetic system 23
  targets for toxic agents 22
  toxic peripheral neuropathy 23
permethrin 197
Personal Protective Equipment (PPE) 4
pesticide contamination of traditional

medicines 210–11
pesticide poisoning 23–4
pesticide toxicology 193–200
  anticholinesterase insecticides 196–7
  carbamate insecticides 196–7
  fungicides 198
  herbicides 198–9
  insecticides 195–8
  moluscicides 199
  nicotine and neonicotinoids 198
  organochlorine insecticides 195–6
  organophosphorus insecticides
    196–7
  pyrethrins and synthetic pyrethroids
    197
  rodenticides 199
pesticides
  acute poisonings worldwide 194
  classification 195
  control of vector-borne diseases
    193–4
  deaths caused worldwide 194
  definition and description 194
  in spices 211
  occupational exposures 194
  suicide by intentional ingestion 194
  uses in disease control 193–4
  uses in food production 194
pharmacokinetics 9
pharmcodynamics 9
phosgene 29, 223, 224, 225, 226
planning and preparation, management
    of chemical incidents 82–3
Pocket Guide to Chemical Hazards
    (NIOSH) 66–7
poisons see toxins
polonium 210 31
polycyclic aromatic hydrocarbons
    (PAHs) 127
pralidoxime 81
pregnancy
  prescription of drugs 33
  traditional medicines to avoid 212
psychological harm 15–16
pulmonary oedemagens (lung damaging
    agents) 225
pulmonary toxins 7
pupil, indicator of toxic effects 33–4

pyrethrins and synthetic pyrethroids 197

**Q**
quinine 205

**R**
radiological weapons 219
Ramazzini, Bernardino, early account of diseases of work 109–10
red blood cells, target of toxic substances 29, 30
relative risk 16
reproductive system
    abnormal function 33
    normal function 33
    target organs 32–3
    study methods 46–8
reproductive toxins 7
respiratory acidosis 29
respiratory disease, SWORD occupational surveillance scheme 119
respiratory system
    abnormal function 29, 30
    external respiration 28–9
    internal respiration 28, 29–30
    normal function 29, 30
    target organs 28–30
retinoblastoma 39
ricin 34
risk, definitions 16
risk assessment
    definition of hazard 15
    definitions of risk 16
    food additives and contaminants 157–8
    harm (physiological and psychological) 15–16
    occupational toxicology 113–14, 115
    relative risk 16
risk assessment model 16–17
    dose-response assessment 17
    exposure assessment 17
    hazard identification 16–17
    risk characterisation 17
risk management 17
    occupational toxicology 115–18
rodenticides 199
routes of exposure to toxic substances 8–9

**S**
safety see risk
Salmonella typhimurium, bacterial reverse mutation test (Ames test) 40–1
sarin 196–7, 222, 223, 224
    Tokyo subway incident (1995) 72, 74, 76, 231, 232
saw palmetto 205
saxitoxin 23
scientific and experimental toxicology 3
sensitisers 7
signs, definition 20 see also symptoms
silica 7
sinoatrial node 25
site-specific assessment criteria (SSAC) 137–9
skin
    absorption of toxic agents 8, 9
    target organ 33, 34
skin irritancy study methods 37
skin sensitisation study methods 37–8
small intestine, target organ 26, 27
socio-economic deprivation, and susceptibility to environmental hazards 93
Soil Guideline Values (SGVs) 130, 136–7, 138–9
soman 196–7, 223, 224
source-pathway-receptor model 89, 90
    exposure assessment 98
    health impact of contaminated land 137
    occupational toxicology 114
spermatozonia, target of toxic substances 32–3
spices, pesticide contamination 211
St John's Wort 204
stomach, target organ 26, 27
Sudan dyes 159–60
sulphur dioxide (SO2) air pollution 125, 126
    case study 95
sulphur mustard 223 see also mustard gas
susceptibility to environmental hazards (vulnerable groups) 87–95
    aspects of vulnerability in subgroups 88
    case study (lead exposure) 93–4

case study (sulphur dioxide air
    pollution) 95
developing foetus 89–92
effects of socio-economic deprivation
    93
elderly people 92
factors affecting vulnerability 88–9
genetic polymorphisms 92–3
infants and young children 89–92
risk assessments for specific groups
    87–8
source-pathway-receptor model 89, 90
traditional medicines to avoid 212–13
uncertainty factors for vulnerable
    groups 87–8
SWORD occupational surveillance
    scheme 119
symptoms
    definition 20
    examples and possible causes 21–2
    see also signs
systemic effects of toxic agents 7

**T**
tabun 196–7, 223, 224
target dose 12
target organ, definition 12
target organs in human body systems
    19–34
    arterial system 25–6
    cardiovascular system 24–6
    central nervous system 20, 22
    definition of signs 20
    definition of symptoms 20
    epithelial system 33–4
    gastro-intestinal system 26–7
    haematopoietic system 30
    heart 25
    immune system 31–2
    liver 27–8
    mechanisms of toxicity 15
    nervous system 20, 22–4
    peripheral nervous system 22–4
    reproductive system 32–3
    respiratory system 28–30
    urinary system 32
tear gas 224
teratogens 7, 33

testes, target organs 32–3
tetrodotoxin 23
thalidomide 7, 33
thallium 23, 81, 185–6
therapeutic index 14
THOR surveillance system 119
threshold dose, definition 13
Tolerable Daily Intake (TDI) for food
    contaminants 158–9
tolerable daily soil intake (TDSI) 135
toluene di-isocyanate 31
total dose, definition 12
Tox Reports 135, 136
TOXALS (life support for CW agent
    casualties) 231
Toxbase on-line information resource
    (NPIS) 82
toxic agents
    absorption in the body 8
    classification by physico-chemical
        properties 5–6
    classification by toxic effects 5–6
    distribution in the body 8
    execretion routes 8
    factors affecting influx and efflux 9–11
    possible fate in the body 9–12
    routes of exposure 8–9
    see also xenobiotics
toxic dose (TD), definition 12, 13
toxic effects see investigation of toxic
    effects
toxic neuropathy 23
toxic peripheral neuropathy 23
toxic substances, definition 2
toxicity
    association between dose and exposure
        3
    mechanisms 15
toxicodynamics 9, 11–12, 57, 222
toxicokinetics 9–11, 55–6, 222
toxicological information
    chemical identification systems 63
    numerical systems of chemical
        identification 63
    users 62
toxicological information sources 62–9
    ATSDR (Agency for Toxic Substances
        and Disease Registry) 67

chemical hazards and poisons 81, 82
chemical identification 63
Committee on Carcinogenicity (CoC)
    67
Committee on Medical Effects of Air
    Pollution (COMEAP) 68
Committee on Mutagenicity (CoM) 67
Compendium of Chemical Hazards
    (HPS) 65
ECETOC (European Centre for
    Ecotoxicology and Toxicology of
    Chemicals) 67
Environment Agency (Contaminated
    Land Exposure Assessment, CLEA) 68
Haz-map occupational toxicology
    database 119
Health and Safety Commission
    (advisory committee on toxic
    substances, ACTS) 68
HSDB (Hazardous Substances Data
    Bank) 66
INCHEM (IPCS) 65
Internet resources 64–7
IRIS (Integrated Risk Information
    System) (US EPA) 66
occupational toxicology 119
Pocket Guide to Chemical Hazards
    (NIOSH) 66–7
primary sources 63
secondary sources 63–4
textbooks 64
TOXNET (US National Library of
    Medicine) 66
UK Agency guidance 68
UK independent advisory committees
    67–8
World Health Organization air quality
    guidelines 68, 129
World Health Organization water
    quality guidelines 68–9, 146
toxicology
    components of the discipline 3
    definition and scope 2–3
    history of development 3–4
    role in health protection 4–5
toxins 222, 225
    definition 2
TOXNET (US National Library of

    Medicine) 66
trace element toxicity
    chromium 187–9
    copper 189–90
    zinc 180–81
trace elements
    definition 174, 175
    list 175
traditional medicines 201–14
    definition 201
    forms of 201–2
    history of 201–2
    regulation in the UK 205–6
    safety and efficacy issues 203–5
    scientific interest in medicinal plants
        204
    spread and extent of use 202–3
    types to avoid during breast-feeding
        212
    types to avoid during pregnancy 212
    types which the elderly should avoid
        213
traditional medicines toxicology
    allopathic adulterants 207–8
    DDT contamination 210
    heavy metal poisoning 206–7
    pesticide contamination 210–11
    pesticides in spices 211
    potentially harmful constituents
        206–12
    risks during breast-feeding 212
    risks during pregnancy 212
    risks for the elderly 213
    risks from animal and human body
        parts 208–9, 212
    toxic plants and toxic plant
        constituents 209–10
    vulnerable groups 212–13
trichlorfon 197
2,4,6-trinitrotoluene 7
triorthocresyl phosphate 23

U
UN number (chemical identifier) 63
uncertainty factors 36, 87–8
urinary system
    abnormal function 32
    normal function see Appendix

target organs 32
urticaria 34

**V**
vagus nerve 25
vasodilators 26
vector-borne diseases, use of insecticides
    193–4
veins see arterial system
vesicant agents 225–6, 227
vinyl chloride monomer 7, 111–13
vulnerable groups see susceptibility to
    environmental hazards
VX (nerve agent) 223, 224

**W**
warfarins 199
water quality see drinking water quality
white blood cells, target of toxic
    substances 30
workplace exposure limits (WELs) 116–18
World Health Organization (WHO)
    air quality guidelines 68, 129
    drinking water quality guidelines 68–9,
        146

**X**
xenobiotics (foreign substances)
    half-life in the body 15
    mechanisms of toxicity 15
    removal by the liver 28

**Z**
zinc
    toxicity 180–81
    trace element 175, 179